The rapid growth of knowledge in molecular biology during the last decade has had far-reaching implications for the understanding, diagnosis and management of haematological malignant disease. The response of many conditions to treatment, and the ease with which patient material can be repeatedly sampled, have made this a fruitful area of study, and in parallel with the expanding contribution of molecular biology there has been growing awareness of the importance of epidemiology, techniques of drug administration, patient support and the evaluation of treatment results.

Haematological Oncology serves as a regular forum for the evaluation and dissemination of this new information, and the topics selected for review range from basic science to clinical applications.

This series provides a comprehensive and up-to-date review of the current state of research and will be an important source of information and knowledge for oncologists, immunologists, postgraduate trainees and other clinical and laboratory workers in the field.

Cambridge Medical Reviews

Haematological Oncology   Volume 2

Cambridge Medical Reviews, a programme of review volumes for the clinical sciences, focuses attention on fields in which rapid and continuing advances in biomedical science have increased significantly our understanding and treatment of disease. Each review series is devoted to a single, clinical discipline. The purpose is to provide a regular evaluation and commentary on the growth of knowledge in that subject. Rigorous standards of selection and editing ensure a reliable and topical series of volumes which will meet the requirements of clinicians and research workers alike.

Haematological Oncology

Series editors

James Armitage
Department of Medicine, University of Nebraska Medical Center,
Omaha, Nebraska, USA

Alan Burnett
Department of Haematology, University of Wales College of Medicine
Cardiff, UK

Armand Keating
Autologous Bone Marrow Transplant Program, The Toronto Hospital, Toronto, Ontario, Canada

Adrian Newland
Department of Haematology, The London Hospital, Whitechapel, London, UK

Cambridge Medical Reviews

Haematological Oncology
Volume 2

EDITORS

ARMAND KEATING
Autologous Bone Marrow Transplant Program
The Toronto Hospital, Toronto, Ontario, Canada

JAMES ARMITAGE
Department of Medicine, University of Nebraska Medical Center
Omaha, Nebraska, USA

ALAN BURNETT
Department of Haematology, University of Wales College of Medicine,
Cardiff, UK

ADRIAN NEWLAND
Department of Haematology, The London Hospital
Whitechapel, London, UK

CAMBRIDGE
UNIVERSITY PRESS

1992

Published by the Press Syndicate of the University of Cambridge
The Pitt Building, Trumpington Street, Cambridge CB2 1RP
40 West 20th Street, New York, NY 10011–4211, USA
10 Stamford Road, Oakleigh, Victoria 3166, Australia

First published 1992

Printed in Great Britain by Redwood Press Limited, Melksham, Wiltshire

A catalogue record of this book is available from the British Library

Library of Congress cataloguing in publication data available

ISBN 0 521 43190 5 hardback

Contents

Contributors

APPELBAUM, FREDERICK R, Professor of Medicine, University of Washington, Member, Fred Hutchinson Cancer Research Center, 1124 Columbia Street, M318, Seattle, WA 98104, USA

BUTTURINI, ANNA, Assistant Professor of Pediatrics, University of Parma, Via A. Gramsci, 14, Parma 43100, Italy

CONNORS, JOSEPH M, Clinical Associate Professor, Internal Medicine, University of British Columbia, British Columbia Cancer Agency, 600 West 10th Avenue, Vancouver, British Columbia V5Z 4E6, Canada

GALE, ROBERT PETER, Associate Professor of Medicine, UCLA School of Medicine Los Angeles, CA 90024-1678, USA

GOSPODAROWICZ, MARY K, Associate Professor, Department of Radiology, University of Toronto, Princess Margaret Hospital, 500 Sherbourne Street, Toronto, Ontario M4X 1K9, Canada

HESS, ALLAN D, Associate Professor of Oncology, Johns Hopkins University School of Medicine, The Johns Hopkins Oncology Center, Room 3-127, 600 North Wolfe Street, Baltimore, Maryland 21205, USA

HOROWITZ, MARY M, Scientific Director, International Bone Marrow Transplant Registry, Medical College of Wisconsin, PO Box 26509, Milwaukee, WI 53226, USA

JONES, RICHARD J, Associate Professor of Oncology, Johns Hopkins University School of Medicine, The Johns Hopkins Oncology Center, Room 2-127, 600 North Wolfe Street, Baltimore, Maryland 21205, USA

MARSH, JUDITH, St George's Hospital Medical School, Department of Cellular and Molecular Sciences, Division of Haematology, Cranmer Terrace, London SW17 0RE, UK

MATTHEWS, DANA C, Acting Assistant Professor, University of Washington, Assistant Member, Fred Hutchinson Cancer Research Center, Pediatric Oncology, 1124 Columbia Street, Seattle, WA 98104, USA

NEMUNAITIS, JOHN J, Director of Hematopoiesis Program, Western Pennsylvania Hospital, Western Pennsylvania Cancer Institute, 4800 Friendship Avenue, Pittsburgh, PA 15224, USA

PHILLIPS, GORDON L, Director, Leukemia/Bone Marrow Transplantation Program of BC, British Columbia Cancer Agency, Vancouver General Hospital, 910 West 10th Avenue, Vancouver, British Columbia V5Z 4E3, Canada

Contributors

POLLIACK, AARON, Professor of Medicine, Head of Lymphoma-
Leukemia Unit, Department of Hematology, Hadassah University
Hospital and Medical School, Jerusalem, Israel 91120

PRESS, OLIVER W, Associate Professor of Medicine, Adjunct Associate
Professor of Biological Structure, University of Washington Medical
Center, Medical Oncology, RC-08, 1959 North East Pacific Street,
Seattle, WA 98195, USA

REECE, DONNA E, Clinical Associate Professor, University of British
Columbia, Member, Leukemia/Bone Marrow Transplantation Program
of B.C., Vancouver General Hospital, 910 West 10th Avenue,
Vancouver, British Columbia V5Z 4E3, Canada

SINGER, JACK W, Professor of Medicine, University of Washington,
Member, Fred Hutchinson Cancer Research Center, Chief, Medical
Oncology, VA Medical Center, Seattle, WA 98108, USA

STOCK, WENDY, University of Chicago, Section of Hematology-
Oncology, MC2115, 5841 South Maryland Avenue, Chicago, IL 60637,
USA

SUTCLIFFE, SIMON B, Vice-President of Oncology Programs, Princess
Margaret Hospital, 500 Sherbourne Street, Toronto, Ontario M4X 1K9,
Canada

WESTBROOK, CAROL A, Associate Professor, University of Chicago,
Section of Hematology-Oncology, MC2115, 5841 South Maryland
Avenue, Chicago, IL 60637, USA

Graft-versus-leukemia effects of bone marrow transplantation

M M HOROWITZ

Introduction

Allogeneic bone marrow transplants can eradicate leukemia in patients with acute myelogenous leukemia (AML), acute lymphoblastic leukemia (ALL), and chronic myelogenous leukemia (CML). Fewer than 20% of patients relapse when transplants are performed in first remission or chronic phase[1-3]. These relapse rates are substantially lower than relapse rates observed with conventional chemotherapy. It is often assumed that the antileukemia efficacy of transplants results from high-dose chemotherapy and radiation given pretransplant. However, both experimental and clinical data indicate that additional mechanisms may operate.

More than 30 years ago, Barnes and Loutit proposed that allogeneic bone marrow transplantation had an antitumor effect not explained by pretransplant chemotherapy or radiation.[4] They compared mice with transplanted leukemia treated with high dose total body radiation followed by either syngeneic or allogeneic bone marrow infusion. The mice receiving syngeneic marrow died of leukemia. Those receiving allogeneic bone marrow survived longer, eventually developed fatal graft-versus-host disease (GVHD) and had no evidence of leukemia at death. Mathé and his colleagues[5] proposed the term adoptive immunotherapy for the antitumor effect of allogeneic bone marrow transplants. This antileukemia effect could be specific, i.e. after sensitization of the donor[6] or the donor's cells[7] with antigens present on the malignant cells, or nonspecific, i.e. associated with GVHD. The term graft-vs-leukemia (GVL) was coined by Bortin and co-workers[8-10] to indicate the adoptive immunotherapeutic effect of transplanted allogeneic bone marrow cells against leukemia cells. GVL can be distinguished from GVH reactions in mice.[8,11-13] The experimental data regarding GVL effects are not described in this chapter but are reviewed by Jones and Hess in their chapter, and also by

All correspondence to: Dr MM Horowitz, Statistical Center for Transplant Research, Medical College of Wisconsin, PO Box 26509, Milwaukee, WI 53226, USA.

Cambridge Medical Reviews: Haematological Oncology Volume 2
© Cambridge University Press 1992

Sosman[14] and Truitt[15]. This review summarizes clinical data supporting an antileukemia effect of allogeneic transplants due to immune-mediated effects of the graft.

Evidence for an antileukemia effect of transplanted allogeneic cells include the following clinical observations: (a) a lower incidence of leukemia relapse in allograft recipients with acute and/or chronic GVHD as compared to those without GVHD; (b) higher relapse rates after identical twin versus allogeneic bone marrow transplants; (c) high relapse rates after T-cell depleted transplants; and (d) the recent report of cytogenetic remissions induced after post-transplant relapse by infusion of donor leucocytes without other specific antileukemia chemotherapy.

The antileukemia effect of GVHD

Numerous single and multi-institution reports demonstrate an inverse correlation between development of GVHD and the risk of leukemia recurrence (Table 1). In 1979, Weiden and colleagues reported that the risk of relapse was 2.5 times less in 79 allograft recipients with moderate-to-severe acute or chronic GVHD than in 117 with no or minimal GVHD.[16] Patients included those transplanted for ALL or AML between 1970 and 1977 with a variety of disease states prior to transplant. Survival was similar with and without GVHD. A 1981 report from the same group described the association between chronic GVHD and relapse in 163 patients with ALL and AML transplanted in remission or relapse and surviving in remission at least 150 days after transplant.[17] The actuarial probability of relapse was 62% among patients without acute or chronic GVHD, 43% among those with only acute GVHD, 34% among those with only chronic GVHD and 12% among those with both acute and chronic GVHD. In multivariate analysis, chronic GVHD was significantly associated with decreased relapse with a relapse rate 0.31 to 0.36 times the rate in patients without GVHD ($P < 0.005$). In these patients who had already survived 150 days posttransplant, survival was significantly higher in patients with chronic GVHD. These data do not provide an accurate estimate of the impact of GVHD on the survival of all transplant recipients since more than 80% of all GVHD-related deaths occur prior to 150 days posttransplant.[18]

A 1981 study from UCLA examined relapse rates in 46 allograft recipients surviving $\geq$ 30 days posttransplant.[19] Actuarial relapse rates were 62% in 22 patients with grade 0–I acute GVHD and 20% in 24 with grade II–IV acute GVHD ($P=0.05$). All patients in this study were in relapse at the time of transplant; 10 had never achieved remission. There was no difference in survival with and without GVHD.

A 1984 study from the European Bone Marrow Transplant Group including 229 patients with AML in first or second remission from 27 centers reported decreased relapse with chronic but not acute GVHD.[20] Similarly, a

Table 1. *Associations between GVHD and relapse after allogeneic bone marrow transplants*

Institution (ref)	N	Acute GVHD	Chronic GVHD	Acute and/or Chronic GVHD	Comments
FHCI, 1979[16]	196	NE*	NE	→	ALL, AML in remission or relapse
FHCI, 1981[17]	163	–	→	→	ALL, AML in remission or relapse; surviving ≥ 150 days
UCLA, 1981[19]	46	→	NE	NE	Acute leukemia in relapse
EBMTG, 1984[20]	229	–	→	NE	AML in remission
Genoa, 1984[21]	78	–	→	NE	ALL, AML, CML
FHCI, 1985[22]	114	–	–	→	Children; ALL in remission or relapse
U Minn, 1987[23]	40	→	NE	NE	ALL in remission or relapse
U Minn, 1987[24]	46	NE	NE	→	ALL in remission
MSK, 1987[25]	97	–	→	NE	Children; ALL, AML in remission or relapse
FHCI, 1989[26]	481	→	–	–	Early ALL, AML, CML
	263	→	–	–	Intermediate ALL, AML, CML
	458	–	–	→	Advanced ALL, AML, CML
IBMTR, 1990[27]	1783	→	→	→	Early ALL, AML, CML

* ↓ indicates decreased relapse; – indicates no association with relapse; NE indicates association with relapse not evaluated.
Abbreviations FHCI: Fred Hutchinson Cancer Institute; UCLA: University of California, Los Angeles; EBMTG: European Bone Marrow Transplant Group; U Minn: University of Minnesota; MSK: Memorial Sloan Kettering; IBMTR: International Bone Marrow Transplant Registry.

report from Genoa of 78 patients with ALL, AML or CML reported probabilities of relapse of 13% and 63% for patients with and without chronic GVHD, respectively (P=0.00004).[21]

A 1985 report of 114 children with ALL (5 in first marrow remission, 46 in second or subsequent remission and 63 in relapse) showed a decreased risk of relapse among patients with acute and/or chronic GVHD (relative risk 0.26, P=0.002).[22] In this study development of chronic GVHD was associated with improved survival (P=0.005).

A 1987 study of 40 patients with high risk ALL reported decreased relapse risk in patients with grade II–IV acute GVHD (73% vs 57%, P=0.04). There was a trend toward improved relapse-free survival among patients with GVHD but this was not statistically significant (P=0.11).[23] A comparison of allogeneic and autologous transplants for high risk refractory ALL at the same institution showed a higher relapse risk after autologous (79%) than allogeneic (56%) transplants.[24] Relapses after autotransplants tended to occur earlier than after allogeneic transplants. Some recurrences after autologous transplants may have been due to reinfusion of leukemia cells in the autologous graft. However, the relapse rate with autologous transplants was similar to that after allografts without GVHD (73%) suggesting that the absence of GVHD-mediated antileukemia activity was an important factor. Transplant-related mortality was higher after allogeneic than autologous transplants; leukemia-free survival was similar at 5 years.

A 1987 study of 97 children with ALL or AML reported an antileukemia effect of chronic but not acute GVHD after adjustment for other risk factors.[25]

Sullivan et al. recently studied 1202 recipients of allografts for AML, ALL and CML.[26] Of these patients 481 patients had early (acute leukemia in first remission or CML in chronic phase) leukemia, 263 intermediate leukemia (acute leukemia in second or subsequent remission or CML in accelerated phase) and the remainder advanced disease. Using multivariate analyses, they were unable to show an effect of acute or chronic GVHD upon relapse in patients with early leukemia except for those with ALL. Acute GVHD was associated with decreased relapse in patients with intermediate ALL and AML. Development of acute or chronic GVHD was associated with decreased relapse in advanced acute leukemia and CML. A study of 2254 recipients of allogeneic transplants for early leukemia (first remission acute leukemia or CML in first chronic phase) reported to the International Bone Marrow Transplant Registry (IBMTR) demonstrated a statistically significant reduction in relapse risk among patients developing GVHD (Fig. 1).[27] In this study, recipients of non-T-cell depleted allografts not developing GVHD had a 3-year probability of relapse of 25 ± 6% (95% confidence interval). Recipients with acute GVHD only, chronic GVHD only or both had 3-year probabilities of relapse of 22 ± 5%, 10 ± 7%, and 7 ± 3% respectively. In multivariate analyses adjusting for other variables affecting relapse, patients

4

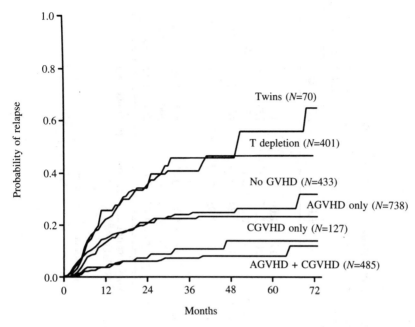

Fig. 1. Actuarial probability of relapse after bone marrow transplantation for early leukemia according to type of graft and development of graft-versus-host disease.[27]

developing only acute GVHD had a relative risk of relapse of 0.68 (P=0.03) compared to patients without acute or chronic GVHD; those with only chronic GVHD had a relative risk of 0.43 (P=0.01); and those with both acute and chronic GVHD had a relative risk of 0.33 (P=0.0001). GVHD was associated with decreased relapse in all three types of leukemia although the relative importance of acute and chronic GVHD differed for the three types of leukemia (Table 2). Chronic GVHD had a stronger antileukemia effect in AML and CML and acute GVHD a stronger effect in ALL. Patients with both acute and chronic GVHD had the lowest risk of relapse. Relapse correlated inversely with severity of GVHD. One hundred and forty-one patients with mild acute and chronic GVHD had a relative risk of relapse of 0.50 (P=0.02) or a 2-fold decrease in relapse risk as compared to those without GVHD; 72 patients with moderate GVHD had a relative risk of 0.22 (P=0.009) or a 4.5-fold decrease in risk; none of 49 patients with severe acute and chronic GVHD relapsed (P=0.04).

Deliberate induction of GVHD by employing either no or abbreviated posttransplant immune suppression, with or without infusion of donor buffy coat cells, has been attempted to decrease leukemia recurrence in patients at high risk of relapse.[28,29] The incidence of acute but not chronic GVHD was

Table 2. *Relative risk of relapse* after bone marrow transplantation for early leukemia (data from reference 27)*

Study Group	ALL 1st CR			AML 1st CR			CML CP			ALL patients		
	N	RR	P	N	RR	P	N	RR	P	N	RR	P
Allogeneic, non-T-depleted												
No GVHD**	90	1.00	–	228	1.00	–	115	1.00	–	433	1.00	–
Acute GVHD only	141	0.36	0.004	330	0.78	0.26	267	1.15	0.75	738	0.68	0.03
Chronic GVHD only	28	0.44	0.16	54	0.48	0.12	45	0.28	0.16	127	0.43	0.01
Acute and chronic GVHD	84	0.38	0.02	237	0.34	0.0003	164	0.24	0.03	485	0.33	0.0001
Syngeneic	12	0.99	0.99	34	2.58	0.0008	24	2.95	0.08	70	2.09	0.005
Allogeneic, T-depleted												
All patients	84	1.20	0.61	163	1.30	0.33	154	5.14	0.0001	401	1.76	0.002
No GVHD	43	1.48	0.33	83	1.57	0.12	74	6.91	0.0001	200	2.14	0.0001
Acute and/or chronic GVHD	41	0.98	0.97	80	0.80	0.60	80	4.45	0.003	201	1.32	0.25

* Relative risks are derived from multivariate Cox regression adjusting for leukocyte count at diagnosis, recipient age, organ impairment pretransplant, donor–recipient sex-match and drug used to prevent GVHD.
** Reference group.

Abbreviations **RR**: relative risk in comparison to reference group; ALL: acute lymphoblastic leukemia; AML: acute myelogenous leukemia; CML: chronic myelogenous leukemia; CR: complete remission; CP: chronic phase; GVHD: graft-versus-host disease.

increased by these maneuvers. Results were disappointing with no significant decreases in relapse observed and overall survival decreased due to higher transplant-related mortality.

Leukemia relapse after identical twin transplants

The importance of allogeneic cells in eradicating leukemia after bone marrow transplants can be studied by comparing relapse rates after allogeneic and identical twin transplants.

Weiden et al. compared the relapse rate in 46 recipients of identical twin transplants for AML or ALL with the relapse rate in 117 recipients of allogeneic transplants with grade 0 or I acute GVHD and no chronic GVHD and 79 recipients of allograft with grade II–IV acute or any chronic GVHD.[16] The relapse rate after syngeneic transplants was about 1.5 times higher than after allogeneic transplants ($P<0.10$). The rate was similar after identical twin transplants and allogeneic transplants without GVHD (relative risk 1.2, $P=NS$) but significantly higher after identical twin transplants than after allogeneic transplants associated with grade II–IV acute or any chronic GVHD (relative risk 2.7, $P=0.0003$) suggesting that the increased anti-leukemia efficacy of allografts was due to GVHD-mediated antileukemia effects. Most of the twins in this study were in relapse at the time of transplant.

In 1984, Gale and Champlin summarized results of 31 identical twin transplants for AML in first remission reported by five centers and one cooperative group and compared these to results of HLA-identical sibling transplants for AML in first remission at the same centers.[30] The actuarial relapse rate was 59 ± 20% for twins compared to 18 ± 4% for HLA-identical siblings. Allogeneic transplants with and without GVHD were not examined separately so the extent to which the difference in relapse rates could be explained by GVHD could not be evaluated.

A 1987 update of the Seattle twin transplant data compared the probability of relapse in 53 recipients of twin transplants for AML or ALL with 785 recipients of allogeneic transplants for AML or ALL.[31] The probability of relapse was 75% after twin transplants and 62% after allogeneic transplants ($P<0.0001$).

The 1990 IBMTR study of 2254 recipients of bone marrow transplants for early leukemia included 70 recipients of transplants from identical twins: 12 with ALL, 34 with AML and 24 with CML (Fig. 1, Table 2).[27] The relative risks of relapse for recipients of identical twin transplants as compared to recipients of allogeneic transplants *without acute or chronic GVHD* was 2.09 ($P=0.005$). When the different leukemias were analyzed separately, a significant increase in relapse risk with identical twin transplants was observed only in AML (relative risk 2.58, $P=0.008$). A trend toward increased relapse with identical twin versus allogeneic transplants without GVHD was also seen in

CML (relative risk 2.95, $P=0.08$). A recent update of this analysis, including information for 92 identical twin transplants, confirmed these results.[32] These data suggest that allogeneic cells have an antileukemia effect independent of GVHD. It may be that leukemia-associated antigens, not recognized by genetically identical immune cells, are recognized by allogeneic immune cells. Alternatively, the different relapse rates may reflect nonspecific effects of subclinical GVHD directed at minor histocompatibility antigens.

It is generally assumed that the development of leukemia in twin transplant recipients represents relapse though this is difficult to formally prove. It is not possible to absolutely exclude increased susceptibility to leukemia or leukemic transformation in the immediate posttransplant period in genetically identical donor cells, however, this seems unlikely since leukemia has not developed in any of the 70 twin donors.

Leukemia relapse after T-cell depleted transplants

Another way of determining whether the bone marrow graft has antileukemia activity is to observe whether manipulating the marrow affects relapse, despite similar pretransplant conditioning. This situation occurs with T-cell depleted transplants.

Extensive data from animal models indicate that T-cells in the transplanted bone marrow cause GVHD. Removing T-cells from the donor marrow decreases acute and chronic GVHD regardless of the method of T-cell depletion.[1,32-42] Because GVHD is a major cause of mortality and morbidity after allogeneic transplants, some centers deplete T-cells from the donor bone marrow prior to infusion. Generally, pretransplant preparative regimens are similar whether or not the donor bone marrow is T-cell depleted, except that some centers use higher doses of radiation or chemotherapy.[36,43] Despite similar or more intense conditioning, the risk of leukemia relapse is substantially higher after T-cell depleted than non-T-cell depleted transplants, indicating that an important mediator of antileukemia activity is removed during the process of T-cell depletion. This increased leukemia relapse has been observed in multiple centers using a variety of methods for T-cell depletion.[1,33,37,44,45]

Since GVHD has an antileukemia effect, increased relapses observed with T-cell depletion may result completely, or in part, from removal of cells responsible for GVHD. However, in a recent IBMTR study of GVL effects in early leukemia, 159 CML patients receiving T-cell depleted transplants, with or without GVHD, had higher probabilities of relapse (relative risks 6.91 and 4.45, respectively, $P=0.0001$) than 115 recipients of non-T-cell depleted allografts without GVHD (Table 2).[27] These data suggest that T-cell depletion alters the antileukemia effect of transplants in CML by a mechanism separate from GVHD.

The IBMTR recently analyzed results of 731 HLA-identical sibling T-cell depleted transplants for all stages of leukemia performed between January 1982 and December 1987.[46] Results were compared to 2480 non-T-cell depleted transplants performed during the same interval. The likelihood of leukemia relapse between T-cell depleted and non-T-cell depleted transplants was compared after stratifying for type of leukemia and disease state (Table 3). There was significantly increased leukemia relapse in all T-cell depleted groups except AML in $\geq$ 2nd remission and CML in blast phase. The adverse effect on relapse in early leukemia was greatest in CML (RR 5.61; P <0.0001), intermediate in AML (RR 1.94; P <0.007), and least in ALL (RR 1.83; P <0.05). After adjusting for the incidence and severity of acute and chronic GVHD, the relative relapse risks for AML and ALL in first remission and CML in chronic phase were 1.66 (P = NS), 1.55 (P = NS), and 4.87 (P <0.0001), respectively. The increased relapse after T-cell depleted transplants for ALL and AML appear to be wholly explained by the decreased incidence of GVHD and, presumably, GVHD-associated antileukemia effects. Other mechanisms appear to operate in CML. This effect is presumably mediated by T-cells but could result from some other cells or factor affected by T-cell depletion. T-cells might interact with leukemia cells directly or by facilitating engraftment or producing lymphokines that affect growth of leukemia cells. In ALL and AML, the risks of relapse with T-cell depletion were similar to non-T-cell depleted transplants without GVHD, suggesting that increased relapse in this setting is due primarily to decreased GVHD-associated antileukemia activity.

Reinfusion of donor buffy coat cells to treat posttransplant relapse

A recent report from Kolb et al. emphasizes the importance of donor cells in maintaining remission after transplants for CML.[47] This paper described three patients with hematologic relapse 1.5–3 years after HLA-identical sibling transplants for CML in chronic phase. Interferon, administered daily for $\geq$ 3 months, failed to induce clinical or cytogenetic remission. These patients then received leukocyte transfusions from their original donors. Between 4.4 and 7.4 $\times$ 10^8/kg mononuclear cells were administered. Two of the three patients developed clinically significant GVHD that responded to immune suppression. All achieved complete clinical and cytogenetic remission with re-establishment of full hematopoietic chimerism. This successful application of adoptive immunotherapy without the use of cytotoxic chemotherapy provides strong evidence for an important role of donor cells in maintaining remission after transplantation.

Conclusions

Considerable clinical data exist supporting the notion of an antileukemia effect of allogeneic bone marrow transplants not fully explained by pretransplant cytotoxic therapy and attributable to transplantation of immune com-

Table 3. Adjusted* 2-year probabilities and relative risks of relapse following T-cell depleted bone marrow transplantation (data from reference 46)

Disease	Status	Non-T-Cell depleted		T-Cell depleted			
		N at risk	Probability of relapse	N at risk	Probability of relapse	Relative risk	P
ALL	1st remission	260	17%	89	29%	1.83	<0.05
AML	1st remission	560	17%	159	30%	1.94	<0.007
CML	Chronic phase	452	10%	172	44%	5.61	<0.0001
Early leukemia		1272	15%	420	37%	2.75	<0.0001
ALL	≥2nd remission	312	39%	61	59%	1.79	<0.03
AML	≥2nd remission	105	41%	28	26%	0.57	NS
CML	Accelerated phase	219	24%	73	51%	2.65	<0.002
Intermediate leukemia		636	34%	162	51%	1.71	<0.003
ALL	Relapse	171	55%	35	75%	1.73	<0.03
AML	Relapse	205	45%	43	66%	1.79	<0.03
CML	Blast phase	81	57%	31	63%	1.17	NS
Advanced leukemia		457	51%	109	70%	1.70	<0.002

* Probabilities adjusted for age of patient, infection present in the week pretransplant, performance score pretransplant, donor age, and year of transplant, using Cox proportional hazard regression.

petent donor cells. This GVL activity may be mediated through a variety of mechanisms and is not always associated with clinically significant GVHD. Further advances in characterization and control of the GVL phenomenon are needed both to improve the results of clinical bone marrow transplantation and to use this effect to treat leukemia outside the transplant setting.

Acknowledgements
Supported by Public Health Service Grant PO1-CA-40053 from the National Cancer Institute and the National Institute of Allergy and Infectious Diseases of the US Department of Health and Human Services; and grants from Alpha Therapeutic Corporation; Armour Pharmaceutical Company; Bristol-Myers; Burroughs-Wellcome Company; Charles E Culpeper Foundation; Cutter Biologicals Inc; Eleanor Naylor Dana Charitable Trust; Eppley Foundation for Research; Hoechst-Roussel Pharmaceuticals Inc; Immunex Corporation; Robert J and Helen C Kleberg Foundation; Eli Lilly and Company; Ambrose Monell Foundation; Noble Foundation; Ortho Biotech Corporation; John Oster Family Foundation, Inc.; Elsa U Pardee Foundation; RGK Foundation; Roerig (a Division of Pfizer Pharmaceuticals); Sandoz Research Institute; Stackner Family Foundation; Starr Foundation; Joan and Jack Stein Charities; Swiss Cancer League; Wyeth-Ayerst Research; and Xoma Corporation.

The author thanks Ms Dottie Jacobson for typing the manuscript and Drs A J Barrett and M M Bortin for their critical review of the manuscript.

References
(1) Goldman JM, Gale RP, Horowitz MM et al. Bone marrow transplantation for chronic myelogenous leukemia in chronic phase: increased risk for relapse associated with T-cell depletion. *Ann Intern Med* 1988; 108: 806–14.
(2) Barrett AJ, Horowitz MM, Gale RP et al. Marrow transplantation for acute lymphoblastic leukemia: factors affecting relapse and survival. *Blood* 1989; 74: 862–71.
(3) Gale RP, Horowitz MM, Biggs JC et al. Transplant or chemotherapy in acute myelogeneous leukaemia. *Lancet* 1989; i: 1119–22.
(4) Barnes DWH, Corp MJ, Loutit JF, Neal FE. Treatment of murine leukaemia with xrays and homologous bone marrow. *Br Med J* 1956; 2: 626–7.
(5) Mathé G, Amiel JL, Schwarzenberg L, Cattan A, Schneider M. Adoptive immunotherapy of acute leukemia: experimental and clinical results. *Cancer Res* 1965; 25: 1525–31.
(6) Woodruff MFA. The experimental basis of immunotherapy. In: Woodruff MFA, ed. *The interaction of cancer and host: its therapeutic significance.* New York, Grune & Stratton, 1980: 164–233.
(7) Cheever MA, Greenberg PD, Fefer A. Specific adoptive therapy of established leukemia with syngeneic lymphocytes sequentially immunized in vivo and in vitro and nonspecifically expanded by culture with interleukin 2. *J Immunol* 1981; 126:1318–22.

(8) Bortin MM, Rimm AA, Saltzstein EC, Rodey GE. Graft versus leukemia. III. Apparent independent antihost and antileukemia activity of transplanted immunocompetent cells. *Transplantation* 1973; 16: 182–8.

(9) Bortin MM, Rimm AA, Saltzstein EC. Graft versus leukemia: Quantification of adoptive immunotherapy in murine leukemia. *Science* 1973; 179: 811–13.

(10) Bortin MM. Graft versus leukemia. In: Bach FH, Good RA, eds. *Clinical immunobiology.* Vol II. New York, Academic Press, 1974: 287–306.

(11) Bortin MM, Truitt RL, Rimm AA, Bach FH. Graft-versus-leukemia reactivity induced by alloimmunization without augmentation of graft-versus-host reactivity. *Nature* 1979; 281: 490–1.

(12) Truitt RL, Shih C-Y, Lefever AV, Tempelis LD, Andreani M, Bortin MM. Characterization of alloimmunization-induced T lymphocytes reactive against AKR leukemia in vitro and correlation with graft-vs-leukemia activity in vivo. *J Immunol* 1983; 131: 2050–8.

(13) Truitt RL, LeFever AV, Shih CC-Y. Manipulation of graft-vs-host disease for a graft-versus-leukemia effect after allogeneic bone marrow transplantation in AKR mice with spontaneous leukemia/lymphoma. *Transplantation* 1986; 41: 301–10.

(14) Sosman JA, Sondel PM. The graft versus leukemia (GVL) effect following bone marrow transplantation (BMT): a review of laboratory and clinical data. *Hematol Rev* 1987; 2: 77–91.

(15) Truitt RL, LeFever AV, Shih CC-Y, Jeske JM, Martin TM. Graft-vs-leukemia effect. In: Burakoff SJ, Deeg HJ, Ferrara J, Atkinson K, eds. *Graft-versus-host disease: immunology, pathophysiology and treatment.* Marcel Dekker Inc, New York, 1990: 177–204.

(16) Weiden PL, Flournoy N, Thomas ED et al. Antileukemic effect of graft-versus-host disease in human recipients of allogeneic-marrow grafts. *N Eng J Med* 1979; 300: 1068–73.

(17) Weiden PL, Sullivan KM, Flournoy N, Storb R, Thomas ED. Antileukemic effect of chronic graft-versus-host disease: contribution to improved survival after allogeneic marrow transplantation. *N Eng J Med* 1981; 304:1529–33.

(18) Bortin MM, Ringdén O, Horowitz MM, Rozman C, Weiner RS, Rimm AA. Temporal relationships between the major complications of bone marrow transplantation for leukemia. *Bone Marrow Transpl* 1989; 4: 339–44.

(19) McIntyre R, Gale RP. Relationship between graft-versus-leukemia and graft-versus-host in man – UCLA experience. In: OKunewick JP, Meredith RF, eds. *Graft-versus-leukemia in man and animal models.* Boca Raton, FL: CRC Press 1981: 1–9.

(20) Zwaan FE, Hermans J, Barrett AJ, Speck B. Bone marrow transplantation for acute nonlymphoblastic leukemia: a survey of the European Group for Bone Marrow Transplantation (EGBMT). *Br J Haematol* 1984, 56: 645–53.

(21) Bacigalupo A, Van Lint MT, Frassoni F, Marmont A. Graft-versus-leukaemia effect following allogeneic bone marrow transplantation. *Br J Haematol* 1985; 61: 749–51.

(22) Sanders JE, Flournoy N, Thomas ED et al. Marrow transplant experience in children with acute lymphoblastic leukemia: an analysis of factors associated

with survival, relapse and graft-versus-host disease. *Med Pediatr Oncol* 1985; 13: 165–72.

(23) Weisdorf DJ, Nesbit ME, Ramsay NKC et al. Allogeneic bone marrow transplantation for acute lymphoblastic leukemia in remission: prolonged survival associated with acute graft-versus-host disease. *J Clin Oncol* 1987; 5: 1348–55.

(24) Kersey JH, Weisdorf D, Nesbit ME et al. Comparison of autologous and allogeneic bone marrow transplantation for treatment of high-risk refractory acute lymphoblastic leukemia. *N Eng J Med* 1987; 317: 461–67.

(25) Brochstein JA, Kernan NA, Groshen S et al. Allogeneic bone marrow transplantation after hyperfractionated total-body irradiation and cyclophosphamide in children with acute leukemia. *N Eng J Med* 1987; 317: 1618–24.

(26) Sullivan KM, Weiden PL, Storb R et al. Influence of acute and chronic graft-versus-host disease on relapse and survival after bone marrow transplantation from HLA-identical siblings as treatment of acute and chronic leukemia. *Blood* 1989; 73: 1720–8.

(27) Horowitz MM, Gale RP, Sondel PM et al. Graft-v-leukemia reactions after bone marrow transplantation. *Blood* 1990; 75: 555–62.

(28) Sullivan KM, Deeg HJ, Sanders J et al. Hyperacute graft-v-host disease in patients not given immunosuppression after allogeneic marrow transplantation. *Blood* 1986; 4: 1172–5.

(29) Sullivan KM, Storb R, Buckner CD et al. Graft-versus-host disease as adoptive immunotherapy in patients with advanced hematologic neoplasms. *N Eng J Med* 1989; 320: 828–34.

(30) Gale RP, Champlin RE. How do bone marrow transplants cure leukemia? *Lancet* 1984; ii: 28–30.

(31) Fefer A, Sullivan KM, Weiden P et al. Graft versus leukemia effect in man: The relapse rate of acute leukemia is lower after allogeneic than after syngeneic marrow transplantation. In: Truitt RL, Gale RP, Bortin MM, eds. *Cellular immunotherapy of cancer*. New York, Alan R. Liss, Inc., 1987: 401–8.

(32) Gale RP, Horowitz MM, Bortin MM. Identical twin transplants for leukemia. *Blood* 1990; 76 (suppl 1): 540a.

(33) Poynton CH. T cell depletion in bone marrow transplantation. *Bone Marrow Transpl* 1988; 3: 265–79.

(34) Kernan NA, Collins NH, Juliana L et al. Clonable T lymphocytes in T-cell depleted bone marrow transplants correlate with development of graft-versus-host disease. *Blood* 1986; 68: 770–3.

(35) De Witte T, Hoogenhout J, de Pauw B et al. Depletion of donor lymphocytes by counterflow centrifugation successfully prevents acute graft-versus-host disease in matched allogeneic marrow transplantation. *Blood* 1986; 67: 1302–8.

(36) Cobbold S., Martin G, Waldmann H. Monoclonal antibodies for the prevention of graft-versus-host disease and marrow graft rejection: the depletion of T cell subsets in vitro and in vivo. *Transplantation* 1986; 42: 239–47.

(37) Maraninchi D, Gluckman E, Blaise D et al. Impact of T-cell depletion on outcome of allogeneic bone-marrow transplantation for standard-risk leukaemias. *Lancet* 1987; 2: 175–8.

(38) Prentice HG. T cell depletion in allogeneic bone marrow transplantation. *Transpl Proc* 1987; 19: 155–6.

13

(39) Herve P, Cahn JY, Flesch M et al. Successful graft-versus-host disease prevention without graft failure in 32 HLA-identical allogeneic bone marrow transplantations with marrow depleted of T cells by monoclonal antibodies and complement. *Blood* 1987; 69: 388–93.

(40) Prentice HG, Hermans J, Zwaan FE. Relapse risk in allogeneic BMT with T cell depletion of donor marrow. *Bone Marrow Transpl* 1988; 3 (suppl 1): 30–2.

(41) O'Reilly RJ, Kernan NA, Cunningham I et al. Allogeneic transplants depleted of T cells by soybean lectin agglutination and E rosette depletion. *Bone Marrow Transpl* 1988; 3 (suppl 1): 3–6.

(42) Martin PJ, Hansen JA, Buckner CD et al. Effect of in vitro depletion of T cells in HLA-identical allogeneic marrow grafts. *Blood* 1985; 66: 664–72.

(43) Sondel PM, Bozdech MJ, Trigg ME et al. Additional immunosuppression allows engraftment following HLA-mismatched T cell-depleted bone marrow transplantation for leukemia. *Transpl Proc* 1985; 17: 460–1.

(44) Apperley JF, Jones L, Hale G et al. Bone marrow transplantation for patients with chronic myeloid leukemia: T-cell depletion with Campath-1 reduces the incidence of graft-versus-host disease but may increase the risk of leukaemic relapse. *Bone Marrow Transpl* 1986; 1: 53–66.

(45) Butturini A, Gale RP. The role of T-cells in preventing relapse in chronic myelogenous leukemia. *Bone Marrow Transpl* 1987; 2: 351–4.

(46) Marmont AM, Horowitz MM, Gale RP, et al. T-cell depletion of HLA-identical transplants in leukemia. *Blood* 1991; 78: 2120–30.

(47) Kolb HJ, Mittermüller J, Clemin CH et al. Donor leukocyte transfusions for treatment of recurrent chronic myelogenous leukemia in marrow transplant patients. *Blood* 1990; 76: 2462–5.

Therapy of hematologic malignancies using radioimmunotherapy (RAIT)

F R APPELBAUM, D C MATTHEWS AND O W PRESS

Introduction

Recently, a number of clinical studies of the use of radiolabeled antibodies as treatment for hematologic malignancies have been initiated. The impetus for these studies comes from two different directions. First, there are the experiences already gained with the use of unmodified antibodies. The lessons learned here are that antibodies reactive with tumor-associated or tumor-specific antigens can be administered without appreciable toxicity, but result in, at best, only temporary and partial remissions.[1-4] Studies in both animal models and man have found that the failure of unmodified antibody to eliminate tumor is due both to the existence of variant tumor cells which lack the targeted antigen as well as an inability of the tumor-bearing host to eliminate all tumor cells which react with the antibody.[5-8] Both of these limitations might be overcome with the use of radiolabeled antibodies. Radionuclides which deliver their energy locally over several cell diameters should provide the antibody with a potent effector mechanism to eliminate the targeted antigen-positive cells. Since the energy is deposited over a short distance, antigen-negative variant cells within the antigen-positive tumor mass should also be effectively irradiated.

A second argument for the use of RAIT for hematologic malignancies comes from experiences gained with the use of systemic radiotherapy for these diseases. Relatively low-dose total body irradiation (TBI) in the range of 150 cGy is an effective agent for the treatment of indolent lymphomas, resulting in a high incidence of responses, albeit temporary and partial.[9] Efforts to escalate the dose of TBI have been limited by marrow toxicity. High-dose TBI, in the range of 12 to 15 Gy, given in the context of marrow transplantation, is much more effective and results in curative therapy for many patients with hematologic malignancies.[10] However, disease recurrence after

All correspondence to: Dr FR Appelbaum, Fred Hutchinson Cancer Research Center, 1124 Columbia Street, Room M318, Seattle, Washington 98104, USA.

Cambridge Medical Reviews: Haematological Oncology Volume 2
© Cambridge University Press 1992

marrow transplantation remains a significant problem and, in most settings, is the most common reason for failure of this approach. Published studies demonstrate that transplant regimens employing higher doses of TBI can lower recurrence rates, but these higher doses are associated with an increase in non-relapse deaths leading to no overall survival benefit. For example, 2 prospective randomized studies, 1 in acute myelogenous leukemia (AML) and 1 in chronic myelogenous leukemia (CML), comparing preparative regimens which include 12 Gy versus 15.75 Gy found a markedly decreased incidence of relapse with the higher dose of TBI, but also a higher incidence of non-relapse mortality resulting in similar long-term disease-free survivals for the 2 radiation doses.[11,12] These observations raise the possibility that by targeting radiotherapy specifically to sites of disease, treatment outcomes might be improved by increasing the dose to tumor, decreasing the relapse rate, and avoiding toxicities to normal organs.

This chapter includes a discussion of some of the animal studies which have led to the current clinical trials of RAIT for hematologic malignancies and a summary of the current status of these trials. Because there are substantial differences in the way RAIT has been applied to the treatment of leukemia versus lymphoma, these 2 situations will be discussed separately.

RAIT for leukemia

Preclinical studies

Many of the principles underlying the use of radiolabeled antibodies as treatment for leukemia have been defined in murine, canine and primate models.[13-16] We have based our clinical studies on work conducted in a canine transplant model. The initial canine studies were designed to determine the concentrations of labeled antibodies directed against marrow precursors which ended up in marrow and various other organs after i.v. infusion. For these studies, selected antibodies were labeled with trace amounts of ^{131}I using the Chloramine T method, and infused intravenously at a dose of 1 mg/kg. Animals were imaged using a gamma camera over 48 hours and then sacrificed. The amount of radionuclide in separate organs was determined and biodistribution curves were derived by scaling the gamma camera measured activity curves to the radioiodine concentrations in those organs as determined at autopsy. From these biodistribution curves the absorbed dose expressed as cGy/mCi administered to each organ was determined using methods developed by the MIRD Committee.

Among the different antibodies studied, including an anti-IA antibody, an anti-CD44 antibody, and an antimyeloid antibody termed DM5, the results obtained with DM5 are most relevant to the current discussion. As shown in Fig. 1(a), shortly after injection there was rapid specific uptake of the antibody–radionuclide conjugate in the marrow. There was some early uptake of

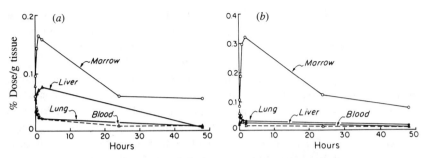

Fig. 1. Mean activity curves for ^{131}I-DM5 for organs of interest (marrow, liver, lung and blood pool) generated by scaling the gamma camera-derived time activity curves for each organ to the ^{131}I concentration per gram of tissue measured directly from necropsy samples. Panel A describes 4 dogs given 1 mg/kg ^{131}I-DM5 without pretreatment. Panel B represents 4 dogs given 1 mg/kg cold DM5 2 hours before the labeled dose.

the radionuclide in the liver which, we reasoned, might have been due to binding of the antibody to circulating cells and clearance of these cells by the liver. Therefore, a study was conducted to test whether a dose of unlabeled antibody given directly before the labeled dose might improve biodistribution and, as shown in Fig. 1(b), this was, in fact, the case.[17] Based on the results shown in Fig. 1(b), ^{131}I-DM5 would deliver more than 10-fold more radiation to the marrow than to any normal organ. In these studies the residence time of the radionuclide was limited because, after binding, some of the antibody conjugate was internalized, metabolized and the ^{131}I then released from the cell. Studies from a number of laboratories including our own have shown that the residence of the radionuclide at its target can be prolonged by administration of propylthiouracil, through the use of alternative methods of iodinating antibodies, or by using other radionuclides.[18–20] Before beginning the human studies, it was further shown in this animal model that after administration of an anti-myeloid antibody labeled with large amounts of ^{131}I, marrow could be ablated and that with marrow transplantation this effect could be reversed.[14]

Studies of radiolabeled anti-CD33 antibody as treatment for AML in man

Based on the encouraging results obtained in the canine model, we initiated a trial of ^{131}I-anti-CD33 antibody in man.[21] CD33 is an antigen principally restricted to immature myeloid cells being found on roughly 50% of marrow cells, but not on mature hematopoietic cells in the peripheral blood or on nonmyeloid tissue. It is found on the blasts of more than 90% of cases of AML. The design of the study was to first test the biodistribution of ^{131}I-anti-CD33 in patients with AML scheduled for marrow transplantation by infusing antibody labeled with trace doses of ^{131}I followed by external imaging and multiple blood and marrow specimens. In this way, biodistribution curves could be constructed much as already described for the canine studies and dosimetric estimates to separate organs determined. If these biodistribution studies predicted that more radiation would be delivered to marrow than to normal organs, the patients were then entered onto a dose escalation study in which increasing doses of ^{131}I conjugated to anti-CD33 were combined with a standard preparative regimen of cyclophosphamide (60 mg/kg $\times$ 2 days) followed by 12 Gy TBI. To date, 9 patients with AML have been studied. In 4 of the 9, the biodistribution studies predicted that up to 3-fold more radiation would be delivered to marrow than to normal organs. In the other 5 patients, more radiation would be delivered to a nonmarrow organ than to marrow. This outcome was less impressive than expected given the preclinical animal data. The major reason for the decreased marrow dose in humans compared to the animal models appeared to be that although ^{131}I was rapidly taken up by the marrow, the residence time of the radionuclide in the marrow was very brief, presumably because after binding, the antibody–radionuclide complex was rapidly internalized and then underwent catabolism or enzymatic and/or hydrolytic digestion with subsequent release of iodine from the marrow space. Additional differences between the human experience and that seen in the animal model were that with doses of antibody much above 0.1 mg/kg marrow sites were saturated resulting in less favorable biodistribution, whereas in the animal studies higher doses of antibody were tolerated. This outcome presumably reflects the very limited expression of CD33 in man. A final difference was that preclearance with cold antibody had little effect on subsequent antibody behavior probably because the circulating cells did not express CD33. The 4 patients with favorable biodistribution went on to therapy with ^{131}I-anti-CD33 followed by cyclophosphamide and TBI and marrow transplantation. The treatment in all 4 cases was well tolerated and no dose limiting toxicities were seen. Therefore, this dose escalation study continues. This study to date has demonstrated that in some patients ^{131}I-anti-CD33 can target marrow relatively specifically and that high doses of ^{131}I can be added to a standard transplant preparative regimen. This study also demonstrates some of the limitations of this approach, principally the short residence of the radionuclide within the marrow space.

A second study of radiolabeled anti-CD33 has recently been reported by Scheinberg et al.[22] Unlike the previously mentioned trial, this study was not intended as treatment, but rather to determine the distribution of the antibody conjugate and so only trace labeled antibodies were infused. As in the previously mentioned study, after infusion of antibody there was rapid uptake of the radionuclide conjugate in marrow. Uptake as a percent of the injected dose was best with the lowest amounts of antibody administered and retention in the marrow space was brief, presumably because the majority of the bound antibody was internalized and subsequently metabolized. These 2 studies then are consistent in their findings concerning the use of conventionally labeled anti-CD33 antibodies.

A number of strategies are being developed to overcome the limitations so far seen using an anti-CD33 antibody labeled conventionally with ^{131}I in the treatment of AML. One strategy is to develop labeling techniques which allow stable retention of the radionuclide in the cell after the antibody radionuclide binds to its target. A second approach is to target a different antigen which is stable and not internalized. A number of alternative labeling methods exist which may allow for sustained retention of the radionuclide within the targeted cell. The use of bifunctional chelates such as DTPA is one potential approach. Nude mice injected with a human erythroleukemia cell line will develop a subcutaneous tumor. If these mice are injected with an anti-CD33 antibody labeled with ^{131}I using chloramine T or with ^{111}In using DTPA there will be 7-fold greater retention of the DTPA label at 48 hours than of the chloramine T label.[19] There is, however, prolonged retention of the DPTA label in the liver as well. Another approach is to label antibodies with iodine using a nonmetabolizable cellulose fragment in the form of tyramine cellobiose (TCB). In the same nude mouse model retention of TCB labeled anti-CD33 resulted in retention of the iodine in the tumor at least as long as seen with the indium labeled antibody but with less uptake in nonmarrow organs. Based on these encouraging results a trial using TCB labeled anti-CD33 is currently underway in selected patients with myeloid leukemias.

Another approach to the treatment of leukemia with RAIT is to select a target antigen which is cell surface stable. CD45 (T200) is such an antigen which is present on virtually all lymphohematopoietic cells in relatively high numbers and is not found on nonhematopoietic cells. Experiments in mice and more recently in primates have shown that following intravenous administration of 0.5 mg/kg of conventionally labeled anti-CD45 there is marked uptake in spleen, lymph nodes, and marrow and that the label is retained at these sites with relative stability.[15,16] Estimation of radiation absorbed doses demonstrated that these antibodies would deliver up to 5 times more radiation to spleen and lymph nodes and up to 3-fold more to marrow than to liver or lung.

Use of RAIT in the treatment of other leukemias

Based on the results obtained in primates mentioned above, a trial of radiolabeled anti-CD45 antibody in patients with ALL undergoing marrow transplantation has been initiated. The design of this study is similar to that previously described for CD33. To date, 2 patients have been studied and both have demonstrated biodistribution results very similar to that predicted from the primate studies. Both have gone on to the transplant phase and have tolerated the procedure well.

The use of ^{90}Y-labeled anti-Tac is currently being evaluated for the treatment of HTLV-1 associated, Tac-expressing acute T-cell leukemia.[23] Patients are being treated with relatively low doses of radionuclide (5 to 10 mCi per patient) without marrow support. Results of this trial are not yet published.

Studies of RAIT for lymphoma

Preclinical murine experiments

Many of the principles underlying the use of radiolabeled antibodies to treat lymphoma come from experiments in murine models. A number of different investigators have contributed to this field, but in this chapter only one series of experiments performed by Badger et al. will be reviewed as an example of what has been learned. In this series of experiments, the biodistribution and therapeutic effects of radiolabeled antibodies were studied in mice bearing transplanted lymphomas.[5,6] Two situations were examined, one in which the antibody was truly tumor specific and a second in which the antibody reacted with a differentiation antigen expressed both by the tumor and by a proportion of normal murine lymphocytes. These experiments demonstrated that using the tumor specific antibody, up to 5-fold more radiation could be delivered to the tumor than to normal tissues and that ^{131}I antibody could induce complete regression of tumor masses where unmodified relevant antibody or labeled irrelevant antibody had no effects. Marrow suppression proved to be the dose limiting toxicity and without marrow support animals could not be cured. With marrow support, however, complete eradication of tumor was possible. When a tumor-associated rather than a tumor-specific antibody was used, similar results could be achieved. The only major difference was that optimal biodistribution depended on infusing higher doses of antibody, presumably because these higher doses were able to saturate sites on normal lymphocytes and thereby allow continued binding of radiolabeled antibody to tumor cells. In additional experiments, mixtures of antigen positive and antigen negative tumor cells were inoculated into mice in order to test whether radiolabeled antibodies could eliminate antigen negative tumor cells within an antigen positive tumor mass.[24] These experiments demonstrated that complete eradication of tumor was possible even though the tumor mass contained up to 10% antigen negative tumor cells. Based on these and other experiments, several groups have initiated studies of radioimmunotherapy for lymphoma.

Studies of radioimmunotherapy for lymphoma in man

Cutaneous T-cell lymphoma Rosen et al. have studied the use of ^{131}I labeled T101 antibody in patients with cutaneous T-cell lymphomas.[25] The first 6 patients entered on study were treated at a dose of 10 mg of antibody trace labeled with ^{131}I in order to determine the biodistribution of the labeled antibody. Five of these 6 patients then went on to therapy with antibody labeled with between 100–150 mCi of [131]I. When the amount of radionuclide localizing to tumor was compared to that in normal skin, only modest lesion to nonlesion ratios were obtained, ranging from 0.9–2.1. Similarly, lesion to bone marrow ratios ranged from 0.3–1.5. However, all 5 treated patients responded to therapy with partial responses lasting from 3 weeks to 3 months. The contribution of specific radiation, nonspecific radiation, and the effects of antibody alone were impossible to distinguish. The dose limiting toxicity seen in this study was significant marrow suppression at the 150 mCi dose level.

A second study involving cutaneous T-cell lymphoma and radiolabeled antibodies was performed by Carrasquillo et al.[26] As opposed to the study by Rosen, this study was solely for the purpose of immunodetection rather than actual treatment. In this study, antibody T101 was labeled with ^{111}In using the DTPA method. Although precise dosimetric estimates were not made, this study did demonstrate that lesions could be visualized and that as opposed to the experience with ^{131}I labeled T101, prolonged retention of the label at the site of tumor was seen. Further, less nonspecific uptake in the liver was seen when higher doses of antibody (in the range of 50 mg) were used as opposed to lower doses. These findings are consistent with those in animal models of T-cell lymphoma referred to earlier. Together, these studies from Carrasquillo and Rosen suggest that radioimmunotherapy of cutaneous T-cell lymphoma is possible, that substantial doses of antibody may be required to achieve the best biodistribution and that deiodination of conventionally labeled T101 is a problem which might be overcome with alternative methods of antibody labeling.

Non-Hodgkin's lymphomas A number of studies of the use of radiolabeled pan-B cell antibodies in the treatment of non-Hodgkin's lymphoma have recently been published. Scheinberg et al., for example, performed a dosimetry study using an antibody termed OKB7 which is reactive with both malignant and normal B-cells.[27] In this study, 18 patients were given trace labeled antibody at 6 different doses ranging from 0.1–40 mg with 3 patients treated at each level. Following infusion, biodistribution of the trace label antibody was determined by patient imaging and biopsies of tumored masses. The antibody infusions were well tolerated with no toxicities found. The antibody exhibited an early serum half-life of 1.9 hours and a later phase of 21.7 hours which was not dose dependent within the antibody dose range studied. Similarly, the amount of radionuclide that ended in the tumor mass was also unrelated to dose within this dose range, but rather was determined in part by the amount of antigen expressed by the tumor and in part by the size of the tumor mass. Thus, patients with small tumors and large amounts of antigen had the greatest uptake of antibody whereas patients with bulky tumors and low expression of antigen had much less uptake. Precise dosimetric estimates were not provided for all patients, but in at least 2 of the 18 patients very high tumor to total body ratios were reported. No patient had a therapeutic response to the antibody infusion.

Another ^{131}I labeled pan-B cell antibody termed LL2 has been studied by Goldenberg et al.[28] This trial involved 16 patients who were given trace labeled antibody followed by dosimetric studies. The blood clearance of LL2, like that of OKB7, was biphasic with an early halflife of 2.1 hours and a later halflife of 32.0 hours. In 6 of the 16 patients, the biodistribution studies suggested that higher doses of radiation would be delivered to tumor than to normal organs using radiolabeled antibodies. In the best of these circumstances, the ratio was found to be 5 : 1. Seven of the 16 patients then went on to the treatment phase of the study using antibody labeled with between 7–50 mCi of [131]I. Partial responses were seen in 2 of the 7 patients.

[131]I labeled LYM1, an antibody reactive with a class II variant, has been studied by DeNardo et al. in several clinical trials.[29–32] In the first trial patients were given 5 mg of cold antibody as preclearance followed by 1–10 mg LYM1 labeled with 30–60 mCi of [131]I. Thereafter, patients were treated with a repeat dose every 2–6 weeks to a total of cumulative ^{131}I dose of 300 mCi. Among the 18 patients, 2 complete responses and 8 partial responses were seen. In a subsequent study, the amount of ^{131}I labeled to LYM1 was increased to determine the maximum tolerated dose without marrow support. Nine patients have been entered into that study, and it appears that the maximum tolerated dose will be approximately 150 mCi of ^{131}I with thrombocytopenia being dose limiting.

In Seattle, we have been studying several different B-cell associated antibodies.[33–35] These studies have a biodistribution and a therapy phase. Initially, patients with recurrent B-cell lymphomas have undergone biodistribution studies at 0.5, 2.5, and 10 mg/kg of the antibody trace labeled with ^{131}I to determine the impact of antibody dose on localization of radionuclide to tumor and normal organs. If the biodistribution studies demonstrate that all measurable tumor sites would receive more radiation than any critical normal organ (lung, liver, and kidneys), the patients were then treated with high-dose [131]I. The treatment arm of the study was designed to test the toxicities of increasing doses ^{131}I with autologous marrow support. To date we have found that, in 13 of 27 patients, these biodistribution studies showed that greater amounts of radiation could be delivered to tumor compared to kidney, lung or liver. This 'favorable' distribution of antibody was only seen in patients with relatively small tumor burden. Thus, of the patient population studied, 13 of 18 patients who had tumor burdens less than 0.5 kg showed favorable biodistribution, whereas favorable biodistribution did not occur in any of 9 patients who had tumor burdens greater than 0.5 kg. The ability to achieve favorable biodistribution also appeared to be dependent upon the amount of antibody infused. This was most apparent in studies of the anti-CD37 antibody where favorable biodistribution was not seen at the lowest dose tested (0.5 mg/kg) and was most often seen at the highest dose tested (10 mg/kg) where favorable biodistribution was observed in 7 of 16 patients. In these studies, several different antibodies were compared one to another. It was found that anti-idiotypic antibodies had no apparent advantage over pan-B cell antibodies, although these studies are admittedly preliminary. In addition, we found that the use of the anti-CD20 antibody may be less dependent on antibody dose than use of the anti-CD37 antibody.

Twelve patients have been treated on this study to date. Doses of ^{131}I have ranged from 232–628 mCi and have been designed to deliver from 500–2025 cGy to the normal organ receiving the most radiation. The calculated dose to tumor in these patients was between 615–6400 cGy. Myeloid suppression has been the only significant toxicity encountered so far with a white cell and platelet count nadir at approximately 3 weeks after therapy. With the use of cryopreserved autologous marrow, the extent of this toxicity has been limited and no treatment-related fatalities have been seen. Among the first 10 patients treated so far, there have been 1 partial and 9 complete responses with the complete responses lasting from 4 to more than 30 months. Four patients are currently in continuous complete remission.

Hodgkin's disease   The use of a polyclonal antiferritin antibody radiolabeled with ^{131}I for the treatment of Hodgkin's disease has been pioneered by the Johns Hopkins group.[36,37] After their initial phase I studies they expanded this therapy to a phase II study in 38 patients with advanced progressive Hodgkin's disease. These patients received ^{131}I antiferritin intravenously at a dose of 30 mCi on day 1 and 30 mCi on day 5. Objective partial remissions of measurable disease were recorded in 40% of patients. Toxicities, once again, were essentially hematopoietic. The group from Johns Hopkins has gone on to study the use of alternative labels such as ^{90}Y and, although only preliminary results have been published, responses have clearly been seen in this setting as well. More recently, they have increased the dose of ^{90}Y with autologous marrow support and report complete responses in 4 of 8 Hodgkin's patients so treated.

Conclusions
The clinical trials so far published of the therapeutic use of radioimmunoconjugates define a number of important principles and also highlight the

promise and problems of this treatment modality. For example, important interactions of disease type and extent with antibody dose have been seen. In the setting of leukemia, very rapid uptake of the radiolabel in the target organ has been observed even at low antibody dose; this is distinct from the setting of lymphoma where slower uptake has been seen and higher doses of antibody have been required to achieve optimal tumor to normal tissue ratios. Further, in leukemia the ability to target marrow has not been dependent on the extent of disease whereas with lymphoma it has proven difficult to achieve therapeutic ratios in patients with large tumor burdens. These differences presumably relate to the greater accessibility of the marrow to the blood stream and therefore, to the infused antibody. Approaches under study to improve the accessibility of lymphoma masses to the infused antibody include the use of antibody fragments which might diffuse into the tumor more rapidly and the use of IL-2 or other agents which might improve vascular permeability.

Depending on the antigen targeted, both in leukemia and lymphoma internalization with subsequent metabolism and release of the radionuclide from the target is a problem when using antibodies conventionally labeled with [131]I. This problem can be diminished with the use of alternative labeling chemistries, with other radionuclides or by choosing targets which are cell surface stable. All 3 approaches are being explored in current dosimetry trials.

In every therapy study of RAIT for hematologic malignancy which has involved dose escalation, marrow toxicity has been dose limiting. The marrow suppressive effects of radiolabeled antibodies in the treatment of leukemia are obviously due to direct targeting of the marrow. In the setting of lymphoma, the mechanisms of marrow suppression are more complex and probably vary depending on the radionuclide used. With the use of the radionuclides so far studied in man, that is ^{131}I or ^{90}Y, marrow suppression has clearly been dose limiting and is probably the result primarily of radiation from the blood as source organ. In the treatment of lymphoma, the highest doses of ^{131}I tolerable without marrow support appear to be around 100–150 mCi and result in partial responses in many patients. Repetitive dosing at 100–150 mCi of ^{131}I can be accomplished in some patients but marrow suppression tends to be cumulative and limits the utility of this approach. Studies in animal models demonstrate that hematopoietic growth factors such as G-CSF can decrease the marrow suppressive effects of systemic radiation without marrow support by several hundred cGy.[38] With marrow transplantation support, the dose of radionuclide that can be given for the treatment of lymphoma is as yet undetermined since dose escalation studies have not yet reached the maximum tolerated dose (MTD). It is encouraging, however, that at doses considerably less than the MTD, complete responses (some of which are enduring in excess of 3 years) have already been seen. It is also encouraging to note that, in the treatment of leukemia, substantial doses of radiotherapy targeted to the marrow can be combined with standard transplant preparative regimens without undue toxicity. As in the lymphoma studies, the maximum tolerated dose has not yet been reached.

Acknowledgements
This work was supported in part by National Institutes of Health grants numbers: CA18029, CA47748, CA44991, and CA18105.

References
(1) Meeker TC, Lowder J, Maloney DG et al. A clinical trial of anti-idiotype therapy for B cell malignancy. *Blood* 1985; 65: 1349–63.

(2) Press OW, Appelbaum F, Ledbetter JA et al. Monoclonal antibody 1F5 (anti-CD20) serotherapy of human B cell lymphomas. *Blood* 1987; 69: 584–91.

(3) Brown SL, Miller RA, Horning SJ et al. Treatment of B-cell lymphomas with anti-idiotype antibodies alone and in combination with alpha interferon. *Blood* 1989; 73: 651–61.

(4) Hale G, Dyer MJ, Clark MR et al. Remission induction in non-Hodgkin lymphoma with reshaped human monoclonal antibody CAMPATH-1H. *Lancet* 1988; ii: 1394–9.

(5) Badger CC, Krohn KA, Peterson AV, Shulman H, Bernstein ID. Experimental radiotherapy of murine lymphoma with ^{131}I-labeled anti-Thy 1.1 monoclonal antibody. *Cancer Res* 1985; 45: 1536–44.

(6) Badger CC, Krohn KA, Shulman H, Flournoy N, Bernstein ID. Experimental radioimmunotherapy of lymphoma with ^{131}I-labelled anti-T-cell antibodies. *Cancer Res* 1986; 46: 6223–8.

(7) Cleary ML, Meeker TC, Levy S et al. Clustering of extensive somatic mutations in the variable region of an immunoglobulin heavy chain gene from a human B cell lymphoma. *Cell* 1986; 44: 97–106.

(8) Meeker T, Lowder J, Cleary ML et al. Emergence of idiotype variants during treatment of B-cell lymphoma with anti-idiotype antibodies. *N Eng J Med* 1985; 312: 1658–65.

(9) Young RC, Johnson RE, Canellos GP et al. Advanced lymphocytic lymphoma: randomized comparisons of chemotherapy and radiotherapy, alone or in combination. *Cancer Treat Rep* 1977; 61: 1153–9.

(10) Thomas ED. Bone marrow transplantation – past, present and future. In: *The Nobel prizes*. Stockholm, The Nobel Foundation, 1990.

(11) Clift RA, Buckner CD, Appelbaum FR et al. Allogeneic marrow transplantation in patients with acute myeloid leukemia in first remission. A randomized trial of two irradiation regimens. *Blood* 1990; 76: 1867–71.

(12) Clift RA, Buckner CD, Appelbaum FA, Bryant E et al. Allogeneic marrow transplantation in patients with chronic myeloid leukemia in the chronic phase. A randomized trial of two irradiation regimens. *Blood* 1991; 77: 1660–5.

(13) Scheinberg DA, Strand M. Kinetic and catabolic considerations of monoclonal antibody targeting in erythroleukemic mice. *Cancer Res* 1983; 43: 265–72.

(14) Appelbaum FR, Brown P, Sandmaier B et al. Antibody-radionuclide conjugates

as part of a myeloblative preparative regimen for marrow transplantation. *Blood* 1989; 73: 2202–8.

(15) Matthews DC, Appelbaum FR, Eary JF et al. Radiolabeled anti-CD45 monoclonal antibodies target hematolymphoid tissue in murine and macaque models. *Antibody Immunoconjugates and Radiopharmaceuticals* (in press).

(16) Matthews DC, Appelbaum FR, Eary JF et al. Radiolabeled Anti-CD45 monoclonal antibodies target lymphohematopoietic tissue in the macaque. *Blood* 1991; 78 (7): 1864–74.

(17) Bianco JA, Sandmaier B, Brown P et al. Specific marrow localization of an ^{131}I-labeled anti-myeloid antibody in normal dogs: effects of a 'cold' antibody pretreatment dose on marrow localization. *Exp Hematol* 1989; 17: 929–34.

(18) Bianco JA, Brown PA, Durack L et al. Effects of propylthiouracil on the biodistribution of an ^{131}I-labeled anti-myeloid antibody in normal dogs: dosimetry and clinical implications. *J Nucl Med* 1990; 31: 1384–9.

(19) van der Jagt RHC, Badger CC, Appelbaum FR. Tumor localization of radiolabled anti-myeloid antibodies in a human erythroleukemia xenograft model. *Cancer Research* 1992; 52 (1): 89–94.

(20) Ali SA, Eary JF, Warren SD, Badger CC, Krohn KA. Synthesis and radioiodination of tryamine cellobiose for labeling monoclonal antibodies. *Nucl Med Biol* 1988; 15: 557–61.

(21) Appelbaum FR, Matthews DC, Eary J et al. Use of radiolabelled anti-CD33 antibody to augment marrow irradiation prior to marrow transplantation for AML. *Transplantation* (in press).

(22) Scheinberg DA, Lovett D, Divgi CR et al. A phase I trial of monoclonal antibody M195 in acute myelogenous leukemia: specific bone marrow targeting and internalization of radionuclide. *J. Clin Oncol* 1991; 9: 478–90.

(23) Waldmann TA. Monoclonal antibodies in diagnosis and therapy. *Science* 1991; 252: 1657–62.

(24) Nourigat CL, Badger CC, Bernstein ID. Treatment of lymphoma with radiolabeled antibody: elimination of tumor cells that lack the target antigen. *J Natl Cancer Inst* 1990; 82: 1.

(25) Rosen ST, Zimmer AM, Goldman-Leikin R et al. Radioimmunodetection and radioimmunotherapy of cutaneous T cell lymphomas using an ^{131}I-labeled monoclonal antibody: an Illinois Cancer Council Study. *J Clin Oncol* 1987; 5: 562–73.

(26) Carrasquillo JA, Bunn PA, Jr., Keenan AM et al. Radioimmunodetection of cutaneous T-cell lymphoma with ^{111}In-labeled T101 monoclonal antibody. *N Eng J Med* 1986; 315: 673–80.

(27) Scheinberg DA, Straus DJ, Yeh SD et al. A phase I toxicity, pharmacology, and dosimetry trial of monoclonal antibody OKB7 in patients with non-Hodgkin's lymphoma: effects of tumor burden and antigen expression. *J Clin Oncol* 1990; 8: 792–803.

(28) Goldenberg DM, Horowitz JA, Sharkey RM. Targeting, dosimetry, and radioimmunotherapy of B-cell lymphomas with ^{131}I-labeled LL2 monoclonal antibody. *J Clin Oncol* 1991; 9 (4): 548–64.

(29) DeNardo GL, DeNardo SJ, O'Grady LF, Mills SL, Lewis JP, Macey DJ.

Radiation treatment of B cell malignancies with immunoconjugate. *Front Radiat Ther Oncol* 1990; 24: 194–201.

(30) DeNardo SJ, DeNardo GL, O'Grady LF et al. Treatment of a patient with B cell lymphoma by ^{131}I LYM-1 monoclonal antibodies. *Int J Biol Markers* 1991; 2: 49–53.

(31) DeNardo SJ, DeNardo GL, O'Grady LF. Pilot studies of radioimmunotherapy of B cell lymphoma and leukemia using ^{131}I Lym-1 monoclonal antibody. *Antibody, Immunoconjugates, and Radiopharmaceuticals*, 1988; 1:17.

(32) DeNardo SJ, DeNardo GL, O'Grady LF et al. Treatment of B cell malignancies with ^{131}I Lym-1 monoclonal antibodies. *Int J Cancer* 1988; 3: 96–101.

(33) Eary JF, Press OW, Badger CC et al. Imaging and treatment of B-cell lymphoma. *J Nucl Med* 1990; 31: 1257–68.

(34) Press OW, Eary JF, Badger CC et al. Treatment of refractory non-Hodgkin's lymphoma with radiolabeled MB-1 (anti-CD37) antibody. *J Clin Oncol* 1989; 7: 1027–38.

(35) Press OW, Eary JF, Badger CC et al. High-dose radioimmunotherapy of B cell lymphomas. *Front Radiat Ther Oncol* 1989; 24: 204–13.

(36) Lenhard RE, Jr., Order SE, Spunberg JJ, Asbell SO, Leibel SA. Isotopic immunoglobulin: a new systemic therapy for advanced Hodgkin's disease. *J Clin Oncol* 1985; 3: 1296–300.

(37) Vriesendorp HM, Herpst JM, Leichner PK, Klein JL, Order SE. Polyclonal ^{90}Yttrium labeled antiferritin for refractory Hodgkin's disease. *Int J Radiat Oncol Biol Phys* 1989; 17: 815–21.

(38) Schuening FG, Storb R, Goehle S et al. Effect of recombinant human granulocyte colony-stimulating factor on hematopoiesis of normal dogs and on hematopoietic recovery after otherwise lethal total body irradiation. *Blood* 1989; 74: 1308–13.

Autologous graft-versus-host disease

R J JONES AND A D HESS

Introduction

Autologous bone marrow transplantation (BMT) has become effective therapy for patients with high-risk lymphomas[1-4] and acute leukemias,[5-7] with long-term disease-free survival and probable cure in 20–50% of patients. Tumor recurrence remains the major cause for failure of autologous BMT, accounting for nearly 90% of the failures. However, animal models suggest that a 25–50% improvement in relapse rate, as would be needed to cure the majority of patients with high-risk hematologic malignancies who now relapse after autologous BMT, probably requires no more than an average of 1–2 logs of additional tumor cell kill.[8,9] Nevertheless, this small amount of additional tumor cell kill likely represents the most drug-resistant population of cells. In addition, current cytotoxic preparative regimens for BMT are at or near non-hematologic dose-limiting toxicity. Thus, a further increase in the intensity of, or the addition of, new cytotoxic agents to these preparative regimens has not been very fruitful. Other approaches for improving the antitumor activity of autologous BMT are therefore needed. Immunologic approaches for eradicating tumor should be particularly effective after autologous BMT for hematologic malignancies, as they would be used in a period of minimal residual disease, and should be truly non-cross resistant with the cytotoxic therapy.

Graft-versus-host-disease (GVHD) develops in about 50–70% of patients undergoing allogeneic BMT, and is the main cause of toxicity in these patients. However, GVHD also seems to produce a clinically significant antileukemia effect.[6,10-13] Although initial reports were unable to establish a similar graft-versus-lymphoma effect after allogeneic BMT,[1,14] recent studies have also established the existence of a clinically significant antilymphoma effect associated with allogeneic BMT that is similar in magnitude to the graft-versus-leukemia effect.[15] Attempts to prevent GVHD by T lymphocyte

All correspondence to: Dr RJ Jones, The Bone Marrow Transplantation Program, The Johns Hopkins Oncology Center, Room 2–127, 600 North Wolfe Street, Baltimore, Maryland 21205, USA.

Cambridge Medical Reviews: Haematological Oncology Volume 2

depletion of allogeneic marrow grafts have led to increased relapse rates following allogeneic BMT.[12,13] Therefore, control of GVHD has not significantly improved survival after allogeneic BMT, as the decreased mortality resulting from GVHD is offset by increased relapse rates. Likewise, although autologous or syngeneic BMT avoid the toxicity of GVHD, the graft-versus-tumor effect is also absent; this appears to be a major reason for the higher relapse rates after autologous and syngeneic BMT compared to allogeneic BMT.[6,10]

A syndrome similar to GVHD develops spontaneously in 5–10% of patients undergoing autologous or syngeneic BMT.[16–18] This syndrome clinically resembles GVHD, but it is a mild, self-limited disease that generally involves only the skin. Histologic changes of this 'autologous GVHD' are also identical to those of allogeneic GVHD. Because spontaneous autologous GVHD is a relatively uncommon phenomenon, it has not been possible to establish if it is associated with an antitumor effect. Autologous GVHD was controversial until the development of animal models for the syndrome.[19–21] In these models, GVHD developed in rats or mice treated with cyclosporine (CsA) after syngeneic BMT.

GVHD after syngeneic BMT in rats appears to be mediated by autoreactive lymphocytes directed against class II histocompatibility (HLA-DR or Ia) antigens.[22] GVHD after syngeneic BMT in animals also exhibits antitumor activity, similar to allogeneic GVHD, against tumors that express Ia antigen.[23,24] Since most lymphomas (including Reed–Sternberg cells of Hodgkin's disease) and acute leukemias express Ia antigens,[25] autologous GVHD could potentially produce a clinical immunologic antitumor effect without increasing posttransplant toxicity. The authors have found that autologous GVHD can be induced with CsA in patients undergoing autologous BMT,[26] and preliminary results suggest that CsA-induced autologous GVHD also manifests clinical antitumor activity.

Animal models

Immunologic mechanisms of syngeneic GVHD

Glazier et al. reported that rats treated with CsA for 30–40 days after syngeneic BMT developed a T lymphocyte dependent autoimmune syndrome 14–28 days after discontinuation of the CsA.[19] Initially, this syndrome resembled acute GVHD with erythema and dermatitis, and histologic lesions indistinguishable from the pathology of allogeneic GVHD were observed in the skin and liver.[27] This syngeneic GVHD in rats rapidly progressed to a more chronic form of GVHD with its relevant histologic features.[28] This syndrome can also be induced in mice with the use of CsA.[20,21] Both CD4+ and CD8+ T lymphocytes are required for the full development of syngeneic GVHD.[29] The transfer of large numbers of CD8+ cells from animals with syngeneic GVHD results in just an acute form of syngeneic GVHD in the recipients, that resolves within 2 weeks. The addition of CD4+ T-cells from the animals with syngeneic GVHD both augmented the transfer of the acute form of syngeneic GVHD and also allowed progression to the chronic form. The effector T-cells of syngeneic GVHD appear to recognize Ia antigen on target cells.[22,30] Moreover, the effector cells appear to recognize a public determinant of Ia since the effector cells are capable of lysing Ia-bearing cells from multiple strains of rats in addition to self.[22]

Several factors have been shown to be essential for the induction of syngeneic GVHD. This syndrome can only be induced in rats that were treated with CsA for a minimum of 28 days.[31] Total body irradiation, or other regimens that can ablate the lymphohematopoietic system, are generally necessary for the syndrome to be induced,[19,20] although normal, nontransplanted animals may develop syngeneic GVHD if treated with CsA for extended periods of time (over 6 months).[32] An intact thymus that is included within the irradiation field is also required, as shielding the thymus during total body irradiation results in failure to induce the syndrome.[27] Taken together, it appears that ablation of the lymphohematopoietic system is needed to damage the thymus and to eliminate peripheral host autoregulatory mechanisms. The damaged thymus gives rise to the effector cells of syngeneic GVHD. CsA appears to augment the development of autoreactive lymphocytes by blocking mechanisms that delete autoreactive T-cells in the thymus.[33]

Antitumor activity of syngeneic GVHD

To determine if syngeneic GVHD exhibited antitumor activity, as is seen with allogeneic GVHD, studies were initiated using the CRL1662 myeloma cell line derived from the LouM strain of rat.[23] This tumor was chosen because it expressed Ia antigen. Syngeneic GVHD had been reported to show no antileukemia activity against a rat leukemia;[34] however, this leukemia does not express Ia and therefore would not be expected to be a target of syngeneic GVHD. Splenic T-cells from LouM rats that developed syngeneic GVHD were able to lyse CRL1662 tumor cells in vitro.[23] Cytolytic activity of the lymphocytes against the tumor cells declined to baseline as the syngeneic GVHD resolved. Lysis of tumor cells was blocked by preincubation of the tumor cells with antibodies specific for Ia antigen but not with antibodies against class I antigens. The interferons, both gamma and alpha, have been shown to upregulate Ia expression on hematologic malignancies.[35,36] Incubation of the tumor cells with γ-interferon increased expression of Ia antigen and also enhanced the lysis of the cells by the lymphocytes obtained from rats with syngeneic GVHD.[23] These studies demonstrated that syngeneic GVHD manifested antitumor activity in vitro, and confirmed that the effector cell was a T lymphocyte specific for the Ia antigen.

Our preliminary data also confirms that syngeneic GVHD produces anti-tumor activity in vivo. Syngeneic GVHD in mice will kill L1210 leukemia cells (which also express class II antigens) in vivo. An advantage of using this leukemia is that it can be used as a model of minimal residual disease, as just one L1210 cell can kill a mouse.[8,37] This allowed us to demonstrate that syngeneic GVHD will actually cure mice injected with small numbers of L1210 cells. It appeared that syngeneic GVHD was able to kill 1–2 logs of L1210 cells in vivo. Syngeneic GVHD in rats will also produce antitumor activity in vivo.[24] Syngeneic GVHD results in about a 1 log kill of CRL1662 myeloma cells injected into rats. However, both γ-interferon[24] and α-interferon appear to enhance the antitumor effect of syngeneic GVHD by 1–2 logs in the rat model. The magnitude of the immunologic antitumor activity generated by syngeneic GVHD appears similar to that produced by allogeneic GVHD.[9]

Human studies
Based on the results of the animal studies, the authors designed a study to determine whether GVHD could be induced in patients undergoing autologous BMT for hematologic malignancies.[26] They treated 5 consecutive patients with aggressive non-Hodgkin's lymphoma (3 patients) or Hodgkin's disease (2 patients) in resistant relapse (no longer responsive to conventional salvage therapy) with autologous BMT and CsA. The preparative regimen was busulfan plus cyclophosphamide in 3 patients who had received prior irradiation and cyclophosphamide plus total body irradiation in the other 2 patients. CsA was started on the day of BMT and was continued for 28 days at 1 mg/kg per day. Histologically proven grade II GVHD of the skin developed in all 5 patients at a median of 11 days (range 9–13) after BMT, at the time of initial evidence of hematologic recovery. An erythematous maculopapular rash affecting the face, ears, upper trunk, and extremities (palms and soles) developed in all 5 patients, and involved the entire body of 2 patients. No patient developed evidence of extracutaneous GVHD. One patient died of fungal sepsis on day 12 after BMT, and the autologous GVHD resolved in 1 to 3 weeks in the other 4 patients, spontaneously in 2 patients and with corticosteroids in 2. The antigenic specificities of cytotoxic lymphocytes from 1 of the patients were tested in a cell mediated lysis assay. The lymphocytes collected during autologous GVHD were cytotoxic for the patient's own pretransplant lymphocytes and for lymphocytes from a healthy volunteer. The cytotoxicity was blocked by incubating the target cells with anti-Ia monoclonal antibodies. Lymphocytes obtained after resolution of clinical autologous GVHD would no longer react against the patient's own pretransplant lymphocytes or the healthy donor's lymphocytes. As in the animals with syngeneic GVHD, autoreactive lymphocytes recognizing a public epitope of the Ia antigen appear to mediate clinical autologous GVHD. Other groups

have now confirmed the authors' clinical results with inducing autologous GVHD, including finding Ia-restricted autoreactive lymphocytes in patients with autologus GVHD.[38,39]

In order to evaluate the potential antitumor activity of autologous GVHD, a phase II trial was undertaken to study induced autologous GVHD in patients with intermediate or high-grade non-Hodgkin's lymphoma in sensitive relapse (still responsive to conventional salvage therapy prior to BMT).[40] Although very few of these patients can be cured with conventional salvage therapy, about 50% of these patients appear to be curable wtih autologous BMT.[3,4] Nearly all of the failures following autologous BMT are a consequence of relapse. A 1–2 log additional tumor cell kill (as is seen with syngeneic GVHD in animals) over that provided by the preparative regimen, would be expected to decrease the relapse rate to less than 25%.[8,9] On this protocol 20 patients have been treated. About 80% of the patients have developed histologically proven cutaneous GVHD. The majority of the patients developed autologous GVHD during initial hematologic recovery, while on the CsA. About a quarter of the patients developed autologous GVHD after stopping the CsA, usually within 2 weeks of stopping the drug. The autologous GVHD resolved without incident in all patients. Lymphocytes obtained from patients at the time of autologous GVHD showed Ia-restricted autoreactivity. The preliminary results also suggest that there may be a clinically significant antitumor effect, similar to that seen in the animal models, associated with autologous GVHD. The authors have also been able to induce GVHD in patients undergoing autologous BMT with 4-hydroperoxycyclophosphamide purging for acute myeloid leukemia, and the initial antileukemia results likewise look promising.

Conclusions

BMT is effective treatment for patients with high-risk lymphomas and acute leukemias, and appears to be the treatment of choice for patients with these diseases at relapse. The main cause for failure of autologous BMT is tumor recurrence. Allogeneic BMT is one approach for decreasing the relapse rate associated with autologous grafts. The improved tumor control associated with allogeneic results in large part from a graft-versus-tumor effect. However, in general, allogeneic BMT has not substantially improved the disease-free survival of patients with high-risk lymphomas and acute leukemias compared to autologous BMT, because the decreased relapse rate associated with allogeneic BMT is offset by an increased mortality resulting from GVHD.[6,15]

The mechanisms responsible for the immunologic antitumor effect associated with allogeneic BMT are not completely understood. Most of the graft-versus-tumor activity following allogeneic BMT appears to result from chronic GVHD,[11,13] although there may be an antitumor effect associated with allogeneic GVHD that is independent of clinically apparent GVHD.[13] T-cells from mice with acute GVHD primarily display host antigen-specificity, while T-cells from mice with chronic GVHD exhibit Ia-specific autoreactivity.[41] Therefore, lymphocytes obtained during CsA-induced syngeneic or autologous GVHD have a pattern of reactivity similar to lymphocytes in chronic GVHD. Since most hematologic malignancies express Ia antigen,[25] it is not surprising that both chronic GVHD and autologous GVHD appear to manifest clinical antitumor activity.

CsA-induced autologous GVHD appears to generate immunologic antitumor activity without increased posttransplant toxicity. Whether this antitumor activity will translate into improved disease-free survival after autologous BMT is currently being studied in clinical trials. Furthermore, it should be possible to enhance the clinical antitumor activity of autologous GVHD by modulating either the effector cells or the target cells or both. Stimulation of the effector T-cells of autologous GVHD should improve their antitumor activity. A number of cytokines, i.e. IL-2 and IL-6,[42] stimulate cytotoxic T-cells and can induce antitumor activity. The interferons could be used to upregulate Ia expression on tumor cells and make these cells more sensitive to the cytotoxic effects of the effector T-cells of autologous GVHD. IL-2 has been examined as a means to enhance the graft-versus-tumor effect associated with allogeneic BMT, and, not unexpectantly, produced severe, fatal GVHD.[43,44] However, since autologous GVHD is a mild, self-limited disease, it is possible that the antitumor effect associated with this syndrome could be amplified without substantially increasing toxicity. In fact, preliminary data suggest that γ interferon will increase the antitumor effect of CsA-induced syngeneic GVHD in rats.[24] Clinical trials have begun to investigate the toxicity and efficacy of the interferons combined with CsA-induced autologous GVHD.

References
(1) Jones RJ, Piantadosi S, Mann RB et al. High-dose cytotoxic therapy and bone marrow transplantation for relapsed Hodgkin's disease. *J Clin Onc* 1990; 8: 527–37.
(2) Carella AM, Congiu AM, Gaozza E et al. High-dose chemotherapy with autologous bone marrow transplantation in 50 advanced resistant Hodgkin's disease patients: an Italian study group report. *J Clin Onc* 1988; 6: 1411–16.
(3) Philip T, Armitage JO, Spitzer G et al. High-dose therapy and autologous bone marrow transplantation after failure of conventional chemotherapy in adults with intermediate-grade or high-grade non-Hodgkin's lymphoma. *N Eng J Med* 1987, 316: 1493–8.
(4) Takvorian T, Canellos GP, Ritz J et al. Prolonged disease-free survival after autologous bone marrow transplantation in patients with non-Hodgkin's lymphoma with a poor prognosis. *N Eng J Med* 1987; 316: 1499–505.

(5) Yeager AM, Kaizer H, Santos GW et al. Autologous bone marrow transplantation in patients with acute nonlymphocytic leukemia, using ex vivo marrow treatment with 4-hydroperoxycyclophosphamide. *N Eng J Med* 1986; 315: 141–7.

(6) Kersey JH, Weisdorf D, Nesbit ME et al. Comparison of autologous and allogeneic bone marrow transplantation for treatment of high-risk refractory acute lymphoblastic leukemia. *N Eng J Med* 1987; 317: 461–7.

(7) Sallan SE, Niemeyer CM, Billett AL et al. Autologous bone marrow transplantation for acute lymphoblastic leukemia. *J Clin Onc* 1989; 7: 1594–601.

(8) Skipper HE, Schabel FM Jr, Wilcox WS. Experimental evaluation of potential anticancer agents. XIII. On the criteria and kinetics associated with 'curability' of experimental leukemia. *Cancer Chemotherapy Reports* 1964; 35: 1–111.

(9) Hageenbeek A, Martens ACM, Schultz FW. The graft-versus-leukemia reaction after allogeneic bone marrow transplantation only adds one log of leukemia cell kill. *Blood* 1988; 72: 390a. (Abstract)

(10) Weiden PL, Flournoy N, Thomas ED et al. Antileukemic effect of graft-versus-host disease in human recipients of allogeneic-marrow grafts. *N Eng J Med* 1979; 300: 1068–73.

(11) Weiden PL, Sullivan KM, Flournoy N, Storb R, Thomas ED. Antileukemic effect of chronic graft-versus-host disease. *N Eng J Med* 1981; 304: 1529–33, 1981.

(12) Butturini A, Bortin MM, Gale RP. Graft-versus-leukemia following bone marrow transplantation. *Bone Marrow Transpl* 1987; 2: 233–42.

(13) Horowitz MM, Gale RP, Sondel PM et al. Graft-versus-leukemia reactions after bone marrow transplantation. *Blood* 1990; 75: 555–62.

(14) Appelbaum FR, Sullivan KM, Buckner CD et al. Treatment of malignant lymphoma in 100 patients with chemotherapy, total body irradiation, and marrow transplantation. *J Clin Onc* 1987; 5: 1340–7.

(15) Jones RJ, Ambinder RF, Piantadosi S, Santos GW. Evidence of a graft-versus-lymphoma effect associated with allogeneic bone marrow transplantation. *Blood* 1991; 77: 649–53.

(16) Rappeport J, Mihm M, Reinherz E, Lopansri S, Parkman R. Acute graft-versus-host disease in recipients of bone-marrow transplants from identical twin donors. *Lancet* 979; ii: 717–20.

(17) Hood AF, Vogelsang GB, Black LP, Farmer ER, Santos GW. Acute graft-vs-host disease. Development following autologous and syngeneic bone marrow transplantation. *Arch Dermatol* 1987; 123: 745–50.

(18) Einsele H, Ehninger G, Schneider EM et al. High frequency of graft-versus-host like syndromes following syngeneic bone marrow transplantation. *Transplantation* 1988; 45: 579–85.

(19) Glazier A., Tutschka PJ, Farmer ER, Santos GW. Graft-versus-host disease in cyclosporin A-treated rats after syngeneic and autologous bone marrow reconstitution. *J Exp Med* 1983; 158: 1–8.

(20) Cheney RT, Sprent J. Capacity of cyclosporine to induce auto-graft-versus-host disease and impair intrathymic T cell differentiation. *Transpl Proc* 1985; 178: 528–30.

(21) Bryson JS, Jennings CD, Caywood BE, Kaplan AM. Induction of a syngeneic graft-versus-host disease like syndrome in DBA/2 mice. *Transplantation* 1989; 48: 1042–7.

(22) Hess AD, Horwitz L, Beschorner WE, Santos GW. Development of graft-vs-host disease like syndrome in cyclosporine-treated rats after syngeneic bone marrow transplantation. *J Exp Med* 1985; 161: 718–30.

(23) Geller RB, Esa AH, Beschorner WE, Frondoza CG, Santos GW, Hess AD. Successful in vitro graft-versus-tumor effect against an Ia-bearing tumor using cyclosporine-induced syngeneic graft-versus-host disease in the rat. *Blood* 1989; 74: 1165–71.

(24) Noga S, Horwitz L, Hess A. Gamma interferon (INF) augments the graft-vs-tumor effect of syngeneic graft-vs-host-disease (SGVHD) in the rat. *J Leukocyte Biol* 1990; Suppl 1: 36. (Abstract)

(25) Foon KA, Todd RF III. Immunologic classification of leukemia and lymphoma. *Blood* 1986; 68: 1–31.

(26) Jones RJ, Vogelsang GB, Hess AD, Farmer ER, Mann RB, Geller RB et al. Induction of graft-versus-host disease after autologous bone marrow transplantation. *Lancet* 1989; i: 754–7.

(27) Glazier A, Tutschka PJ, Farmer ER. Studies on the immunobiology of syngeneic and autologous graft-versus-host disease in cyclosporine treated rats. *Transpl Proc* 1983; 15: 3035.

(28) Beschorner WE, Shinn CA, Fischer AC, Santos GW, Hess AD. Cyclosporine-induced pseudo-graft-versus-host disease in the early post-cyclosporine period. *Transplantation* 1988; 46: 112–17.

(29) Hess AD, Fischer AC, Beschorner WE. Effector mechanisms in cyclosporine A-induced syngeneic graft-versus-host disease: role of CD4+ and CD8+ T lymphocyte subsets. *J Immunol* 1990; 145: 526–33.

(30) Sorokin R, Kimura H, Schroder K, Wilson DH, Wilson DB. Cyclosporine-induced autoimmunity: conditions for expressing disease, requirement for intact thymus, and potency estimates of autoimmune lymphocytes in drug-treated rats. *J Exp Med* 1986; 164: 1615.

(31) Hess AD, Fischer AC. Immune mechanisms in cyclosporine-induced syngeneic graft-versus-host disease. *Transplantation* 1989; 48: 895–900.

(32) Shinozowa T, Beschorner WE, Hess AD. Prolonged administration of cyclosporine and the thymus: Irreversible immunopathologic changes associated with autologous pseudo-graft-versus-host disease. *Transplantation* 1991 (in press)

(33) Jenkins MK, Schwartz RH, Pardoll DM. Effects of cyclosporine A on T cell development and clonal deletion. *Science* 1988; 241: 1655–8.

(34) Tutschka PJ, Berkowitz SD, Tuttle S, Klein J. Graft-versus-leukemia in the rat – the antileukemic efficacy of syngeneic and allogeneic graft-versus-host disease. *Transpl Proc* 1987; XIX: 2668–73.

(35) Baldini L, Cortelezzi A, Polli N et al. Human recombinant interferon α-2C enhances the expression of class II HLA antigens on hairy cells. *Blood* 1986; 67: 458–64.

(36) Gressier VH, Weinkauff RE, Franklin WA, Golomb HM. Modulation of the expression of major histocompatibility antigens on splenic hairy cells – differen-

tial effect upon *in vitro* treatment with alpha-2b-interferon, gamma-interferon, and interleukin-2. *Blood* 1988; 72: 1048–53.

(37) Jones RJ, Colvin OM, Sensenbrenner LL. Prediction of the ability to purge tumor from murine bone marrow using clonogenic assays. *Cancer Res* 1988; 48: 3394–7.

(38) Dale BM, Atkinson K, Kotasek D, Biggs JC, Sage RE. Cyclosporine-induced graft vs host disease in two patients receiving syngeneic bone marrow transplants. *Transpl Proc* 1989; 21: 3816–17.

(39) Carella AM, Gaozza E, Piatti G. Induction of graft versus host disease (GvHD) after ABMT for high risk ALL in first CR and second chronic phase of chronic myeloid leukemia. *Exp Hematol* 1990 (in press)

(40) Jones RJ, Santos GW. New conditioning regimens for high risk marrow transplants. *Bone Marrow Transpl* 1989; 4: 15–17.

(41) Parkman R. Clonal analysis of murine graft-versus-host disease: I. Phenotypic and functional analysis of T lymphocyte clones. *J Immunol* 1986; 136: 3543–8.

(42) Mule JJ, McIntosh JK, Jablons DM, Rosenberg SA. Antitumor activity of recombinant Interleukin 6 in mice. *J Exp Med* 1990; 171: 629–36.

(43) Sprent J, Schaefer M, Gao E-K, Korngold R. Role of T cell subsets in lethal graft-versus-host disease (GVHD) directed to class I versus class II H-2 differences. *J Exp Med* 1988; 167: 556–69. (Abstract)

(44) Jadus MR, Peck AB. Lethal murine graft-versus-host disease in the absence of detectable cytotoxic T lymphocytes. *Transplantation* 1983; 36: 281–9. (Abstract)

Pathophysiology and treatment of acquired aplastic anaemia

J C W MARSH

Introduction

The aims of this critique are first to review recent progress in the understanding of the pathogenesis of acquired aplastic anaemia (AA), derived not only from ongoing clinical studies, but also from the availability of new laboratory methodology and the application of pre-existing in vitro techniques to the further study of this disorder. Studies on the nature of the haemopoietic failure in AA provide a unique opportunity to analyze the interaction of the haemopoietic stem cell with haemopoietic growth factors and the marrow microenvironment. Secondly, a critical update on the management of AA will be presented, demonstrating that the outcome of severe AA continues to improve since the mid 1970s when a mortality rate of 80% was reported with supportive care alone. In patients treated with antilymphocyte globulin (ALG) or androgens, but not in transplanted patients, the late development of clonal disease is being recognized due to the improved long-term survival associated with 'immunosuppressive' therapy. This has raised difficult new management problems in such patients, as well as contributing new insights into the pathogenesis and natural history of AA.

Definition

AA represents the failure of haemopoiesis. Because its pathogenesis has been poorly understood, definitions have been based on the end result of a reduction in haemopoietic activity of myeloid lineages in the bone marrow. A working definition is peripheral blood pancytopenia in the presence of a hypocellular bone marrow and without an excess of blasts. Normal marrow haemopoietic tissue is replaced by fat cells, but reticulin fibres are not increased.

All correspondence to: Dr JCW Marsh, St George's Hospital Medical School, Department of Cellular and Molecular Sciences, Division of Haematology, Cranmer Terrace, London SW17 0RE, UK.

Cambridge Medical Reviews: Haematological Oncology Volume 2
© Cambridge University Press 1992

Incidence

AA is not a common disorder. Its incidence varies considerably worldwide, probably reflecting different exposures to drugs, chemicals and viruses. In Europe, an estimate of < 3 cases per million population per year has recently been reported, based on a careful study from 8 separate regions using strict diagnostic criteria for AA.[1] Other studies reporting a higher incidence in Europe ranging from 5–25 per million per year, come from the 1960s and early 1970s when less rigid diagnostic criteria were used, and probably included cases of myelodysplastic syndrome (MDS) especially in the older patients.[2–4] A high incidence of AA in the Far East, Japan and China may be due to more frequent hepatitis, use of chloramphenicol, and greater exposure to insecticides.[5] In Europe, equal numbers of males and females are affected, with 2 peaks in age incidence for males (15–25 years and >60 years) and 1 peak for females (>60 years).

Classification

AA has been classified in many ways, reflecting the heterogeneous nature of the disorder. Fig. 1 represents an attempt to summarize most of the currently used classifications. In congenital AA, such as Fanconi anaemia and dyskeratosis congenita, failure of haemopoiesis may result in pancytopenia due to a presumed stem cell defect. In amegakaryocytic thrombocytopenia, congenital red cell aplasia and congenital neutropaenia, a proportion of patients with the corresponding monocytopenia later develop pancytopenia with generalized marrow failure. Recent reviews summarize diagnosis and treatment of the congenital bone marrow failure syndromes.[6–7]

Inevitable, transient and idiosyncratic AA

Acquired AA may be subdivided into inevitable, transient and idiosyncratic AA.[8] Inevitable AA is caused by cytotoxic drugs or radiation occurring within 2–4 weeks of exposure. The aplasia is dose dependent and usually recovers in 2–4 weeks unless supralethal doses of radiation or cytotoxic drugs are given. Transient AA may occur after certain viral infections such as infectious mononucleosis or systemic lupus erythematosis (SLE), although prolonged aplasia may also occur in these situations. This shortlived aplasia may have an immune origin or may be due to direct infection of haemopoietic cells. Idiosyncratic AA is the category of disease usually considered in reports and reviews of the AA syndrome. It develops unpredictably in a small minority of individuals after exposure to certain agents which may or may not be identified. The disease is prolonged, and spontaneous recovery is unusual. The remainder of this review is concerned with idiosyncratic AA.

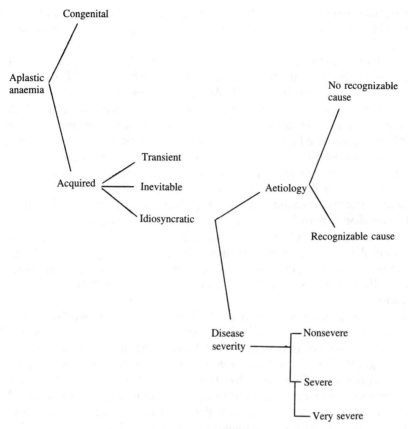

Fig. 1. Classification of aplastic anaemia.

Aetiology

In approximately 75–80% of cases of idiosyncratic AA, no obvious cause can be identified; these are termed idiopathic. Recognizable causes include viruses, drugs, chemicals, paroxysmal nocturnal haemoglobinuria (PNH), SLE and possibly pregnancy.

Many drugs have been implicated in the aetiology of AA, and possible mechanisms in AA recently reviewed by Gordon-Smith.[9] The International Agranulocytosis and AA study of 1986[10] showed that the evidence for many cases of drug induced AA is not strong and is often based on a small number of reported cases. The best documented drugs that may cause AA include chloramphenicol, phenylbutazone (and to a lesser extent indomethacin) and gold. Chemicals that have been associated with AA include benzene, aniline dyes and organic solvents. Benzene more commonly gives rise to MDS or

41

acute leukaemia with nonspecific or clonal cytogenetic changes, in addition to reversible cytopenias and AA, although these may not all be separate entities.[11]

AA is a rare complication of hepatitis. Most often it is associated with non-A, non-B hepatitis[12], although hepatitis A[13], hepatitis B[14] and Epstein Barr virus[15] have also been implicated. An agent ('hepatitis C') responsible for most cases of non-A, non-B hepatitis has recently been identified.[16] Pol examined the prevalence of hepatitis C in patients with AA, but found no significant difference between those with post hepatitic AA and patients with idiopathic disease or AA of known cause (15.8 vs 9.1% respectively).[17] Pol suggested that the low prevalence in non-A, non-B hepatitic AA may be due to a non-A, non-B, non-C virus, or defective immune function in such patients. The true incidence of post hepatitic AA is unclear on account of relatively few reported cases and incomplete serological investigations in earlier reported studies. Longstanding claim of a poor prognosis for post hepatitis AA has been made. However it may be that patients with post hepatitic AA have a poor prognosis because of very severe aplasia characteristically seen in this subgroup, rather than a direct association with the hepatitis.

Proving an association between a rare disease such as AA, and the common occurrence of pregnancy is difficult. Nevertheless there are well-documented reports of spontaneous remission of AA occurring at time of delivery[18] or following abortion[19-21], and recurrence of aplasia with subsequent pregnancies.[21] This controversial topic has been reviewed by Aitchison with some recommendations for management based on recent patient presentations.[21] In contrast the association of AA with PNH is well documented, and this is discussed later in relation to pathogenesis of AA.

Disease severity

The criteria for severe AA drawn up by International Aplastic Anaemia Study Group are widely used in management decisions (Table 1).[22] They not only have prognostic value but also permit comparisons of different treatment modalities and a particular form of therapy between centres with patients of similar disease severity. Patients who do not fulfil these criteria have non-severe AA. A recent modification to these criteria has been to include a particularly severe form of AA termed 'very severe AA' defined by neutrophil count $< 0.2 \times 10^9/l$, since these patients have a very poor prognosis unless treated by allogeneic bone marrow transplantation (BMT).[23] In approximately one-third of cases, the bone marrow may be more cellular than expected from peripheral blood counts, due to patchy marrow involvement. In these cases ferrokinetic studies using ^{52}Fe or ^{59}Fe whole body marrow scans may reflect the true disease severity, however, the peripheral blood count remains the best single indicator of disease severity.[24]

Table 1. *Criteria for severe aplastic anaemia**

1. Bone marrow hypocellularity:	<25% of normal or 25–50% of normal and <30% residual haemopoietic cells
2. Peripheral blood criteria:	Neutrophils <0.5 × 10^9/l Platelets <20 × 10^9/l Reticulocytes <1% (corrected for haematocrit)
3. For severe AA, 1 bone marrow and 2 of 3 peripheral blood criteria required.	

* International Aplastic Anaemia Study Group.[22]

Diagnosis

Physical examination of a patient with acquired AA should be normal apart from clinical signs attributable to the pancytopenia. Skeletal or skin abnormalities would raise the possibility of a congenital form of AA, although in Fanconi anaemia these anomalies may be absent in up to 30% of patients.[25] Therefore in younger patients presenting with AA (perhaps those less than 20 years of age, or older if some phenotypic abnormality is suspected) it is mandatory to exclude Fanconi anaemia by peripheral blood chromosome analysis using the diepoxybutane stress test[26] and by family studies, first because of the necessity to use much lower doses of cyclophosphamide and irradiation prior to BMT in view of an increased sensitivity to chemoradiotherapeutic agents, and secondly because genetic counselling is required for affected families. A Hams Dacie test and examination of the urine for haemosiderin should be performed to exclude PNH. (The presence of a reticulocytosis is also suggestive of PNH, as is a low neutrophil alkaline phosphatase score.) Both bone marrow aspirate and trephine biopsy (preferably from more than one site) are essential. The trephine provides a better assessment of marrow cellularity and may also detect clusters of blast cells which might be missed on aspiration. This is particularly relevant in those cases that later transform to MDS or acute leukaemia, and also in children in whom acute lymphoblastic leukaemia (and more rarely acute myeloblastic leukaemia) can occasionally present in a hypoplastic phase.[27,28] The differentiation of AA from hypoplasia MDS[29] may also be difficult, since it is not uncommon to see some dysplastic features especially dyserythropoiesis and even dysmegakaryocytopoiesis in patients with typical AA.[30] Bone marrow cytogenetic analysis may help to differentiate between the two in some cases, although they may not represent separate entities.[31]

J C W Marsh

Pathogenesis

Stromal cell mediated haemopoiesis – a model for normal haemopoiesis

Since AA represents the failure of normal haemopoiesis in vivo, it is relevant to present a currently favoured model for the control of normal haemopoiesis, to illustrate areas where defects could theoretically result in bone marrow failure. Such a model, namely stromal cell mediated haemopoiesis (Fig. 2), is based on the following evidence. First, clonogenic cultures of bone marrow have shown the importance of the haemopoietic growth factors, and more recently, negative regulatory factors such as transforming growth factor-β (TGF-β)[32] and stem cell inhibitor/macrophage inflammatory protein-Iα (MIP-Iα),[33,34] in the maintenance of normal haemopoietic homeostasis. Secondly, long-term bone marrow cultures (LTBMC) have demonstrated that direct cell–cell contact between stromal cells and haemopoietic cells is critical.[35,36] Thirdly, a link between these two approaches comes from studies of proteoglycans which bind haemopoietic growth factors[37,38] and present them to the target stem cells which can then undergo self-renewal or differentiation. The attachment of the haemopoietic cells to stromal cells probably involves a specific interaction as well as a separate nonspecific interaction site which strengthens the binding.[39] Proposed pathogenetic mechanisms of bone

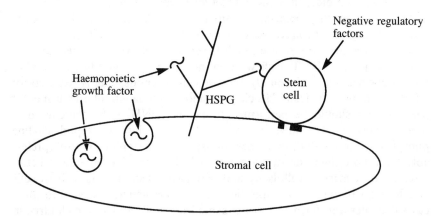

Fig. 2. Stromal cell mediated haemopoiesis – a model for normal haemopoiesis.

Haemopoietic growth factors (such as GM-CSF and IL-3) are produced and released by stromal cells and become bound to heparan sulphate residues of the extracellular matrix proteoglycans (HSPG). The heparan sulphate residues 'present' the growth factors to the target haemopoietic cells which can then proliferate or differentiate. Haemopoietic negative regulators such as TGF-β and MIP-1α appear to act in concert with the haemopoietic growth factors to permit rapid and reversible changes in hemopoietic activity according to demand.

marrow failure in AA to date involve certain components of this model system and include a stem cell deficiency or defect, which may be either intrinsic or secondary to abnormal cellular or humoral regulation, and a defect in the stromal cell microenvironment.

Pathogenetic mechanisms in AA

The evidence from clinical studies for an intrinsic stem cell defect in AA is becoming increasingly convincing, and combined with recent in vitro data, less emphasis can be placed on immunological and stromal defects as primary pathogenetic mechanisms. Evidence for this point of view is presented as follows:

Intrinsic stem cell defect   It is recognized that 30–50% of syngeneic transplants for AA are successful when a simple marrow infusion is given without prior immunosuppressive preconditioning, supporting the theory of a primary stem cell deficiency.[40,41] A small proportion (4%) of patients with AA at diagnosis and without haematological evidence of MDS or leukaemia, have an acquired clonal cytogenetic abnormality.[42] PNH is an acquired premalignant clonal disorder which may later evolve to generalized bone marrow failure (in 25% of patients), but in addition approximately 5–10% of AA patients later acquire the PNH clone. Acute leukaemia develops in a small proportion of patients with PNH.[43] Other clonal disorders, namely MDS and acute myeloid leukaemia (AML) are being recognized increasingly with long follow-up of patients with a clear cut diagnosis of AA at presentation following the advent of specific therapy for AA with antilymphocyte globulin (ALG). The risk of developing a clonal disorder such as PNH, MDS or AML increases progressively with time after ALG treatment with a 57% risk of any one of these disorders at 8 years, resulting in late deaths.[44] No obvious plateau for survival is seen at present for ALG treated patients. A separate study reports a risk of 10% for AML in AA patients treated with ALG and surviving 2 or more years.[45] It is uncertain whether or not ALG increases the risk of clonal evolution in patients with AA. The same findings have also been reported in patients treated with supportive care or androgens alone.[46]

There are two genetically anaemic strains of mice, the Sl/Sl^d and W/W^v. Mutations at either locus lead to macrocytic anaemia, mast cell deficiency, sterility and coat colour abnormalities.[47] The Sl/Sl^d strain is characterized by a marrow stromal defect and the W/W^v strain with a stem cell defect.[48] The stem cell defect of the W/W^v mouse is due to a defective receptor (c-kit)[49,50] for stem cell factor.[51–53] The Sl/Sl^d microenvironmental defect is due to decreased production of stem cell factor.[51–53] In vitro LTBMC studies have recently been performed to assess stem cell and stromal cell function in AA.[54–56] Bone marrow from most patients with AA forms a normal stromal layer in LTBMC but haemopoiesis is severely defective with evidence of little

45

or no generation of haemopoietic progenitors (Fig. 3(a)). To ascertain whether this haemopoietic defect is due to abnormal stem cell or stromal cell function, crossover experiments have been done inoculating/adherent cell depleted haemopoietic cells from AA bone marrow onto normal preformed

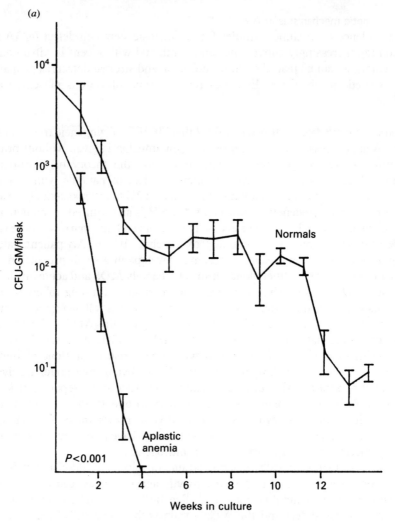

Fig. 3. Long-term bone marrow culture studies in aplastic anaemia (Fig. 3(a) from Marsh et al., 1990 with permission, and Fig. 3(b) from Marsh et al., 1991 with permission).

(a) Growth of bone marrow from normals (n=20) and 26 patients with treated AA in LTBMC. A similar pattern was seen in 5 untreated patients. Haemopoiesis was quantitated by assaying for CFU-GM in the non-adherent layer weekly.

46

irradiated LTBMC stromas to assess stem cell function in AA and 2 haemopoietic cells from normal bone marrow onto preformed irradiated AA stromas to assess stromal function in AA. In one series of 32 patients treated with immunosuppressive therapy, stem cell function was defective in all of 20 cases studied, including 6 untreated cases. A stromal defect was detected in

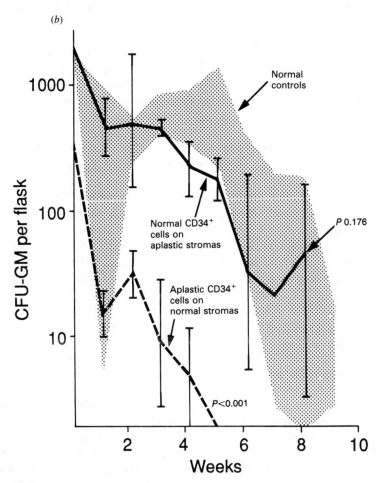

(b) Analysis of stromal and 'stem cell' function in AA using crossover-LTBMC. Stippled area represents 95% confidence intervals from normal controls (from 4 experiments growing normal CD34+ cells on different normal irradiated LTBMC stromas. A similar pattern of stromal and stem cell function in AA was seen when adherent cell depleted marrow were used instead of CD34+ marrow cells as the inoculating population of cells. Results shown for patients in a and b represent mean ± ISE.

47

only 1 of 14 patients.[56] Similar results of abnormal stem cell function with normal stromal function were reported in all 5 patients by Gibson,[57] although Hotta[58] reported abnormal stromal function in 3 out of 9 patients with acute severe AA (stem cell function was not assessed in these patients). However, none of these studies distinguishes between an intrinsic or secondary stem cell defect. Since most cases of AA studied in vitro thus far using the LTBMC of system demonstrate stem cell defects, it is theoretically possible that this may be due to an abnormality of the *c-kit* proto-oncogene or receptor, although this has yet to be investigated.

Analysis of marrow mononuclear cells expressing the CD34 antigen in a small series of patients with treated non-severe AA has shown a significant reduction in the proportion labelling with the CD34 monoclonal antibody MY10. The CD34 positive cells demonstrated reduced clonogenic potential in short-term culture and morphologically the small blasts of lymphocyte size, which in normal bone marrow express the phenotype CD33− CD34+,[59] were either absent or severely deficient.[60] Using CD34+ marrow cells instead of adherent cell-depleted cells in the crossover/LTBMC experiment described above, the severe stem cell defect was confirmed (see Fig. 3(b)) even after allowing for the reduced (5-fold) clonogenic potential of AA CD34+ cells by comparing the data with normal controls where one fifth the number of inoculating normal CD34+ cells were grown on normal stromas (Fig. 3(c)).[60] Because transplantation of normal CD34+ marrow cells in lethally irradiated baboons results in lymphohaemopoietic reconstitution,[61] this fraction probably contains the putative stem cell, and since the CD33−/CD34+ cells represent the subfraction of precursors of colony-forming cells with marrow repopulating ability,[59] it is likely that the stem cell is to be found within this subfraction. Although not fully quantitated, morphological analyses performed suggest that the CD33−/CD34+ cell fraction is reduced or absent in the AA patients studied. Absence or severe reduction of such cells with marrow repopulating ability could explain the defect in haemopoietic cell function in vitro detected in LTBMC studies.[60]

Assessment of clonality based on X chromosome analysis to determine whether haemopoiesis is monoclonal or polyclonal is now possible in a large proportion of females. Previously, using glucose 6 phosphate dehydrogenase (G6PD) isoenzyme analysis this approach was limited to only a few female patients on account of the low incidence of G6PD heterozygotes in the Caucasian population. Using such an approach, Abkowitz described a patient heterozygous for G6PD with non-severe AA, without evidence of MDS or acute leukaemia and with a normal marrow karyotype, whose red cells, neutrophils, platelets, granulocyte-macrophage colony forming cells (CFU-GM), most early erythroid progenitors (BFU-E) and T cells, expressed only one G6PD isotype inferring that these cells were derived from a single stem cell clone.[62] The availability of DNA probes for 2 polymorphic genes

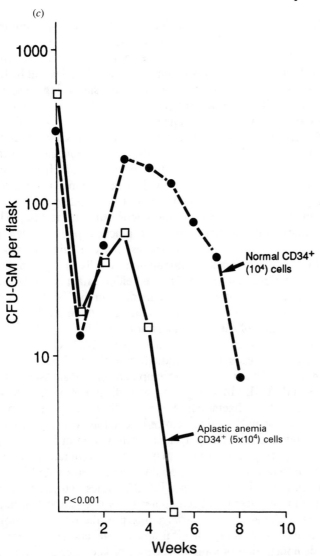

(c) Analysis of 'stem cell' function in AA using comparable numbers of inoculated CFU-GM. To allow for the 5-fold reduced clonogenic potential of AA C D34+ marrow cells compared with normal CD34+ cells, which meant that fewer CFU-GM (and BFU-E and by implication fewer marrow repopulating cells) within the AA CD34+ cells were inoculated at initiation of LTBMC compared with numbers from normal CD34+ cells, results from using 5×10^4 AA CD34+ cells on normal stromas have been compared with those using only 10^4 normal CD34$^+$ cells inoculated onto normal stromas. When this is taken into account, a significant 'stem cell' defect still remains suggesting a deficiency in the very primitive progenitors with marrow repopulating ability.

(hypoxanthine phosphoribosyl transferase, HPRT and phosphoglycerate kinase, (PGK)[63] on the X chromosome has permitted analysis of clonality, based on the same principles as for G6PD enzyme variant analysis, in a much larger proportion of females. Approximately 50% of females will be heterozygous for either or both the respective polymorphic sites using these 2 probes. Another X linked DNA probe, M27β;[64] which recognizes multiallelic variation, is now available with reported heterozygosity rates of > 90%. Using the HPRT and PGK probes, the Leiden group have recently reported that 4 out of 8 patients with AA at diagnosis showed a monoclonal pattern of haemopoiesis.[65] This contrasts with another small study from Manchester reporting only one of 6 AA patients with a monoclonal pattern following immunosuppressive therapy ([66] and unpublished update of results). The finding of a monoclonal pattern of haemopoiesis using this technique however requires cautious interpretation. From the practical point of view extreme degree of lyonization must be excluded as this can mimic a monoclonal pattern. Also a small monoclonal population of cells may be masked by a larger population of normal cells. From the Leiden data it is of interest to note that a monoclonal pattern was also demonstrated in the T-cells in 3 patients, although extreme lyonization was not excluded in these patients. This is in contrast to the findings of Mehta demonstrating the absence of T-cell receptor β and γ gene arrangements in 21 patients with AA.[67] Obviously a larger number of patients needs to be studied, but the finding of clonality at diagnosis may be relevant to later development of clonal disorders such as PNH, MDS and AML. In the setting of a diagnosis of AA, however, a monoclonal pattern of haemopoiesis may reflect stem cell depletion or emergence of a resistant defective stem cell clone following an earlier episode of severe marrow damage. The polyclonal pattern seen in 5 out of 6 patients after immunosuppressive treatment may reflect regeneration of several or many defective stem cell clones, especially as these patients all have a functional stem cell defect in vitro from LTBMC studies. To clarify further the significance of these patterns of haemopoiesis, it will be important to perform serial analysis of clonality and to always interpret the results in conjunction with more conventional morphological and cytogenetic assessment. Nevertheless the demonstration of a high incidence of later clonal disease in long-term survivors after ALG suggests that clonal cytogenetic abnormalities and possibly also apparent clonality seen in studies of X-linked polymorphisms, represent pre-malignant changes in these patients with otherwise typical AA. Perhaps an intrinsic stem cell defect is a prerequisite for this later complication.

Other possible pathogenetic mechanisms Complete autologous haemopoietic reconstitution following allogeneic BMT has been reported in a small proportion of AA patients to support the theory of immune mediated AA.[41] The demonstration that 50–70% of syngeneic transplants for AA are unsuccessful unless immunosuppressive preconditioning therapy is given does not necessarily prove that the aplasia is due to immunological factors alone, since these may be secondary to a stem cell defect leading to an autoimmune response against phenotypically abnormal stem cells. Response to immunosuppressive therapy such as ALG is also cited to support an immunological mechanism in AA. Its reported immunosuppressive action is based on a lymphocytotoxic effect in the presence of complement which may act against an abnormal population of circulating activated T suppressor cells present in a proportion of patients with AA.[68] However, ALG may also stimulate haemopoiesis by its mitogenic effect on lymphocytes[69] leading to release of haemopoietic growth factors, for example IL-3, IL-4, and IL-6. In addition, ALG may directly stimulate haemopoietic progenitors,[70] and influence natural killer (NK) cells.[71] The increase in circulating activated T suppressor cells in some AA patients has not been confirmed by all groups of workers and is probably due to immune dysregulation secondary to multiple blood transfusion rather than being a major pathogenetic pathway for AA. Increase in interferon γ and interleukin-2 (IL-2) have also been described in some patients[69,70] but likewise results are not universally reproducible.[72] Many of the early immunological in vitro studies looking for cellular and humoral inhibition of haemopoiesis in AA were not controlled to exclude transfusion-induced sensitization that may result in inhibition of marrow progenitors. Interestingly, Kaminski has shown that alloreactive CD8$^+$ cytotoxic T lymphocytes are generated by blood transfusions in contrast to low numbers found in untransfused patients.[73] Finally, correlation between these studies and clinical response to ALG is poor. Response to ALG is usually incomplete, suggesting either an ongoing immune process or a persistent primary stem cell defect.

Levels of colony stimulating factors and erythropoietin are generally increased in AA.[74,75] However, Nakao has reported in some patients with AA, decreased production of interleukin-1 (1L-1) by monocytes,[76] but again one cannot distinguish between cause and effect in this situation.

A review of Fig. 2 would indicate that other potential defects could occur within this model of normal haemopoiesis and theoretically result in bone marrow failure. For example, there could be defective adhesion of stem cells to stroma, defective production of proteoglycans resulting in abnormal presentation of haemopoietic growth factors to the target haemopoietic cells, increased production of one or more negative regulatory factors or increased sensitivity of haemopoietic cells to their effects. There are no reports to date of such studies in AA.

Treatment

Supportive treatment

During the last 10–15 years, the quality of supportive care has improved considerably, including appropriate use of new antibiotics, increased availability of platelet transfusions (including single donor transfusions), use of leucocyte-depleted transfusions and increased awareness of the need to avoid using blood products from family members prior to planned BMT. These factors need to be taken into account when retrospectively analyzing treatment outcome in AA. Back in the mid 1970s it was shown that severe AA carried an 80% mortality when treated with only supportive care.[22] It is likely that this figure has been reduced with the improvements in supportive care outlined above but for obvious ethical reasons it would not now be possible to repeat this study to verify or refute this point. It is important to try and avoid alloimmunization from multiple blood transfusions which may result in a greater chance of graft rejection following BMT for AA, as well as causing refractoriness to random donor platelet transfusions. However, a balance needs to be achieved between preventing life-threatening haemorrhage and avoiding unnecessary transfusions to prevent alloimmunization.

Bone marrow transplantation (BMT)

The pioneering work in BMT for AA was done by ED Thomas and colleagues in Seattle with the first successful transplant for AA using an HLA identical sibling donor reported in 1970,[77] and their contribution to further developments in this field is widely acknowledged.

Syngeneic BMT   Of 19 patients wth AA transplanted from syngeneic donors recently reported by the International BMT Registry[41] 18 are alive with full haemotological recovery. Six were transplanted with immunosuppression initially, and there were 9 out of 13 who required a second transplant with immunosuppression following no engraftment or transient engraftment with marrow infusion alone.

Prior in vitro co-cultures of donor and recipient bone marrow do not always predict whether syngeneic BMT will be successful or not without immunosuppressive (high dose cyclophosphamide) preconditioning.[40] In general, the presence of a detectable inhibitor (whether cellular or humoral) of donor haemopoiesis in the recipient indicates the need for preconditioning, but in the absence of an inhibitor, a single marrow infusion given without cyclophosphamide is not always successful. If the patient is clinically well, and such an inhibitor is not detectable, it may be reasonable to give initially a marrow infusion alone, since 30–50% of unselected patients will respond. In theory, if no inhibitor is present, a greater proportion should respond. Syngeneic marrow with cyclophosphamide can be used if this approach is unsuccessful, or given initially in patients unlikely to survive a second transplant if the first fails. Those patients with very severe AA are best treated with high dose cyclophosphamide initially as rapid neutrophil recovery is essential in these cases. There have been case reports of recurrent graft failure following syngeneic BMT, despite the use of high dose cyclophosphamide even with the addition of irradiation.[78–80] It has been suggested that this may be due to re-emergence of an abnormal population of T-cells responsible for the original disease,[78] and Goss reported recipient NK cell mediated inhibition of donor marrow in this setting.[81] The demonstration that syngeneic BMT in 2 elderly patients (aged 62 and 69 years respectively) was well tolerated using full dose cyclophosphamide (and additional total lymphoid irradiation in 1 of these cases),[82] is consistent with the idea that the increased mortality among older patients (>45 years) transplanted for severe AA using HLA identical sibling donors, is mainly due to a higher incidence of acute graft-versus-host disease (GVHD) and not to toxicity from the conditioning regimen.

BMT using HLA identical sibling donors   The superiority of BMT carried out soon after presentation of severe AA using high dose cyclophosphamide (with methotrexate as prophylaxis against GVHD) over conventional therapy (supportive measures and androgens) was first reported by Camitta.[22] Other groups subsequently reported series of patients where BMT was delayed and a high incidence of graft failure of 30–60% occurred, associated with sensitization by multiple pre-BMT transfusions.[83] Various manoeuvres were employed during the second half of the 1970s to overcome the problem of graft failure in transfused patients. These included increased pretransplant immunosuppression with modified total body irradiation (TBI),[84] thoraco-abdominal[85] or total lymphoid irradiation,[86] the use of unirradiated donor buffy coats in the early post transplant period,[87] and the use of cyclosporin (CSA).[88] As a result, the incidence of graft failure was reduced to around 15%, but GVHD remained a problem. Indeed, TBI has now been abandoned for HLA identical sibling transplants for AA on account of an unacceptably high incidence of GVHD and interstitial pneumonitis. A further decrease in the incidence of graft failure due to other factors has occurred during the last decade and these will be discussed as part of the current status of BMT for severe AA.

It is widely accepted that patients with severe AA <45 years of age who have an HLA identical sibling donor are best treated with early BMT. Although recent data from the European Group for Bone Marrow Transplantation (EBMT) suggest that patients >20 years of age and with neutrophils $0.2–0.5 \times 10^9/l$ do better with ALG than with BMT,[23] the data were analyzed without sufficiently long follow-up to detect later complications of clonal disease among the ALG-treated group. Such patients are also at risk for relapse of their aplasia and LTBMC studies suggest that ALG does not cure the disease (see pathogenesis). These observations suggest that early transplantation of all severe AA patients between the ages of 20 and 45 years is preferable to ALG treatment. Additional information can now be obtained to predict whether an individual patient would benefit from BMT or immunosuppressive therapy in this situation. Bacigalupo, on behalf of the EBMT Severe Aplastic Anaemia Working Party,[89] has devised an individualized prognostic scoring system for survival based on the following risk factors: neutrophil count, clinically significant haemorrhage, refractoriness to random platelets and patient age. By matching the patient with a similar group of patients in the validation programme, the survival of the patient can be predicted for BMT and immunosuppressive therapy. (A Bacigalupo, personal communication).

Long-term actuarial survival following BMT using genotypically identical sibling donors is currently 60–75% for multiply transfused patients, and at least 80% for untransfused patients[90] and transfused or untransfused children.[91]

The incidence of graft rejection is now around 10%. The importance of giving a marrow cell dose of $>3.0 \times 10^8$/kg has been confirmed as an important variable for engraftment.[92] Other variables predicting graft rejection are positive in vitro tests of cell mediated immunity,[93] the number of blood transfusions, and year of transplant.[94] The latter probably reflects changing transfusion practices as discussed previously. A correlation has also been shown between graft failure and length of pre-BMT history, confirming the importance of early BMT prior to sensitization.[95] To reduce further the risk of graft failure in heavily sensitized patients with a long history ($>$ 1 year), the Hammersmith team have recently used intravenous Campath IG given for 5 days pre-BMT in addition to their standard regimen of cyclophosphamide and CSA. All 5 patients successfully engrafted (J Hows, personal communication). Seattle are now using ALG as increased preconditioning to help prevent rejection in heavily sensitized patients.[96] The use of buffy coats in sensitized patients has been abandoned because of the increased risk of chronic GVHD.[97] The use of T-cell depletion of donor marrow to reduce acute GVHD is no longer used for HLA identical sibling BMT in AA on account of a very high incidence of graft rejection.[41] The importance of successful engraftment to outcome is reflected by survival figures following second BMT for graft failure, varying from 25–50%.[41,95,96]

Factors associated with acute GVHD are increasing age, the use of irradiation and previous donor pregnancy.[98,99] The use of laminar air flow rooms was previously shown also to be a factor but this now appears to be less important.[99] Until very recently the incidence of significant acute GVHD ($\geq$ grade 2) remained high at between 30 and 60%. A decrease to 18% has been reported from Seattle with a combination of CSA and methotrexate[99] (compared with 53% using methotrexate alone). However, this has not resulted in improved survival on account of an increase in chronic GVHD seen in 55% of patients and resulting in late deaths in 27% of these patients.

Increasing age, acute GVHD, the use of unirradiated donor buffy coats,[100] and irradiation,[101] are also associated with increased chronic GVHD. This is in striking contrast to the virtual absence of significant chronic GVHD using CSA alone.[95]

In summary, the most important single factor that has improved survival over the last 10 years has been the use of CSA instead of methotrexate as anti-GVHD prophylaxis.[101,102] Cyclosporin has resulted in a low rate of graft failure and chronic GVHD and has improved the long-term quality of life of those transplanted especially in terms of normal development and fertility. The occurrence of late graft failure previously reported with the use of CSA has been eliminated by extending the period of CSA administration post transplant from 6 to 9 months.[95] In contrast, changes in pretransplant conditioning regimen to reduce graft rejection have had no impact on survival.[101] The use of radiation is associated with increased GVHD, interstitial pneumonitis and long-term complications of delayed growth, sterility, and second malignancies. Unirradiated donor buffy coats have increased the incidence of chronic GVHD. An important unanswered question is whether the use of combined CSA and MTX confers any advantage or disadvantage compared with CSA alone. This can only be answered with a prospective randomized study of a large number of patients. Such a study is currently being set up by the EBMT.

BMT using unrelated and partially HLA matched family donors   Only about 30% of patients in Western Europe and North America with severe AA who are <45 years old have an HLA genotypically-identical sibling donor. Hence the need to consider alternative donors especially for those with very severe AA and who are <20 years old. Of these, 1–2% will have an HLA phenotypically identical family member, and results of BMT using these donors with the same pretransplant conditioning regimen are similar to HLA genotypic sibling transplants (See Table 2). Early results of BMT using unrelated or mismatch family donors were very disappointing and worse than results of immunosuppressive therapy.[103,104] There were few survivors due to a much higher incidence of graft failure and acute GVHD. Many patients could be described as end-stage being heavily transfused and often infected at the time of transplant. In many cases, insufficient pretransplant immunosuppression was used. Recent data, however, have shown that progress has been made in this area, on account of several factors.

1. More intensive conditioning protocols have been used in addition to high dose cyclophosphamide, namely TBI (Seattle protocol)[105] or

Table 2. *BMT for severe aplastic anaemia using alternative donors*

	FAMILY			UNRELATED	
	HLA phenotypic match	HLA mismatch		HLA 'match'	HLA mismatch
		one antigen	>one antigen		
Seattle[+] 1970–1990	7/9 (a) (b)	1/13 3/7	0/3 2/5	4/11	1/5
Milwaukee[0] 1982–1990	1/1	3/4	1/6	1/2	3/3
EBMT[*] 1978–1991	6/11	3/7	0/24	2/7	1/8
Hammersmith[×] 1981–1990	1/2	1/4	0/2	1/4	2/9
GEGMO[#]	0/3	0/9	2/8	3/12	–

Figures represent number of survivors out of total number transplanted.

(a) represents results of patient transplanted from 1970–1982 (using cyclophosphamide alone) (b) from 1984–1990 (using TBI and cyclophosphamide). Updated results of published reports are shown, B Camitta [0], C Anasetti [+], J Hows [×], E Gluckman [#], and A Bacigalupo[*] personal communications.

GEGMO: Groupe Français d'Etude de la Greffe de Moelle Osseuse.

cytosine arabinoside and TBI (Milwaukee protocol)[106] to reduce graft failure.

2. Increased anti-GVHD prophylaxis with either T-cell depletion of donor marrow and methyl prednisolone (Milwaukee protocol) or a combination of CSA and methotrexate (Seattle protocol).

3. Improved transfusion practices such as CMV seronegative blood products for those cases where both donor and recipient are CMV seronegative. This practice has virtually eliminated the risk of CMV pneumonitis in such transplants.

4. More rapid and accurate HLA typing is now possible using DNA restriction fragment length polymorphism[107] or oligonucleotide analysis.[108] The very recently described HLA typing by polymerase chain reaction (PCR) fingerprinting can produce a result less than 8 hours after DNA isolation.[109]

5. Better patient selection means that only young patients, preferably with a short history of aplasia (emphasizing the importance of early BMT) should be considered, although Camitta has successfully transplanted multiply transfused children.[106] Transplants in .patients with sepsis should be avoided since they are most unlikely to survive the procedure. Potentially, haemopoietic growth factors such as granulocyte-colony stimulating factor (G–CSF) may have a role in treating infected patients prior to BMT.

6. Better donor selection is possible with the recent availability of a test based on cytotoxic T-cell analysis that can predict before BMT both the severity of acute GVHD[110] and the potential of the donor to reject a particular graft.[73]

A summary of the updated results of BMT for severe AA using unrelated and family donors from the major transplant centres is shown in Table 2. The results from Milwaukee demonstrate a high incidence of successful outcome from BMT in children using unrelated or one antigen mismatch family donors. More than a one antigen mismatch family donor BMT in children and adults is associated with an unacceptably poor outcome. The IMUST (International Marrow Unrelated Search and Transplant) study,[111,112] a prospective international multicentre study, was commenced in 1989 to evaluate problems with donor search procedure and the outcome following unrelated BMT for leukaemia, MDS and AA compared with HLA identical sibling transplants. A recent interim analysis from this study has shown that poor risk disease is the strongest predictor of search failure,[113] indicating the need to find unrelated donors more quickly. One may be able to accept some degree of mismatch using intensive conditioning protocols and T-cell depletion in the interest of speed, as shown for children in the report from the Milwaukee group.

A scheme for the role of BMT in the treatment of acquired severe AA proposed by Hows (1990)[114] is depicted in Fig. 4. For the reasons discussed earlier, BMT from an HLA identical sibling donor (or an HLA phenotypically identical parent) may be considered the treatment of choice for patients with severe AA who are <45 years old. For those patients who lack an HLA identical sibling donor, BMT from an unrelated or one antigen mismatch family donor should perhaps at present be restricted to children with severe AA and young adults (<30 years old) with very severe AA (neutrophils <0.2 ×10⁹/l). The results from the IMUST study should help to determine whether unrelated BMT is a justifiable approach to the treatment of AA or not. The recent results from Milwaukee would currently support its use in children.

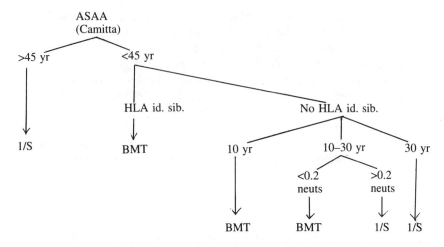

Fig. 4. Which patients should be transplanted for acquired severe aplastic anaemia (ASAA)? Management chart for patients presenting with ASAA, as defined by the Camitta criteria (from Hows 1990 with permission). I/S = immunosuppressive treatment with antilymphocyte globulin. Neuts >0.2 = neutrophil count $>0.2 \times 10^9/l$. HLA-id sib = HLA identical sibling donor.

Immunosuppressive treatment

For convenience, treatment of AA patients with ALG/ATG, androgens, high dose methylprednisone (HDMP) and CSA, has been grouped together under the heading of immunosuppressive treatment although this term may not accurately reflect the mode of action in AA. The first prospective randomized study demonstrating an improvement in response to ALG compared with supportive care in AA was reported by Champlin in 1983.[115] He obtained a partial or complete remission rate of 52% at 3 months after ALG compared with no remission in the latter group.[115] It has been difficult to compare results for ALG therapy between different centres, however, on account of different treatment protocols using different sources of ALG with variable duration of treatment, variation between batches of ALG in terms of protein content and specific activity, concomitant use of androgens and/or steroids and differences in criteria of response to ALG. There is also a wide variation in the standard of supportive care given at different centres. This is reflected by response and survival rates varying from 30 to 70%.[23,116-118] Androgens were shown previously not to influence response to ALG by Champlin,[115] but a prospective randomized study of the EBMT is currently reevaluating this, by comparing ALG plus HDMP with ALG, HDMP and androgens. An interim analysis shows a trend (not significant) towards better survival for severe AA patients in the androgen group (A Bacigalupo, personal communication).

Recent studies suggest that CSA may also have a useful role in the treatment of AA, either on its own[119] or in combination with ALG, androgens and/or prednisone.[120,121] Several of these prospective studies are still in progress, although a German study comparing ALG and HDMP with ALG, HDMP and CSA has demonstrated recently an improved response to the latter combination at 6 months. No improvement in survival was observed, however, in the CSA treated group.[121] Future studies including haemopoietic growth factors such as G–CSF or interleukin-3 (IL-3) with ALG and CSA are currently being explored. In general, it would seem that multiple agents produce better responses than ALG used alone. It is not known, however, whether the use of multiple immunosuppressive agents will increase the risk of clonal evolution in these patients.

Several factors are predictive of response and survival after ALG treatment. The effect of disease severity is reflected by a significantly higher response and survival in non-severe AA compared with severe AA[23,118] although other centres have failed to show that mild AA is associated with a more favourable outcome after ALG.[115,122] Although no study has shown that ALG treatment of non-severe AA effectively changes the natural history of that disease (B Camitta, personal communication), it would be difficult ethically to justify a prospective study to address this point. For patients with very severe AA (neutrophils $< 0.2 \times 10^9/l$) the outcome after ALG is particularly poor and these patients should be considered for early BMT. Response to ALG is worse in children than in adults (discussed later). The patient's sex and the aetiology of the aplasia do not affect survival. Two studies reported that patients treated early after diagnosis had a better response rate,[115,118] although Doney showed that disease duration had no effect on survival.[123] Relapse of the disease frequently occurs following ALG therapy, varying between 25 and 30%.[124,125] A second course of ALG, from a different animal source, can be given to these patients as well as to those who show no response to a first course. Approximately 22% of nonresponders will show a response to a second course of ALG.[118] The high incidence of later clonal disorders and relapse after ALG therapy suggests that ALG does not cure the aplasia but permits recovery of peripheral blood counts enabling a proportion of patients to become transfusion independent and to survive longer.

Haemopoietic growth factors

The recent availability of an increasing number of recombinant human haemopoietic growth factors has already resulted in the clinical use of G–CSF, granulocyte–macrophage-CSF (GM–CSF) and IL-3 in aplastic anaemia (AA). These studies were prompted by results demonstrating improvement in haemopoietic function with GM–CSF, G–CSF and IL-3 in patients with acquired immune deficiency syndrome,[126] myelodysplastic syndrome,[127] following chemotherapy[128] or BMT.[129] Prior knowledge of the action of these growth factors in vitro on AA bone marrow was not available.

The use of GM–CSF in AA has been reported by several groups[130–134] and the results can be summarized as follows: GM–CSF results in an increase in neutrophils, monocytes, eosinophils and sometimes lymphocytes. There is usually no effect on platelet or reticulocyte counts. The effect on myelopoiesis is transient and a response is dependent on the degree of residual haemopoiesis, so that patients with non-severe AA show the greatest response whereas those with very severe disease rarely show any significant response. Serious side effects from GM–CSF have been seen in AA patients using doses ⩾ 16 µg/kg/day notably pulmonary infiltrates, capillary leak syndrome, pericarditis, thrombosis of a central venous catheter, and thrombocytopenia. These side effects usually occur when both the neutrophil and eosinophil counts are elevated. One patient developed inferior vena cava thrombosis shortly after treatment when severely neutropenic. Life-threatening bleeding, namely cerebral haemorrhage, has also been reported during GM–CSF infusion. Children appear to respond to lower doses of GM–CSF, have fewer side effects and experience fewer infective episodes during treatment compared with adults. One of 9 children in the study reported by Guinan[134] and colleagues had a trilineage response which has been maintained for over a year after therapy although this may have been due to spontaneous recovery. In vitro clonogenic cultures of bone marrow have shown variable results from these studies. Guinan[134] and Vadhan Raj[132] separately demonstrated no increased progenitor cell numbers following GM–CSF, and colony numbers pretreatment were not predictive of a response, whereas Champlin[133] showed an increase in CFU–GM and BFU–E after treatment. Moreover, progenitor cell assays can be misleading since only the concentration and not the absolute number of progenitor cells can be assessed in vitro, and little or no account is taken of total marrow cellularity.

Ganser has recently reported the use of IL-3 in 9 patients with AA, most of whom had severe AA.[135] A transient increase in neutrophils, eosinophils, monocytes and lymphocytes was seen in most patients, although the degree of elevation of the cell counts was less than that seen with GM–CSF in AA. Only one patient had a transient increase in platelet count, and a small increase in reticulocytes was documented in 4 patients. The lack of significant stimulation of erythropoiesis with IL-3 (or GM–CSF) probably reflects an absence or severe deficiency or defective response of erythroid progenitors since in AA one would perhaps anticipate that the high circulating levels of erythropoietin would result in synergy with IL-3 or GM–CSF in stimulating erythropoiesis (as seen in normal bone marrow). One patient in their study developed thrombocytopenia during IL-3 treatment and a further patient died of cerebral haemorrhage 5 days after finishing treatment.

As single agents of treatment of AA, GM–CSF and IL-3 appear to have no long lasting effects on haemopoiesis. The significance of an occasional sustained response with one of these factors is difficult to interpret in the light of multiple prior therapies or concomitant treatment with ALG[136] for example. Furthermore, although GM–CSF may have a role in the treatment of severe infection in AA or as part of combination therapy to reduce the period of neutropenia before a response to ALG may be anticipated, this growth factor is associated with significant side effects at high doses. In this respect, trials with G–CSF should be encouraged since clinical studies following chemotherapy have demonstrated fewer side effects of G–CSF.[137,138] In contrast to GM–CSF, G–CSF does not inhibit neutrophil function or induce neutrophil aggregation,[139] and the side effects are usually limited to fever or bone pain. Also, although it is difficult to compare the two growth factors dose for dose, the increase in neutrophil counts is more dramatic with G–CSF and there is no increase in eosinophils. The combination of fewer side effects and a greater effect on neutrophils perhaps favours the use of G–CSF in preference to GM–CSF in AA. It is therefore of interest that Sonoda[140] recently reported preliminary results of long-term administration (2–10 months) of G–CSF in 5 patients with severe AA. All 5 demonstrated a substantial increase in neutrophils and 2 patients were reported to show a dramatic improvement in anaemia associated with a decrease in plasma erythropoietin levels. During treatment there were no infective episodes. CFU–GM recovered in all patients, BFU–E in 3 out of 5 and CFU–Meg were detectable in one patient after treatment.

It is clear that the use of individual haemopoietic growth factors in AA will not reverse the underlying stem cell defect. In vitro studies using purified populations of haemopoietic progenitors have shown that marked synergism occurs with many of the growth factors, for example, IL-3 with GM–CSF or IL-6, and G–CSF with GM–CSF.[141,142] Furthermore, so-called lineage-restricted factors such as G–CSF or M–CSF can stimulate multipotent stem cells in combination with IL-1, a factor which on its own has no colony stimulating activity.[143] The use of a combination of haemopoietic growth factors to preferentially stimulate stem cell renewal rather than differentiation of stem cells in AA should perhaps be approached with caution and be preceded by in vitro studies using for example, long-term marrow cultures in order to help predict which combination might be effective. There is the theoretical possibility of inducing stem cell exhaustion in AA with prolonged use of concomitantly given combinations of growth factors which might have more than additive effects and which stimulate stem cell differentiation in preference to stem cell renewal. At present, growth factor therapy alone should not be used as primary treatment for AA but may be useful in treating infected patients.

Treatment of AA in children

Children with AA show important differences compared with adults in their response to the various treatment modalities described. Two studies have shown that children < 6 years of age show significantly worse survival after ALG treatment than adults.[144,145] Although a trend (not significant) for worse survival in older children with severe AA 6–15 years of age has been reported following ALG,[124] one of the studies demonstrated a response rate of only 43% for children < 15 years old with non-severe AA compared with 82% in adults.[144] These results suggest that the disease in children may have a different pathogenesis than in adults and/or fewer recoverable stem cells. The EBMT showed in an uncontrolled study an advantage in survival (77% versus 37%) for children with severe AA treated with ALG and androgens compared with ALG alone.[145] However, the use of androgens should be approached with caution in children since well-documented side effects include hepatocellular carcinoma, peliosis hepatis, virilization and behavioral problems with aggression and irritability.

It is of interest to note that there has been no significant improvement in survival in children with AA treated with ALG over the last two decades,[145] although standards of supportive care have improved. In contrast, there has been progressive improvement in survival following allogeneic BMT for children (as well as adults) over the same time period. Compared with adults, most centres have reported that children < 18 years of age who have been transplanted for severe AA with an HLA identical sibling donor show improved long-term survival of between 80 and >90%. The incidence and severity of acute GVHD is less in children and this may explain their survival advantage over adults. Since the long-term quality of life is particularly important in children, it is in this age group that the use of irradiation should if at all possible be avoided, and other forms of additional preconditioning immunosuppression (such as ALG) used for heavily sensitized patients. Finally, a significantly improved outcome with BMT compared with ALG has been shown in children < 20 or < 15 years of age with severe AA by the EBMT group[145] and Seattle[121] respectively.

Some children with non-severe AA can pose a difficult management problem. Although they may not strictly fulfil the Camitta criteria for severe AA on account of perhaps a relative degree of preservation of myelopoiesis and/or erythropoiesis, they may have severe thrombocytopenia with potentially life threatening haemorrhage. This subgroup of children with non-severe AA appears to represent those who fare badly with ALG treatment.[144] Since the results of allogeneic BMT in children are excellent (95% survival reported recently from Seattle,[91]) a strong case could be made for early transplantation of these children before they become heavily sensitized or die from haemorrhage.

Concluding remarks

Since the introduction of allogeneic BMT in the early 1970s and ALG in the late 1970s as specific therapy for AA, long-term survival is achieved in more than half of treated cases. Survivors following BMT do not appear to be at risk of later clonal disorders, and the risk of secondary solid tumours is low if irradiation is avoided.[146] Therefore the majority of these patients can be considered to be cured. In contrast amongst long-term survivors following ALG[44,45] or androgen treatment,[46] the later appearance of clonal disease as well as relapse indicates that neither androgens nor ALG cure the underlying disorder. The emergence of MDS, PNH or AML may represent the natural history of AA which had not been seen before, since non-transplanted patients with severe AA did not usually survive long-term prior to the availability of ALG. This has led to a recent reappraisal of the interrelationship between AA and clonal disorders.[31] The optimal management of AA patients (whether severe or non-severe) who later develop a clonal disorder is at present unclear. The decision as to whether to use more intensive immunosuppressive therapy in the pretransplant conditioning regimen for severe AA patients is controversial. Although Appelbaum reported a high incidence of relapse in AA patients with a clonal cytogenetic abnormality transplanted with high dose cyclophosphamide alone,[42] it is possible some of these patients had MDS rather than severe AA prior to BMT. Szer reported the successful outcome of 2 patients with severe AA arising as a complication of PNH who were transplanted from HLA identical sibling donors using only high dose cyclophosphamide,[147] and another similar case was reported by Hows.[88] A more difficult question is whether patients with nonsevere AA who develop a clonal cytogenetic abnormality should be transplanted. In the absence of haematological evidence of MDS or AML it may be reasonable to monitor these patients regularly, and if there is no HLA identical sibling donor available, a search should be made for an unrelated donor, so that in the event of later progression to MDS or AML, the option for early BMT is available. The continued improved survival following BMT using HLA compatible donors, accompanied by recent improvements in results for BMT using alternative donors, provides an increasing chance for cure of these patients.

Acknowledgements

I thank Dr Jill Hows, Dr Bruce Camitta and Professor Mike Dexter FRS for their learned comments and helpful advice during the preparation of this manuscript, and I am also very grateful to Professor Eliane Gluckman on behalf of GEGMO, Dr Claudio Anasetti, and Dr Andrea Bacigalupo for providing me with updated results from their patients.

References

(1) International agranulocytosis and aplastic anaemia study. Incidence of aplastic anaemia: the relevance of diagnostic criteria. *Blood* 1987; 70: 1718–21.

(2) Wallerstein RO, Condit PK, Kasper CK, Brown JW, Morrison FR. Statewide study of chloramphenicol therapy and fatal aplastic anaemia. *JAMA* 1969; 208: 2045–50.

(3) Bottiger LE. Epidemiology and aetiology of aplastic anaemia. In: Heimpel H, Gordon-Smith E, Heit W, Kubanek B, eds. *Aplastic anaemia – pathophysiology and approaches to therapy.* Springer, 1979: 27–32.

(4) Szlo M, Sensenbrenner L, Markowitz J, Weida S, Warm S, Lineth M. Incidence of aplastic anaemia in metropolitan Baltimore: a population-based study. *Blood* 1985; 66: 115–19.

(5) Young NS, Issaragrisil S, Chieh CW, Takaku F. Aplastic anaemia in the Orient. *Br J Haematol* 1986; 62: 1–6.

(6) Evans DI. Congenital defects of the marrow stem cell. In: Gordon-Smith EC, ed., *Aplastic anaemia. Clinical haematology – international practice and research,* Baillière Tindall, 1989; 2: 163–90.

(7) Gordon-Smith EC, Rutherford TR. Fanconi anaemia – constitutional, familial aplastic anaemia. In: Gordon-Smith EC, ed., *Aplastic anaemia. Clinical haematology – international practice and research.* Baillière Tindall, 1989; 2: 139–52.

(8) Gordon-Smith EC. Aplastic anaemia. *Med Int* 1983; 1195–8.

(9) Gordon-Smith EC. Aplastic anaemia – aetiology and clinical features. In: Gordon-Smith EC, ed., *Aplastic anaemia. Clinical haematology – international practice and research.* Baillière Tindall, 1989; 2: 1–18.

(10) International agranulocytosis and aplastic anaemia study. Risks of agranulocytosis and aplastic anaemia: a first report of their relation to drug use with special reference to analgesics. *JAMA* 1986; 256: 1749–57.

(11) Jacobs A. Benzene and leukaemia. *Br J Haematol* 1989; 72: 119–21. (Annotation).

(12) Zeldis JB, Dienstag JL, Gale RP. Aplastic anaemia and non-A, non-B hepatitis. *Am J Med* 1983; 74: 64–8.

(13) Domenech P, Palomeque A, Martinez-Gutierrez A, Vinolas N, Vela E, Jimenez R. Severe aplastic anaemia following hepatitis A. *Acta Haematol* 1986; 76: 227–9.

(14) McSweeney PA, Carter JM, Green GJ, Romeril KR. Fatal aplastic anaemia associated with hepatitis B viral infection. *Am J Med* 1988; 85: 255–6.

(15) Van Doornik MC, van't Veer-Korthof ET, Wieranga H. Fatal aplastic anaemia complicating infectious mononucleosis. *Scand J Haematol* 1978; 20: 52–6.

(16) Choo QL, Kuo G, Weiner AJ, Overby LR, Bradley DW, Houghton M. Isolation of a cDNA clone derived from a blood borne non-A, non-B viral hepatitis genome. *Science* 1989; 244: 359–62.

(17) Pol S, Driss F, Devergie A, Brechot C, Berthelot P, Gluckman E. Is hepatitis C virus involved in hepatitis-associated aplastic anaemia? *Ann Int Med* 1990; 113: 435–7.

(18) Fleming AF. Hypoplastic anaemia in pregnancy. *Br Med J* 1973; ii: 166–7.

(19) Evans IL. Aplastic anaemia in pregnancy resulting after abortion. *Br Med J* 1968; iii: 166–7.

(20) Knispel JW, Lynch VA, Viele BD. Aplastic anaemia in pregnancy: a case report, review of the literature and a re-evaluation of management. *Obstet and Gynaecol Surveys* 1976; 31: 523–8.

(21) Aitchison RG, Marsh JC, Hows JM, Russell NH, Gordon-Smith EC. Pregnancy associated aplastic anaemia: a report of five cases and review of current management. *Br J Haematol* 1989; 73: 541–5.

(22) Camitta BM, Thomas ED, Nathan DG et al. A prospective study of androgens and bone marrow transplantation for treatment of severe aplastic anaemia. *Blood* 1979; 53: 504–14.

(23) Bacigalupo A, Hows J, Gluckman E et al. Bone marrow transplantation (BMT) versus immunosuppression for the treatment of severe aplastic anaemia (SAA): a report of the EBMT SAA working party. *Br J Haematol* 1988; 70: 177–82.

(24) Lewis SM. Course and progress in aplastic anaemia. *Br Med J* 1965; i: 1027–30.

(25) Auerbach AD, Rogatko O, Schroeder-Kurth TM. International Fanconi anaemia registry: relation of clinical symptoms to diepoxybutane sensitivity. *Blood* 1989; 73: 391–6.

(26) Auerbach AD, Adler B, Chaganti RS. Prenatal and postnatal diagnosis and carrier detection of Fanconi anaemia by a cytogenetic method. *Paediatrics* 1981; 67: 128–35.

(27) Melhorn DK, Gross S, Newmann MS. Acute childhood leukaemia presenting as aplastic anaemia: the response to corticosteroids. *J Pediatr* 1970; 77: 647–52.

(28) Breatnach F, Chessells JM, Greaves MF. The aplastic presentation of childhood leukaemia – a feature of common ALL. *Br J Haematol* 1981; 49: 387–93.

(29) Fohlmeister J, Fischer R, Modder B, Rister M, Schaefer HE. Aplastic anaemia and the hypocellular myelodysplastic syndrome: histomorphological, diagnostic and prognostic features. *J Clin Pathol* 1985; 38: 1218–24.

(30) De Planque MM, van Krieken JM, Kluin-Nelemans HC et al. Bone marrow histopathology of patients with severe aplastic anaemia before treatment and at follow-up. *Br J Haematol* 1989; 72: 439–44.

(31) Marsh JC, Geary CG. Is aplastic anaemia a preleukaemic disorder? *Br J Haematol* 1991; 77: 447–52. (Annotation).

(32) Hampson J, Ponting IL, Cook N et al. The effects of TGFβ on haemopoietic cells. *Growth Factors* 1989; 1: 193–202.

(33) Lord BI, Mori KS, Wright EG, Lajtha LG. An inhibitor of stem cell proliferation in normal bone marrow. *Br J Haematol* 1976; 34: 441–5.

(34) Graham GJ, Wright EG, Hewick R et al. Identification and characterization of an inhibitor of haemopoietic stem cell proliferation. *Nature* 1990; 344: 442–4.

(35) Dexter TM, Allen TD, Lajtha LG. Conditions controlling the proliferation of haemopoietic stem cells in vitro. *J Cell Physiol* 1977; 91: 335–44.

(36) Dexter TM, Coutinho LH, Spooncer E et al. Stromal cells in haemopoiesis. In: *Molecular control of haemopoiesis*. Ciba Foundation Symposium. Wiley, Chichester, 1990; 148: 76–95.

(37) Gordon MY, Riley GP, Watt SM, Greaves MF. Compartmentalization of a haemopoietic growth factor (GM-CSF) by glycosaminoglycans in the bone marrow microenvironment. *Nature* 1987; 326: 403–5.

(38) Roberts R, Gallagher JT, Spooncer E, Allen TD, Bloomfield F, Dexter TM. Heparan sulphate bound growth factors: a mechanism for stromal cell mediated haemopoiesis. *Nature* 1988; 332: 376–8.

(39) Tavassoli M, Hardy CL. Molecular basis of homing of intravenously transplanted stem cells to the marrow. *Blood* 1990; 76: 1059–70.

(40) Champlin RE, Feig SA, Sparkes RS, Gale RP. Bone marrow transplantation from identical twins in the treatment of aplastic anaemia: implication for the pathogenesis of the disease. *Br J Haematol* 1984; 56: 455–63.

(41) Champlin RE, Horowitz MM, van Bekkum DW et al. Graft failure following bone marrow transplantation for severe aplastic anaemia: risk factors and treatment results. *Blood* 1989; 73: 606–13.

(42) Appelbaum FR, Barrall J, Storb R et al. Clonal cytogenetic abnormalities in patients with otherwise typical aplastic anaemia. *Exp Haematol* 1987; 15: 1134–9.

(43) Camitta BM, Storb R, Thomas ED. Aplastic anaemia: pathogenesis, diagnosis, treatment and prognosis. *N Eng J Med* 1982; 306: 645–52.

(44) Tichelli A, Gratwohl A, Wursch A, Nissen C, Speck B. Late haematological complications in severe aplastic anaemia. *Br J Haematol* 1988; 69: 413–18.

(45) de Planque MM, Klein-Nelemans JC, van Krieken HJ. Evolution of acquired severe aplastic anaemia to myelodysplasia and subsequent leukaemia in adults. *Br J Haematol* 1989; 73: 121–6.

(46) Najean Y, Hagvenauer O. For the cooperative group for the study of aplastic and refractory anaemias. Long term (5–20 years) evolution of non-grafted aplastic anaemias. *Blood* 1990; 76: 2222–8.

(47) Bernstein A, Chabot B, Dubreuil P et al. The mouse w/c-kit locus. In: *Molecular control of haemopoiesis*. Ciba Foundation Symposium. Wiley, Chichester, 1990; 148: 158–72.

(48) Dexter TM, Moore MAS. In vitro duplication and 'cure' of haematopoietic defects in genetically anaemic mice. *Nature* 1977; 269: 412–13.

(49) Chabot B, Stephenson DA, Chapman VM, Besmer P, Bernstein A. The protooncogene c-kit encoding a transmembrane tyrosine kinase receptor maps to the mouse W locus. *Nature* 1988; 335: 88–9.

(50) Geissler EN, Ryan MA, Housman DE. The dominant white-spotting (W) locus of the mouse encodes the c-kit protooncogene. *Cell* 1988; 55: 185–92.

(51) Zsebo KM, Williams DA, Geissler EN et al. Stem cell factor is encoded at the Sl locus of the mouse and is the ligand for the c-kit tyrosine kinase receptor. *Cell* 1990; 63: 213–24.

(52) Huang E, Nocka K, Beier DR et al. The haematopoietic growth factor KL is encoded by the Sl locus and is the ligand of the c-kit receptor, the gene product of the W locus. *Cell* 1990; 63: 225–33.

(53) Williams DE, Eisenman J, Baird A et al. Identification of a ligand for the c-kit proto-oncogene. *Cell* 1990; 63: 167–74.

(54) Juneja HS, Lee S, Gardner FH. Human long-term bone marrow cultures in aplastic anaemia. *Int J Cell Clon* 1989; 7: 129–35.

(55) Gibson FM, Gordon-Smith EC. Long-term culture of aplastic anaemia bone marrow. *Br J Haematol* 1990; 75: 421–7.

(56) Marsh JC, Chang J, Testa NG, Hows JM, Dexter TM. The haematopoietic

defect in aplastic anaemia assessed by long-term marrow culture. *Blood* 1990; 76: 1748–57.

(57) Gibson FM, Scopes J, Laurie A, Gordon-Smith EC. Contribution of the marrow stroma to the pathogenesis of aplastic anaemia. *Exp Haematol* 1990; 18: 303a. (abstract).

(58) Hotta T, Kato T, Maeda H, Yamao H, Yamada H, Saito H. Functional changes in marrow stromal cells in aplastic anaemia. *Acta Haematol* 1985; 74: 65–9.

(59) Andrews RG, Singer JW, Bernstein ID. Precursors of colony-forming cells in humans can be distinguished from colony-forming cells by expression of the CD33 and CD34 antigens and light scatter properties. *J Exp Med* 1989; 169: 1721–31.

(60) Marsh JCW, Chang J, Testa NG, Hows JM, Dexter TM. In vitro assessment of marrow 'stem cell' and stromal cell function in aplastic anaemia. *Br J Haematol* 1991; 78: 258–67.

(61) Berenson RJ, Andrews RG, Besinger WI, et al. Antigen CD34 positive marrow cells engraft lethally irradiated baboons. *J Clin Invest* 1988; 81: 951–5.

(62) Abkowitz JL, Fialkow PJ, Niebrugge DJ, Raskind WH, Adamson JW. Pancytopenia as a clonal disorder of a multipotent haematopoietic stem cell. *J Clin Invest* 1984; 73: 258–61.

(63) Vogelstein B, Fearon ER, Hamilton SR et al. Clonal analysis using recombinant DNA probes from the X chromosome. *Cancer Res* 1987; 47: 4806–13.

(64) Abrahamson G, Fraser NJ, Boyd Y, Craig I, Wainscoat JS. A highly informative X-chromosome probe M27β can be used for determination of tumour clonality. *Br J Haematol* 1990; 74: 371–2.

(65) van Kamp H, Landergent JE, de Graaff E, Willemze R, Fibbe WE. Clonality of haematopoiesis in patients with aplastic anaemia and myelodysplastic syndromes. *Blood* 1990; 76(suppl 1): 50a. (abstract).

(66) Marsh JCW, Chang J, Cowling GJ, Testa NG, Hows JM, Dexter TM. Clonality studies and long-term marrow culture to assess haemopoiesis in aplastic anaemia. *Exp Haematol* 1990; 18: 306a. (abstract).

(67) Mehta AB, Chiu E, Harhalakis N et al. A T cell lymphoma of suppressor phenotype arising in a patient with severe aplastic anaemia. *Br J Haematol* 1989; 72: 287–9.

(68) Zoumbos NC, Gascon BP, Djeu JY, Trost SR, Young NS. Circulating activated suppressor T lymphocytes in aplastic anaemia. *N Eng J Med* 312: 257–65, 1985.

(69) Gascon P, Zoumbos NC, Scala G. Lymphokine abnormalities in aplastic anaemia: implications for the mechanism of action of antithymocyte globulin. *Blood* 1985; 65: 407–13.

(70) Hunter RF, Mold NG, Mitchell RB, Huang AT. Differentiation of normal marrow and HL60 cells induced by antithymocyte globulin. *Proc Natl Acad Sci USA* 1985; 82: 4823–7.

(71) Neudorf S, Jones M. The effects of antithymocyte globulin on natural killer cells. *Exp Haematol* 1988; 16: 831–5.

(72) Torok Storb B, Johnson GG, Bowder R, Storb R. Gamma-interferon in aplastic anaemia: inability to detect significant levels in sera or demonstrate haematopoietic suppressing activity. *Blood* 1987; 69: 629–33.

(73) Kaminski ER, Hows JM, Goldman JM, Batchelor JR. Pretransfused patients with severe aplastic anaemia exhibit high numbers of cytotoxic T lymphocyte precursors probably directed at non-HLA antigens. *Br J Haematol* 1990; 76: 401–5.

(74) Nissen C, Moser Y, Weis J, Speck B. Stimulating serum factors in aplastic anaemia. I. serum 'releaser' activity for haemopoietic growth factors, a regulator? *Br J Haematol* 1985; 61: 491–8.

(75) Yen YP, Zabala P, Doney K et al. Haematopoietic growth factors in human serum: erythroid burst-promoting activity in normal subjects and in patients with severe aplastic anaemia. *J Lab Clin Med* 1985; 106: 384–92.

(76) Nakao S, Matshushima K, Young N. Decreased interleukin-1 production in aplastic anaemia. *Br J Haematol* 1989; 71: 431–6.

(77) Thomas ED, Buckner CD, Storb R et al. Aplastic anaemia treated by marrow transplantation. *Lancet* 1972; i: 284–9.

(78) Appelbaum FR, Cleever M, Fefer A, Storb R, Thomas ED. Recurrence of aplastic anaemia following cyclophosphamide and syngeneic bone marrow transplantation: evidence for two mechanisms of graft failure. *Blood* 1985; 65: 553–6.

(79) Marsh JC, Harhalakis N, Dowding C, Laffan M, Gordon-Smith EC, Hows JM. Recurrent graft failure following syngeneic bone marrow transplantation for aplastic anaemia. *Bone Marrow Transpl* 1989; 4: 581–5.

(80) Matsue K, Niki T, Shiobara S et al. Transient engraftment of syngeneic bone marrow after conditioning with high dose cyclophosphamide and total abdominal irradiation in a patient with aplastic anaemia. *Am J Haematol* 1990; 33: 56–60.

(81) Goss GD, Wittwer MA, Bezwoda WR et al. Effects of natural killer cells on syngeneic bone marrow; in vitro and in vivo studies demonstrating graft failure due to NK cells in an identical twin treated by bone marrow transplantation. *Blood* 1985; 66: 1043–6.

(82) Laffan M, Durrant S, Harhalakis N, Economou K, Hows JM, Gordon-Smith EC. Bone marrow transplantation in the elderly. *Bone Marrow Transpl* 1987; 2(suppl 1): 105. (abstract).

(83) Storb R, Prentice RL, Thomas ED. Marrow transplantation for treatment of aplastic anaemia. An analysis of factors associated with graft rejection. *N Eng J Med* 1977; 296: 61–6.

(84) Gale RP, Ho W, Feig S et al. Prevention of graft rejection following bone marrow transplantation. *Blood* 1981; 57: 9–12.

(85) Gluckman E, Devergie A, Meletis J et al. Bone marrow transplantation in severe aplastic anaemia. *Bone Marrow Transpl* 1987; 2(suppl 1): 101.

(86) Ramsay NK, Trewan K, Nesbith ME et al. Total lymphoid irradiation as preparation for bone marrow transplantation for severe aplastic anaemia. *Blood* 1980; 55: 344–6.

(87) Storb R, Doney KC, Thomas ED et al. Marrow transplantation with or without donor buffy coat cells for 65 transfused aplastic patients. *Blood* 1982; 59: 236–41.

(88) Hows JM, Palmer S, Gordon-Smith EC. Use of cyclosporin A in allogeneic

bone marrow transplantation for severe aplastic anaemia. *Transplantation* 1982; 33: 382–6.

(89) Bacigalupo A, van Lint MT, Congiu A, Oneto R, for the EBMT SAA Working Party. Report of the EBMT working party on severe aplastic anaemia. *Bone Marrow Transpl* 4(suppl 2): 7. (abstract).

(90) Anasetti C, Doney KC, Storb R et al. Marrow transplantation for severe aplastic anaemia: long-term outcome in fifty 'untransfused' patients. *Ann Intern Med* 1986; 104: 461–6.

(91) Sanders J, Storb R, Thomas ED et al. Marrow transplantation for children with severe aplastic anaemia: improved survival with a combination of methotrexate and cyclosporine given for graft versus host disease prophylaxis. *Exp Haematol* 1990; 18: 311a. (abstract).

(92) Niederwieser D, Pepe M, Storb R, Longhran Jr T, Longton G, for the Seattle Marrow Transplant Team. Improvement in rejection, engraftment rate and survival without increase in graft versus host disease by high marrow cell dose in patients transplanted for aplastic anaemia. *Br J Haematol* 1988; 69: 23–8.

(93) Storb R. Graft rejection and graft versus host disease in marrow transplantation. *Transpl Proc* 1989; 21: 2915–18.

(94) Deeg HJ, Self S, Storb R et al. Decreased incidence of marrow graft rejection in patients with severe aplastic anaemia: changing impact of risk factors. *Blood* 1986; 68: 1363–8.

(95) Hows JM, Marsh JC, Yin JL et al. Bone marrow transplantation for severe aplastic anaemia using cyclosporin: long-term follow-up. *Bone Marrow Transpl* 1989; 4: 11–16.

(96) Storb R, Weiden PL, Sullivan KM et al. Second marrow transplants in patients with aplastic anaemia rejecting the first graft: use of a conditioning regimen including cyclophosphamide and antithymocyte globulin. *Blood* 1987; 70: 116–21.

(97) Storb R, Prentice RL, Buckner CD et al. Graft versus host disease and survival in patients with aplastic anaemia treated by marrow grafts from HLA identical siblings. Beneficial effect of a protective environment. *N Eng J Med* 1983; 308: 302–7.

(98) Flowers ME, Pepe MS, Longton G et al. Previous donor pregnancy as a risk factor for acute graft versus host disease in patients with aplastic anaemia treated by allogeneic marrow transplantation. *Br J Haematol* 1990; 74: 492–6.

(99) Storb R, Deeg HJ, Pepe M et al. Graft versus host disease prevention by methotrexate combined with cyclosporin compared to methotrexate alone in patients given marrow grafts for severe aplastic anaemia: long-term follow-up of a controlled trial. *Br J Haematol* 1989; 72: 567–72 .

(100) Storb R, Prentice RL, Sullivan KM et al. Predictive factors in chronic graft versus host disease in patients with aplastic anaemia treated by marrow transplantation from HLA identical siblings. *Ann Intern Med* 1983; 98: 461–6.

(101) Gluckman E, Champlin RE, Horowitz MM, Camitta B, for the International Bone Marrow Transplant Registry. Impact of treatment regimen on transplant outcome in severe aplastic anaemia (SAA). *Exp Haematol* 1990; 18: 312. (abstract).

J C W Marsh

(102) Hows JM, Bacigalupo A, Gluckman E on behalf of the EBMTG severe aplastic anemia working party. Impact of conditioning protocols on improved outcome of BMT for severe aplastic anemia (SAA). *Bone Marrow Transpl* 1990; 5(suppl 2) 52a. (abstract).
(103) Hows JM, Yin JL, Marsh J et al. Histocompatible unrelated volunteer donors compared with HLA nonidentical family donors in marrow transplantation for aplastic anaemia and leukaemia. *Blood* 1986; 68: 1322–8.
(104) Beatty PG, Di Bartolomeo P, Storb R et al. Treatment of aplastic anaemia with marrow grafts from related donors other than HLA genotypically-matched siblings. *Clin Transplantation* 1987; 1: 117–24.
(105) Storb R, Anasetti C, Appelbaum F et al. Allogeneic marrow transplantation for aplastic anaemia: major issues. In: Champlin RE, Gale RP (eds). *New strategies in bone marrow transplantation*. Wiley-Liss, 1991: 73–85.
(106) Camitta B, Ash R, Menitove J et al. Bone marrow transplantation for children with severe aplastic anaemia: use of donors other than HLA-identical siblings. *Blood* 1989; 74: 1852–7.
(107) Bidwell JL, Bidwell EA, Savage DA, Middleton D, Klouda PT, Bradley BA. A DNA-RFLP typing system that positively identifies serologically well defined and ill defined HLA-DR and DQ alleles, including DRW10. *Transplantation* 1988; 45: 640–6.
(108) Tiercy JM, Zwahlen F, Betuel H, Jeannet M, Mach B. Improved HLA class 11 matching in bone marrow transplantation with unrelated donors by DNA oligonucleotide probing. *Exp Haematol* 1989; 17: 705a. (abstract).
(109) Clay TM, Bidwell JL, Howard MRM, Bradley BA. On behalf of collaborating centres in the IMUST study. PRC fingerprinting for selection of HLA matched unrelated marrow donors. *Lancet* 1991; 337: 1049–52.
(110) Kaminski E, Hows J, Man S et al. Prediction of graft versus host disease by frequency analysis of cytotoxic T cells after unrelated donor bone marrow transplantation. *Transplantation* 1989; 48: 608–13.
(111) Bradley BA, Gore SM, Howard MR, Hows JM. International marrow unrelated search and transplant (IMUST) study. *Bone Marrow Transpl* 1989; 4(suppl 2): 44. (abstract).
(112) Howard MR, Hows JM, Gore SM et al. Unrelated donor marrow transplantation between 1977 and 1987 at four centres in the United Kingdom. *Transplantation* 1990; 49: 547–53.
(113) Howard MR, Bradley BA, Gore SM, Hows JM. Predicting the outcome of unrelated marrow donor (UD) searches: a preliminary IMUST study report. *Blood* 1990; 76(suppl 1): 546a. (abstract).
(114) Hows JM. Results of bone marrow transplantation for nonmalignant disorders. *Transpl and Immunol Lett* 1990; 4: 2–4.
(115) Champlin R, Ho W, Gale RP. Antithymocyte globulin treatment in patients with aplastic anaemia. *N Eng J Med* 1983; 308: 113–18.
(116) Speck B, Gratwohl A, Nissen C et al. Treatment of severe aplastic anaemia with antilymphocyte globulin or bone marrow transplantation. *Br Med J* 1981; 282: 860–3.
(117) Camitta B, O'Reilly RJ, Sensenbrenner L et al. Antithoracic duct lymphocyte globulin therapy of severe aplastic anaemia. *Blood* 1983; 62: 883–8.

(118) Marsh JC, Hows JM, Bryett KA, Al-Hashimi S, Fairhead SM, Gordon-Smith EC. Survival after antilymphocyte globulin therapy for aplastic anaemia depends on disease severity. *Blood* 1987; 70: 1046–52.

(119) Devergie A, Bordeau-Esperou H, Gluckman E. Comparison of cyclosporin A (CyA) and horse antithymocyte globulin (H-ATG) for treatment of severe aplastic anaemia (SAA): a multicentre prospective randomized study. *Bone Marrow Transpl* 1990; 5(suppl 2): 29. (abstract).

(120) Leonard EM, Raefsky E, Griffith P, Kinball J, Nienhuis AN, Young NS. Cyclosporin therapy for aplastic anaemia, congenital and acquired red cell aplasia. *Br J Haematol* 1989; 72: 278–84.

(121) Frickhofen N, Kaltwasser JP, Schrezenmeier H et al. Treatment of aplastic anaemia with antilymphocyte globulin and methyl prednisolone with or without cyclosporine. *N Eng J Med* 1991; 324: 1297–304.

(122) Young NS, Griffith P, Brittain E et al. A multicentre trial of antithymocyte globulin in bone marrow failure. *Blood* 1988; 72: 1861–9.

(123) Doney KC, Weiden PL, Buckner CD, Storb R, Thomas ED. Treatment of severe aplastic anaemia using antilymphocyte globulin with or without an infusion of HLA haploidentical marrow. *Exp Haematol* 1981; 9: 829–34.

(124) Doney K, Kopecky K, Storb R et al. Long-term comparison of immunosuppressive therapy with antithymocyte globulin to bone marrow transplantation in aplastic anaemia. In: Shahidi NT (ed.), *Aplastic anaemia and other bone marrow failure syndromes*. Springer-Verlag, 1990: 104–114.

(125) Marin P, Schrezenmeier H, Bacigalupo A, van Lint MT, for the EBMT SAA Working Party. Relapse of aplasia following ALG treatment: a report of the SAA working party. *Bone Marrow Transpl* 1990; 48a, 28. (abstract).

(126) Groopman JE, Mitsuyasu RT, De Leo MJ, Oette J, Golde DW. Effect of recombinant human granulocyte–macrophage colony-stimulating factor on myelopoiesis in acquired immunodeficiency syndrome. *N Eng J Med* 1987; 317: 593–8.

(127) Vadhan-Raj S, Keating M, LeMaistre A et al. Effects of recombinant human granulocyte-macrophage colony stimulating factor in patients with myelodysplastic syndromes. *N Eng J Med* 1987; 317: 1545–52.

(128) Antman KS, Griffin JD, Elias A et al. Effect of recombinant human granulocyte-macrophage colony stimulating factor on chemotherapy induced myelosuppression. *N Eng J Med* 1988; 319: 593–8.

(129) Nemunaitis J, Singer JW, Buckner CD et al. Use of recombinant human granulocyte-macrophage colony stimulating factor in autologous marrow transplantation for lymphoid malignancies. *Blood* 1988; 72: 834–6.

(130) Antin JH, Smith BR, Holmes W, Rosenthal DS. Phase I/II study of recombinant human granulocyte macrophage colony stimulating factor in aplastic anaemia and myelodysplastic syndrome. *Blood* 1988; 72: 705–13.

(131) Nissen C, Tichelli A, Gratwohl A et al. Failure of recombinant human granulocyte-macrophage colony stimulating factor therapy in aplastic anaemia patients with very severe neutropenia. *Blood* 1988; 72: 2045–7.

(132) Vadhan-Raj S, Buescher S, Broxymeyer HE et al. Stimulation of myelopoiesis in patients with aplastic anaemia by recombinant human granulocyte macrophage colony stimulating factor. *N Eng J Med* 1988; 319: 1628–34.

(133) Champlin RE, Nimer SD, Ireland P, Oette DH, Golde DW. Treatment of refractory aplastic anaemia with recombinant human granulocyte macrophage colony stimulating factor. *Blood* 1989; 73: 694–9.

(134) Guinan EC, Sieff CA, Oette DH, Nathan DG. A phase I/II trial of recombinant granulocyte-macrophage colony stimulating factor for children with aplastic anaemia. *Blood* 1990; 76: 1077–82.

(135) Ganser A, Lindemann A, Seipelt G et al. Effects of recombinant human interleukin-3 in aplastic anaemia. *Blood* 1990; 76: 1287–92.

(136) Potter MN, Mott MG, Oakhill A. The successful treatment of a case of very severe aplastic anaemia with granulocyte macrophage colony stimulating factor and anti-lymphocyte globulin. *Br J Haematol* 1990; 75: 618–19.

(137) Bronchud MH, Potter MR, Morgensten G et al. In vitro and in vivo analysis of the effect of recombinant human granulocyte colony stimulating factor in patients. *Br J Cancer* 1988; 58 (i): 64–9.

(138) Morstyn G, Souza LM, Keech J et al. Effect of granulocyte colony stimulating factor on neutropenia induced by cytotoxic chemotherapy. *Lancet* 1988; i: 667–72.

(139) Nicola NA. Granulocyte colony-stimulating factor. In: Dexter TM, Garland GM, Testa NG, eds. *Colony stimulating factors. Molecular and cellular biology.* Marcel Decker 1990: 77–109.

(140) Sonoda Y, Fujii H, Yashige H et al. Treatment of refractory aplastic anaemia with long-term administration of recombinant human granulocyte colony stimulating factor. *Blood* 1990; 76(suppl 1): 49a. (abstract).

(141) Donahue RE, Seehra J, Metzger M et al. Human interleukin-3 and granulocyte-macrophage colony stimulating factor act synergistically in stimulating haematopoiesis in primates. *Science* 1988; 241: 1820–3.

(142) Leary A, Ikebuchi K, Hirai Y et al. Synergism between interleukin-6 and interleukin-3 in supporting proliferation of human haemopoietic stem cells. *Blood* 1988; 71: 1759–63.

(143) Heyworth CM, Ponting IL, Dexter TM. The response of haemopoietic cells to growth factors: developmental implications of synergistic interactions. *J Cell Sci* 1988; 91: 239–47.

(144) Marsh JC, Hows JM, Bryett KA, Gordon-Smith EC. Young age and outcome of treatment with antilymphocyte globulin for aplastic anaemia. *Bone Marrow Transpl* 1988; 3(suppl 1): 238. (abstract).

(145) Locasciulli A, van't Veer L, Bacigalupo A. Treatment with marrow transplantation or immunosuppression of childhood severe aplastic anaemia: a report from the EBMT SAA working party. *Bone Marrow Transpl* 1990; 6: 211–17.

(146) Withespoon RP, Fisher LD, Schoch G et al. Secondary cancers after bone marrow transplantation for leukaemia or aplastic anaemia. N Eng J Med 1989; 321: 784–9.

(147) Szer J, Deeg HJ, Witherspoon RP et al. Long-term survival after marrow transplantation for paroxysmal nocturnal haemoglobinuria with aplastic anaemia. *Ann Intern Med* 1984; 101: 193–5.

The role of hematopoietic growth factors in bone marrow transplantation: current status and future prospects

J L NEMUNAITIS AND J W SINGER

Introduction

The use of high intensity chemotherapy and/or radiotherapy followed by infusion of bone marrow or peripheral blood stem cells enables long-term disease-free survival in patients with hematologic malignancies or other hematologic disorders (aplastic anemia, myelodysplastic syndrome, immune deficiency syndrome, etc) that are incurable by standard therapy.[1,2] However, complications related to toxicity of the preparative regimen, such as hemorrhage, mucositis, pneumonitis, venoocclusive disease and infection cause significant morbidity and mortality. These complications may be further exacerbated by immunodeficiency related to graft-versus-host disease (GVHD) and therapy to control GVHD if the infused stem cells are derived from an allogeneic donor.[3,4] Hematopoietic growth factors stimulate the proliferation, differentiation and enhance the function of hematopoietic cells.[5-8] The purpose of this chapter is to review recent studies of the application of hematopoietic growth factors in bone marrow transplant (BMT) patients and to suggest some future directions for investigation.

Preclinical studies

More than 20 cytokines involved in hematopoietic cell signalling have been identified and cloned. Several have been produced in sufficient quantity for clinical use and three have been approved in the United States as recombinant drugs; erythropoietin,[9] granulocyte-(G-) colony stimulating factor (CSF)[10] and granulocyte–macrophage (GM)-CSF.[6]

Cytokines are produced by hematopoietic and non-hematopoietic cells and selectively stimulate the survival, proliferation and differentiation of

All correspondence to: Dr JL Nemunaitis, Western Pennsylvania Cancer Institute 4800 Friendship Ave, Pittsburgh PA 15224 USA.

Cambridge Medical Reviews: Haematological Oncology Volume 2
© Cambridge University Press 1992

hematopoietic cells in a lineage restricted manner. G-CSF primarily stimulates neutrophil growth.[10] Macrophage (M)-CSF stimulates monocyte, macrophage growth.[11,12] GM-CSF primarily stimulates neutrophil, monocyte and macrophage growth, but also affects eosinophils, megakaryocytes and erythroid cells.[6] Interleukin-3 (IL-3) has similar proliferative effects to GM-CSF, although its capacity to stimulate early progenitor cells and megakaryocytes appears to be greater.[13,14] Interleukin-1 (IL-1) has many effects on both hematopoietic and nonhematopoietic cells. It stimulates lymphoid cell growth and enhances the survival of myeloid cells.[15] IL-1 induces production of G-CSF, GM-CSF and IL-6 (a lymphoid and megakaryocyte stimulating factor).[16–18] The proliferative effects of exogenous CSFs are enhanced substantially when they are used in combination.[19–21]

Hematopoietic growth factors were isolated on the basis of their proliferative effects on hematopoietic cells. However, all have other effects. For example, G-CSF enhances neutrophil function[10]; M-CSF enhances monocyte and macrophage function.[12] GM-CSF enhances neutrophil, monocyte and macrophage function.[6] IL-3 enhances the activity of eosinophils and IL-1 increases systemic free radical scavenger activity reducing free oxygen radicals produced by radiation damaged tissues, thereby acting as a radioprotectant.[22] GM-CSF stimulates the expression of IL-6[23] and may decrease the expression of TGF-β[24] (a potent inhibitor of myeloid cell differentation).[25] IL-1 and GM-CSF increase the expression of tumor necrosis factor-α,[26] a cytokine with multifunctional effects, including stimulation of extracellular matrix production, mediation of the inflammatory response and regulation of other growth factor genes. G-CSF, GM-CSF and IL-1 stimulate the growth of nonhematopoietic cells, such as endothelial cells.[27] Not surprisingly, neoplastic cells within the target lineages are also stimulated by these growth factors. Some myeloid leukemia cells proliferate in response to G-CSF, GM-CSF, M-CSF and IL-3.[28–31] Normal and abnormal plasma cells (i.e. multiple myeloma cells) are stimulated by IL-6,[32,33] and both lymphoid and myeloid leukemia cells may be stimulated by IL-1.

Animal trials indicate that M-CSF,[34] G-CSF,[35,36] GM-CSF,[37–40] IL-3[41] and IL-1[42–44] are well tolerated at biologically active doses, enhance neutrophil and/or monocyte recovery following cytotoxic chemo-radiotherapy and improve survival in selected test models. Administration of GM-CSF following autologous (A) BMT induced earlier platelet recovery, although the effects of IL-3 and IL-1 on stimulating platelet recovery were more consistent. When certain cytokines are combined or administered in sequence (i.e. IL-3 or IL-1 prior to GM-CSF or G-CSF),[45–47] the stimulation of recovery was substantially enhanced when compared to single cytokine therapy. Survival of neutropenic mice given an infectious challenge is significantly improved by prophylactic administration of cytokines.[37,48–51] These encouraging, preclinical studies led to the early institution of clinical trials with G and GM-CSF in neutropenic patients at risk for serious infections. Patients with poor neutrophil production due to myelodysplasia, aplastic anemia, congenital neutropenia or following administration of myelosuppressive drugs were the target groups in the initial trials.[52-54] This review is limited to studies of recombinant growth factors in patients undergoing BMT. These patients are at high risk for infectious complications by virtue of both prolonged pancytopenia and deficiencies of both cell-mediated and humoral immunity.

Clinical studies in autologous bone marrow transplantation (ABMT)
Phase I/II trials of rhG-CSF and rhGM-CSF in ABMT patients demonstrated minimal toxicities at doses with probable biologic activity (see Tables 1 and 2).[55-65] Phase I-II trials with rhM-CSF, rhIL-1 β and rhIL-3 after ABMT are ongoing. Preliminary results indicate mild, but tolerable systemic toxicity with rhIL-3 and rhIL-1 in BMT patients (unpublished data), and no systemic toxicity with rhM-CSF other than dose-related thrombocytopenia (unpublished data).[66,67] No data on the phase II aspects of these studies are available.

Trials with rhGM-CSF in ABMT patients
It is important to note that three different preparations of rhGM-CSF have been used in clinical trials. An *E. coli*-produced, non-glycosylated product, mammalian cell-produced, glycosylated product and a yeast-derived glycosylated drug. The specific activity of the *E. coli* product is greater than that of the yeast product. In an early trial with non-glycosylated rhGM-CSF, doses ranging from 2-32 $\mu g/m^2$/day were given to patients with breast cancer undergoing ABMT.[55] Toxicity at higher doses (32 $\mu g/m^2$/d) consisted of serosal effusions, fluid retention and pulmonary edema. At lower doses (2 to 16 $\mu g/m^2$/day), mild fluid retention, rashes and myalgias developed in some patients. The toxicities were not limiting. Patients who received rhGM-CSF manifested less hepatic and renal dysfunction (lower bilirubin and creatinine levels) and had less mucositis than historical patients. Yeast-derived, glycosylated rhGM-CSF was administered at lower doses (15 to 240 $\mu g/m^2$/day by 2 hour infusion) in patients with lymphoid malignancies following ABMT.[56,57] This product was well tolerated. Toxicities were limited to joint pains and myalgias in 4 of 15 patients. A dose-related effect of rhGM-CSF on neutrophil recovery was noted with evidence of biologic activity at doses ≥ 60 $\mu g/m^2$/day. The incidence of severe infections in patients who received either rhGM-CSF preparation appeared reduced compared to historical patients (see Table 1). In subsequent phase I/II trials with rhGM-CSF, the rates of neutrophil recovery and the incidence of infection has been variable. In one study, patients with Hodgkin's disease receiving increasing doses of rhGM-CSF after ABMT had neutrophil recovery 7 days earlier than historical

Table 1. Results of phase I/II trials with rhGM-CSF following autologous BMT compared to historical controls

Number of patients		Day ANC >500/mm³		Day platelet independence		% of patients with infection		Day initial discharge		Comments[e]	Refs.
GMCSF	control	GMCSF	control	GMCSF	control	GMCSF	control	GMCSF	control		
19	24	14	19	NS[a]	NS[a]	16	35	NR[b]	NR[b]	Non-glycosylated rhGM-CSF 2–32 µg/kg/d in patients with breast cancer, melanoma	55
22	86	17	25	28	38	18	30	32	41	Yeast-glycosylated rhGM-CSF 60–250 µg/m²/d in patients with ALL, NHL	56,57
6	86	22	25	30	38	0	30	30	41	Yeast-glycosylated rhGM-CSF 15–30 µg/m²/d in patients with ALL, NHL	56
12	19	18	25	30	28	58	68	30	30	Yeast-glycosylated rhGM-CSF 100–400 µg/m²/d in patients with HD	58
5	27	14	24	NR[b,c]	NR[b,c]	NR[b]	52	36	47	Yeast-glycosylated rhGM-CSF 64–256 µg/m²/d >1.2 × 10⁴ CFUGM/kg infused	59
15	27	28	24	NR[b,d]	NR[b,d]	NR[b]	52	50	47	Yeast-glycosylated rhGM-CSF 64–256 µg/m²/d <0.45 × 10⁴ CFUGM/kg infused	59
5	27	23	24	NR[b,d]	NR[b,d]	NR[b]	52	43	47	Yeast-glycosylated rhGM-CSF 16–32 µg/m²/d ≤0.45 × 10⁴ CFUGM/kg infused	59
6	unk	11	20	NR[b]	NR[b]	NR[b]	NR[b]	NR[b]	NR	Yeast-glycosylated rhGM-CSF 500 µg/m²/d	60
16	52	14	20	24	26	6	NR[b]	NR[b]	NR[b]	Mammalian-glycosylated rhGM-CSF 11 µg/m²/d in patients with NHL	61

NS[a] = values not shown, but reported as not significantly different.
NR[b] = not reported.
c = day of platelet transfusion independence was not reported, but the number of platelet units required were significantly less during the first 28 days (81 vs 149 units) compared to historical controls.
d = number of platelet units infused from day 0–28 of all patients who received ≤0.45 CFUGM/kg ($n = 30$) was 215 in the GM-CSF treated patients and 149 in the control group.
e = ALL: acute lymphocytic leukemia, NHL: non-Hodgkin's lymphoma, HD: Hodgkin's disease.

Table 2. *Results of phase I/II trials with rhG-CSF following autologous BMT compared to historical control patients*

Number of patients		Day ANC >500/mm^3		Day platelet independent		% infection		Day discharged		Comments[b]	Refs.
G-CSF	control	G-CSF	control	G-CSF	control	G-CSF	control	G-CSF	control		
15	18	11	20	33	45	53	61	23	29	20 µg/kg/day with a taper over 28 days in patients with NHL, HD, ALL, GCT	62
18	58	13	22	28	32	17	36	NR[c]	NR[c]	60 µg/kg/day with a taper down over 28 days as ANC increase in patients with HD	63
24	24	S[a]	S[a]	NS	NS	18	35	NR[c]	NR[c]	16–64 µg/kg/day in patients with Mel, Br Ca	64,65

S[a] = values not given, but reported as being significantly earlier in patients who received rhG-CSF.
[b] = ALL: acute lymphocytic leukemia; HD: Hodgkin's disease; NHL: non-Hodgkin's lymphoma; GCT: gem cell tumor; Mel: melanoma; Br Ca: breast cancer.
NR[c] = not reported.

patients.[58] However, the frequency of infections was not reduced. In another dose escalation study, rhGM-CSF was given to patients undergoing ABMT for lymphoid malignancy with chemically purged marrow.[59] Both neutrophil recovery and the incidence of infection were similar to historical rates. However, the subset of patients who received rhGM-CSF at doses > 60 $\mu g/m^2$/day and who received $\geq 1.2 \times 10^4$ CFU-GM/kg, had earlier neutrophil recovery. All studies examining the effects of rhGM-CSF in patients receiving unpurged marrows observed acceleration of neutrophil recovery.[55–58,60,61] The grafts obtained with rhGM-CSF appear durable, however, only one trial has described follow up for more than 1 year.[68] Of patients who received rhGM-CSF early after ABMT for lymphoid cancer 28 were followed a median of 774 days. No late toxicity from rhGM-CSF was observed. The relapse rates and overall survival were similar to comparable historical patients.

The effects of rhGM-CSF on platelet recovery and the duration of initial hospitalization have been variable (see Table 1). The relapse rate and short-term survival were unaffected by rhGM-CSF.

Three randomized, placebo controlled trials evaluating rhGM-CSF in auto-logous BMT patients were recently completed.[69–72] A summary of results are shown in Table 3. In the Seattle/Boston/Omaha trial,[69] yeast glycosylated rhGM-CSF was administered at a dose of 250 $\mu g/m^2$/d by 24 hour IV infusion from day 0 (the day of marrow infusion) to day 20. The incidence of bone and chest pain, fevers and skin rashes suggested as rhGM-CSF-induced toxicities in the I/II trials were not different between the rhGM-CSF and the placebo treated patients. Toxicities, such as serositis and capillary leak syndrome, which were observed when using higher doses of non-glycosylated rhGM-CSF, were not seen. The effect on hematopoietic recovery was pronounced. An ANC > 500/mm^3 and 1000/mm^3 was achieved 7 days earlier in patients who received rhGM-CSF. However, the time to achieve an ANC > 100/mm^3 was only 1 day earlier in patients who received rhGM-CSF (day 14 vs 15). RhGM-CSF treated patients required fewer days of intravenous antibiotics, probably due to earlier neutrophil recovery. Antibiotics were generally discontinued once patients achieved an ANC > 500/mm^3. The duration of hospitalization was 6 days shorter in patients given rhGM-CSF. The number of febrile days (temperature $\geq$ 38 °C) were not different between patients who received rhGM-CSF (8 days) and patients who received placebo (8 days). When infection occurred, it generally occurred before patients achieved an ANC > 100/mm^3. The frequency of significant infections (bacteremia, sepsis or invasive tissue infection) was less in patients who received rhGM-CSF (17% vs 30%). This difference was not statistically significant ($P = 0.096$, Fisher exact, 2-tailed analysis) unless streptococcal infections, most of which were catheter-associated, were excluded. Only 2 (3%) rhGM-CSF treated patients developed non-streptococcal infections compared to 12 (19%) placebo treated patients ($P = 0.004$, Fisher exact, 2-tailed analysis). One hun-

Table 3. *Results of phase III trials with rhGM-CSF following autologous BMT*

Number of patients GM-CSF	control	Day ANC >500/mm³ GM-CSF	control	Day platelet independent GM-CSF	control	% infection GM-CSF	control	Day discharged GM-CSF	control	Comments[b]	Refs.
65	63	19	26	26	29	17	30	27	33	Yeast glycosylated rhGM-CSF 250 µg/m²/d by 2 hour IV infusion in patients with ALL, NHL, HD	69
41	47	14	21	19	19	39	47	23	28	Non-glycosylated rhGM-CSF 250 µg/m²/d by continuous infusion in patients with NHL	70, 71
39	40	15	28	39	31	38	70	30	31	Non-glycosylated rhGM-CSF 250 µg/m²/d by continuous infusion in patients with NHL	70, 72

[a] = ALL: acute lymphocytic leukemia; NHL: non-Hodgkin's lymphoma; HD: Hodgkin's disease.

dred day survival, tumor cell response to cytotoxic therapy and early relapse rates were not different between patients who received rhGM-CSF or placebo. The conclusions from this trial were that rhGM-CSF stimulated earlier neutrophil recovery and was associated with fewer infections and shorter hospitalization time. Since it was non-toxic, it appears to be indicated therapy in patients undergoing ABMT with lymphoid cancer.

Two randomized, European trials used *E. coli*-produced rhGM-CSF[71,72] given by continuous infusion at a dose of 250 μg/m²/day. Preliminary results, shown in Table 3, confirm that neutrophil recovery was enhanced and that platelet recovery was unaffected. No toxicity was observed in the first trial and minimal toxicity was observed in the second trial (fluid retention in 12% of rhGM-CSF treated patients). Infections and duration of hospitalization were reduced in one trial and not different in the other trial.

Trials with G-CSF in ABMT

RhG-CSF has not been extensively studied in ABMT patients. The results of the first 3 trials compared to historical patients indicate that rhG-CSF is well tolerated and suggest accelerated neutrophil recovery.[62–65] The incidence of serious infections decreased in 2 of the 3 studies (see Table 2).

In an Australian study,[62] the dose of rhG-CSF was lower than in the subsequent 2 trials.[63,64] The only toxicity described was minor bruising or hemorrhage at the subcutaneous infusion sites in 7 (47%) of the patients. Although neutrophil recovery was enhanced, the incidence of infection and number of febrile days were similar to historical patients. Fewer days of intravenous antibiotics were given to rhG-CSF-treated patients than to historical patients. This most likely reflected neutrophil recovery, since antibiotics were discontinued in afebrile patients when they reached an ANC > 500/mm³. In the second trial, rhG-CSF was administered over 30 minutes via central intravenous line. Of the patients, 30% developed mild to moderate bone pain and one patient developed serositis evidenced by pericardial tamponade, pleural effusions and ascites. Neutrophil recovery was enhanced and the incidence of bacteremia was lower than in historical cases. Severe mucositis was also decreased (6% vs 23%). Preliminary data from the third trial suggest similar results. Short-term survival or recurrent disease rate was not affected in any of these trials and long-term follow-up has not been reported.

Peripheral blood as adjunctive therapy or as the sole stem cells source

The administration of rhG-CSF and rhGM-CSF after BMT shortens the rate of neutrophil recovery after the count reaches 100/mm³. However, the time to achieve an ANC ≥ 100/mm³ and the time to achieve platelet independence is not improved by either rhG-CSF or rhGM-CSF. A pilot study in 6 patients suggested that when autologous peripheral blood progenitor cells (PBPCs) are infused in combination with autologous bone marrow to patients after myeloablative chemoradiotherapy the time to reach an ANC $\geqslant$ 500/mm^3 (day 12) and platelet transfusion independence (day 9) were earlier than in historical patients who were given marrow without PBPCs (day 17 and 24, respectively).[73] However, the duration of severe neutropenia was not shortened in patients who received adjunctive PBPCs. The investigators subsequently administered rhGM-CSF to 7 patients prior to harvest of PBPCs and dramatically increased the number of committed peripheral blood progenitor cells (CFU-GM) harvested compared to previous experience.[74] The day to achieve an ANC $\geqslant$ 500/mm^3 was shortened to 9 days and the severity of mucositis was reduced. Others have suggested based on results of a phase II study in 17 patients that the time to achieve an ANC $\geqslant$ 100/mm^3 can be reduced (11 days to 8 days) by the administration of rhGM-CSF stimulated PBPCs in combination with autologous bone marrow followed by a second course of rhGM-CSF after BMT. Infection occurred less frequently in patients who received rhGM-CSF than in historical patients who did not receive growth factors or PBPCs (39% vs 12%).[75]

In some patients bone marrow cannot be obtained due to tumor involvement or because marrow was damaged by pelvic radiation. PBPCs have been used as the sole source of stem cells and successful engraftment has occurred.[76-78] However, delayed platelet recovery and late graft failure have occurred, predominantly in patients who received $< 50 \times 10^4$ CFU-GM/kg.[79-81] Both rhGM-CSF and rhG-CSF increase the number of circulating progenitor cells.[82,83] RhGM-CSF was used to increase the progenitor cell pool in 12 patients ineligible for marrow harvest.[84] The number of CFU-GM/ml was increased 8.5 fold. Six of the 12 patients subsequently underwent an autologous transplant using peripheral blood mononuclear cells as the only source of stem cells. One patient did not engraft, however, this was attributed to recurrent disease. The other 5 patients achieved an ANC > 500 on day 29 and platelet transfusion independence on day 39.

In summary, when PBPCs are given in combination with bone marrow and either rhGM-CSF or rhG-CSF there is a strong suggestion that the period of absolute neutropenia, incidence of infection and platelet recovery is reduced. However, no prospective controlled trials have been done.

Future directions
There are two major problems in ABMT that need to be addressed in future studies with recombinant growth factors: (i) the 10–14 days duration of severe neutropenia (ANC < 100/mm^3) which was not affected by rhGM-CSF; (ii) the 4–6 weeks of platelet support required following ABMT. Therapies likely to affect these areas include addition of cytokine stimulated PBSC to bone marrow, use of cytokine-primed bone marrow and use of cytokines in combination after the marrow infusion.[85] Early engraftment may be further

improved if early-acting cytokines, such as IL-3, IL-1, c-kit ligand,[86–88] or IL-3–GM-CSF fusion molecule[89] are administered before marrow harvest. A concern in this manipulation is that it may decrease the number of self-renewing stem cells and lead to late graft failure.[90] Preliminary data suggest that if either rhG-CSF or rhGM-CSF can be used to mobilize progenitor cells prior to harvesting peripheral blood, the period of absolute neutropenia following high intensity chemoradiotherapy can be reduced. Earlier acting cytokines, such as IL-3, IL-1, IL-3–GM-CSF fusion molecule and c-kit ligand, which are synergistic with rhG-CSF and rhGM-CSF may further enhance the capacity to harvest both circulating progenitor cells and bone marrow progenitor cells. Preclinical studies suggest the effects may be dramatic when cytokines are used in combination. The indication for eventual use of cytokines which stimulate early progenitors may differ from that of G- or GM-CSF in that the functional enhancing capacity of these agents on mature cells, except for the IL-3–rhGM-CSF fusion molecule, is less than rhGM-CSF, rhG-CSF and rhM-CSF. Therefore, the agents which stimulate early progenitors may be less effective in prevention of neutropenic infections unless combined with cytokines which enhance function, such as M-CSF, G-CSF, GM-CSF or IL-3–GM-CSF fusion molecule. This is especially true in patients with prolonged neutropenia (> 1 week) in whom tissue macrophages may play a significant role in infection clearance before sufficient neutrophils appear in circulation. Growth factors which stimulate late hematopoietic progenitors rarely induce proliferation of solid tumor cells in vitro.[91,92] However, there is little data on the potential effect of growth factors on mobilization of malignant cells into circulation. If growth factors mobilize malignant cells, their use for PBPC harvesting may be restricted to patients in remission and negate their use in patients who have bone marrow involvement with tumor cells. Careful monitoring of patients treated with cytokines to determine if tumor cells are mobilized needs to be done. Growth factors (i.e. M-CSF, GM-CSF) could also be used to stimulate selected hematopoietic cells, such as macrophages, which may be harvested from the peripheral blood and grown in the presence of growth factor to be reinfused for potential antitumor activity.[93] Administration of growth factors concurrently with cytoreductive therapy may also increase the sensitivity of malignant cells (see Future prospects). Finally, the use of cytokines that stimulate thrombopoiesis and early progenitors, such as leukemia inhibitory factor (LIF),[94] IL-3–GM-CSF fusion molecule[89] and c-kit ligand[86–88] alone or in combination with later growth stimulating cytokines, such as IL-6, IL-3, G-CSF or GM-CSF, may also be of benefit.

Use of cytokines in patients with marrow graft failure

Current status

Nearly 10% of patients who undergo BMT fail to engraft or develop late graft failure. The survival of patients with graft failure is less than 20%.[95,96] Graft failure was defined by the authors as either failure to reach an ANC of 100/mm^3 by day 21 in the presence of infection, not reaching an ANC > 100 by day 28, or a sustained (> 7 day) decrease in ANC to < 500/mm^3 after achieving initial engraftment in patients who were also red cell and platelet transfusion dependent. In an analysis of 155 historical patients at the Fred Hutchinson Cancer Research Center who fit this definition for marrow graft failure and did not receive any cytokine, the actuarial survival was 23% at 1 year [16–29% (95% confidence intervals-CI)]. The majority of patients with graft failure died from infection. Neither second marrow infusion nor a second marrow graft following additional immunosuppression, improved the dismal survival rate.

RhGM-CSF was chosen for a clinical trial in graft failure rather than rhG-CSF because rhGM-CSF also stimulates the function and proliferation of tissue macrophages (Kupffer cells, alveolar macrophages, dermal Langerhans cells, peritoneal macrophages). Host macrophages persist in tissues for up to 6 months after marrow ablation in BMT patients. In a multicenter trial, yeast-derived rhGM-CSF was administered at doses from 60 to 1000 µg/m^2/day to 37 patients with marrow graft failure. Of these, 15 had been transplanted from allogeneic, 1 from syngeneic donor and 21 had autografts. Of the patients, 21 increased their ANC to >500/mm^3 within 2 weeks of starting therapy. No consistent early effects on platelet recovery were seen. However, if patients survived, self-sustaining platelet counts were eventually observed. The survival rate to day 100 after starting rhGM-CSF was 59% (44% to 75%, 95% CI), which is significantly different than the historical rate of 32% (Fig. 1).

This Phase I/II trial was broadened to a multicenter Phase II study. RhGM-CSF was given at 250µg/m^2/day by 2 hour infusion for 14 days. Analysis of the first 101 consecutive patients entered into this trial reveals that an overall actuarial survival at 40% with median follow-up of 2 years,[98] a value that is similar to that of the initial 37 patients. The survival of 50 patients with graft failure treated with rhGM-CSF at the Fred Hutchinson Cancer Research Center is similar to that of patients from other centers. Of the Seattle patients, 42% responded by reaching an ANC > 500/mm^3 within 14 days of initiation of rhGM-CSF and an additional 10% of patients responded to a second course of rhGM-CSF. Occasional patients who did not have sustained granulocyte recovery in response to the first course of rhGM-CSF responded to a second or third course. The response rates are similar for autologous and allogeneic transplant patients. Other studies suggest that

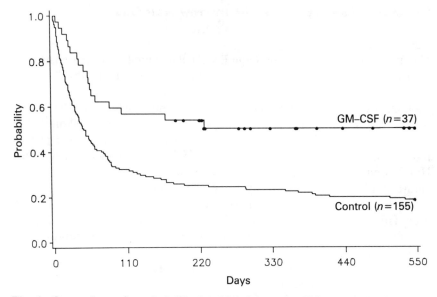

Fig. 1. Comparison of survival (Kaplan–Meier) between 155 consecutive historical patients with graft failure and 37 graft failure patients who received rhGM-CSF. Day 0 in the control patients is day the definition of graft failure was fulfilled and the day 0 of the study patients was the day of initiation of rhGM-CSF[97].

patients with prolonged neutropenia (> 55 days) following BMT may not maintain response to rhGM-CSF.[99] Occasional allogeneic patients who developed graft rejection, responded to rhGM-CSF by recovery of autologous marrow function. No patients with predominantly donor cells prior to receiving rhGM-CSF had autologous recovery. GM-CSF did not worsen GVHD in allogeneic BMT recipients. When compared to historical patients, GM-CSF treatment did not appear to increase the rate of early relapse in patients transplanted for myeloid malignancies. These data suggest that rhGM-CSF may be of benefit to patients who develop graft failure following either autologous or allogeneic BMT.

Future directions
More than half of patients with graft failure treated with rhGM-CSF do not respond to the initial course of treatment with rhGM-CSF. These patients are candidates for trials with other cytokines, such as IL-1, IL-3 and c-kit ligand, which may stimulate more primitive stem cells than GM-CSF. In addition, these patients could be treated with combinations of synergistic growth factors. To continue protection against infection during absolute neutropenia, a cytokine which enhances the function of tissue macrophages should be

included in the combination studies. Tissue macrophages persist for months after BMT and increasing their functional activity may be beneficial. Candidate combinations include rhIL-3 and rhGM-CSF, IL-1 and rhGM-CSF, and c-kit ligand and rhGM-CSF. A trial of the rhGM-CSF-rhIL3 fusion molecule and rhM-CSF may also be of interest.

Studies in patients undergoing allogeneic BMT

Introduction
Three major issues impede the success of allogeneic BMT in neoplastic disease. (1) the morbidty associated with the chemo/radiotherapy; (2) the dualistic problems of graft-versus-host disease (GVHD) and graft rejection; and (3) the difficulty in eradicating the primary disease. If cytokines such as G-CSF or GM-CSF accelerate engraftment and decrease the incidence of serious infections, overall morbidity might be reduced. This could occur through increased tolerance for immunosuppressive therapy. Trials of growth factors in allograft patients require considerable caution since agents that stimulate marrow recovery have the potential to activate T lymphocytes indirectly and thus to exacerbate GVHD. For example, GM-CSF increases the expression of TNF and IL-1 by macrophages[26,100] which in turn activates cytotoxic T-cells[101] and may increase GVHD.[102,103] On the other hand, by reducing infections, rhGM-CSF may be associated with less renal dysfunction and may enable more cyclosporine A to be given, thereby maintaining more effective GVHD prophylaxis. Furthermore, if growth factors decrease circulating endotoxin, a potent stimulus for inflammatory cytokines, it is possible that they might decrease the severity of GVHD. This phenomenon was observed in patients treated in environmental protection rooms and in patients with gastrointestinal tract decontamination. Such patients had a lower incidence of acute GVHD.[3,104] Gnotobiotic mice given major histocompatability complex (MHC) mismatched BMT survived while bacterial replete mice died of graft versus host reaction (GVHR).[105,106] When mice were given rhGM-CSF after allogeneic BMT, survival was improved and the severity of GVHR was either not altered or decreased.[39,107,108] GM-CSF may also affect GVHD through other mechanisms. It reduces the expression of IL-2 receptor on monocytes and stimulates the production of soluble IL-2 receptor and soluble CD8.[109,110] Soluble IL2 receptor may bind circulating molecules of IL-2 making them less available to cell surface receptors.

Clinical studies with rhGM-CSF
To determine the safety of rhGM-CSF in patients with hematologic malignancies undergoing matched, allogeneic BMT from HLA-identical sibling donors, a phase I/II dose escalation trial was done using yeast-derived rhGM-CSF.[111] Since the toxicity of methotrexate (MTX), a drug used for

GVHD prophylaxis, is greatest for rapidly cycling cells, there was concern that concurrent rhGM-CSF might adversely affect hematopoietic reconstitution. Therefore, two independent rhGM-CSF dose escalations were performed; one for patients treated without MTX ($n=28$) and the other for patients who received MTX-containing GVHD prophylactic regimens ($n=19$).

Patients received rhGM-CSF at doses ranging from 30 to 500 µg/m^2/day by 2 hour IV infusion from day 0 to 20 after BMT. RhGM-CSF was well tolerated at doses $\leq$ 250 µg/m^2/day. At doses $\geq$ 500 µg/m^2/day, 3 of 5 patients developed transient myalgias and/or chest pain. Symptoms were relieved by prolongation of the infusion rate of rhGM-CSF and narcotic therapy. The results of the study compared to historical patients are shown in Table 4. The severity of acute GVHD was not adversely affected. Patients who did not receive MTX as part of their GVHD prophylaxis had significantly earlier neutrophil recovery, fewer febrile days (4 vs 9) and earlier time of discharge than similar historical patients and patients who received MTX and rhGM-CSF. In the latter patients, neutrophil recovery was only slightly earlier than that of similar historical patients. The incidence of serious infections was lower than the historical rate in both groups.

Glycosylated rhGM-CSF produced in COS cells was given to patients receiving T-cell-depleted allogeneic BMT in a randomized, placebo controlled, multicenter trial[112] at a dose of 8 µg/kg/day by continuous intravenous (IV) infusion (Table 4). Toxicity was minimal. One patient developed myalgias and required early discontinuation of rhGM-CSF. The severity and incidence of GVHD and the incidence of graft rejection were similar in both groups. Neutrophil recovery was enhanced and infection was decreased in patients who received rhGM-CSF. Short-term relapse and survival were similar in the two groups.

Glycosylated rhGM-CSF from COS cells (8 µg/kg/day as a continuous IV infusion) has also been administered to patients undergoing allogeneic BMT with HLA-matched sibling donors using cyclosporine for GVHD prophylaxis in a phase III trial.[113] No toxicity was ascribed to rhGM-CSF and GVHD was not affected. Neutrophil recovery was earlier, but there was no effect on the duration of hospitalization. Recurrent disease and survival to day 100 were unaffected.

The safety and possible efficacy of yeast-derived rhGM-CSF was tested in 40 patients transplanted from unrelated donors.[114] RhGM-CSF at a dose of 250 µg/m^2/day was administered by 2 hour daily infusion from day 0 to day 20 or day 27 following the marrow infusion. Results were compared the outcomes of 78 historical patients. Consistent with results in sibling donor allografts, minimal toxicity due to rhGM-CSF was observed. The median day the absolute neutrophil count reached 500/mm^3 in patients who received rhGM-CSF was day 21, which is similar to that of historical patients. Never-

Table 4. Results of trials with rhGM-CSF following HLA identical allogeneic BMT

	Number of patients		Day ANC >500/mm³		Day platelet independent		% infection		Day discharged		Comments[e]	Refs.
	GM-CSF	control	GM-CSF	control	GM-CSF	control	GM-CSF	control	GM-CSF	control		
	28	50[a]	14	19	23	21	18	NR[d]	24	31	Yeast glycosylated rhGM-CSF was administered to patients with ALL, ANL, HD, NHL, MDS, CLL, CML who received CSP/Pred for GVHD prophylaxis	111
	19	43[a]	20	24	23	20	22	NR[d]	33	36	Yeast glycosylated rhGM-CSF was administered to patients with ALL, ANL, NHL, MM, CML, who received CSP/Pred for GVHD prophylaxis	111
	29	27[b]	13	18	NS[c]	NS[s]	48	74	NR[d]	NR[d]	Mammalian glycosylated rhGM-CSF was administered to patients with ANL, ALL, CML, NHL, MDS, AA, CLL, MM who received T-cell depleted allogeneic BMT	112
	20	20[b]	13	19	NR[d]	NR[d]	NR[d]	NR[d]	24	24	Mammalian glycosylated rhGM-CSF was administered to patients with ANL, ALL, CML who received CSP for GVHD prophylaxis	113

[a]   = historical control patients.
[b]   = prospective placebo control patients.
NS[c] = values not shown, but reported as not significantly different.
NR[d] = not reported.
[e]   = ALL: acute lymphocytic leukemia; ANL: acute non-lymphocytic leukemia; HD: Hodgkin's disease; NHL: non-Hodgkin's lymphoma; MDS: myelodysplastic syndrome; CLL: chronic lymphocytic leukemia; MM: multiple myeloma; CML: chromic myelogenous leukemia; AA: aplastic anemia; GVHD: graft-versus-host disease; CSP: cyclosporine; Pred: prednisone; MTX: methotrexate.

theless, there were fewer febrile days (4 vs 8), fewer infections (8% vs 24%) and fewer patients developing significant hepatic dysfunction (bilirubin levels ≥ 10 mg/dl) (20% vs 39%) in those who received rhGM-CSF. The overall incidence of acute GVHD in rhGM-CSF and historical patients was similar, but severe acute GVHD (≥ grade III) developed less frequently in patients who received rhGM-CSF (20% vs 37%). Non-relapse mortality was also decreased in patients who received rhGM-CSF (10% vs 33%) (see Fig. 2). Nineteen patients received rhGM-CSF after unrelated marrow graft for CML in chronic phase and survival to day 100 was 100% as compared to 76% in historical controls.

Clinical studies with rhG-CSF

RhG-CSF was used in a phase I/II trial in allogeneic BMT patients transplanted from HLA-identical sibling donors in Japan.[115] At doses ranging from 200 to 800 μg/m²/day by daily 30 minute IV infusion, 3 of 29 patients developed bone pains. Of the patients, 47% developed grade I-II GVHD; 2 patients had severe GVHD. Twenty patients received MTX and cyclosporine for GVHD prophylaxis. The median time to achieve an ANC ≥ 500/mm³ was 16 days. Patients who received cyclosporine without methotrexate ($n=9$) achieved an ANC ≥ 500/mm³ by day 13. Historical patients reached an ANC ≥ 500/mm³

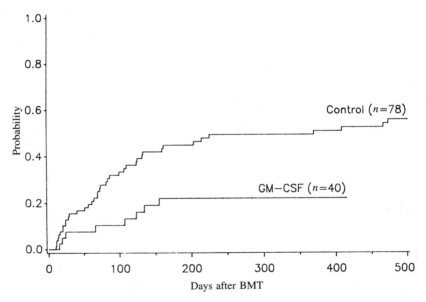

Fig. 2. Comparison of non-relapse mortality (Kaplan–Meier) between 78 consecutive historical patients and 40 rhGM-CSF-treated patients who underwent allogeneic BMT from an unrelated donor.

27 days after marrow infusion. Short term survival and rate of recurrent disease were not compared to historical control patients and the duration of hospitalization and infection were not reported.

Future directions

Randomized, placebo controlled trials must be done to confirm phase II data that suggests that both G-CSF and GM-CSF can decrease the morbidity associated with allografts. A future use of growth factors may be to further decrease the morbidity of marrow donation by administering a short course of a cytokine to a marrow donor to mobilize peripheral blood mononuclear cells to be used as an additional or as a sole source for stem cells. Combining cytokine primed marrow or blood cells with a posttransplant growth factor may further decrease hematopoietic recovery time and thus decrease morbidity. Lastly, the use of growth factors may allow an increase in cytoreductive regimen intensity, thereby decreasing leukemic relapse.

Use of growth factors to treat life-threatening infections

Introduction

A number of growth factors may increase the ability of phagocytic cells to kill microorganisms. As yet, few clinical studies have attempted to exploit these properties. Administration of rhGM-CSF to infected patients with marrow graft failure occasionally resulted in resolution of infection without neutrophil recovery. In order to test the hypothesis that a growth factor that activates cells may be of value in controlling infections, we studied the ability of rhM-CSF to clear established fungal disease in BMT patients.

Clinical studies with rhM-CSF in BMT patients with invasive fungal infection

Invasive fungal disease represents a major clinical problem in BMT patients.[116] In a recent retrospective review of BMT patients treated in Seattle, patients with either 2 or more positive blood cultures for a fungal organism or with histologically proven invasive fungal disease had a 100 day survival of only 20% despite the use of anti-fungal drugs and granulocyte transfusions when appropriate (unpublished data). Of patients undergoing allogeneic BMT 5–15% developed invasive fungal infections, usually in the setting of prolonged neutropenia or severe GVHD.

RhM-CSF is a cytokine which stimulates the proliferation of monocytes and macrophages, and enhances functional activities including phagocytosis, migration, production of oxygen reduction products, intracellular killing of microorganisms and antibody dependent and independent cell-mediated cytotoxicity.[12,117] Survival was improved in animals given rhM-CSF before challenge with live candida organisms. This finding has been duplicated with other cytokines.[118] Unlike other cytokines, M-CSF also improves survival in animals given rhM-CSF after infection with candida species. Improved survival was attributed primarily to enhanced function of monocytes and tissue macrophages. In animal trials of recombinant human M-CSF, thrombocytopenia was identified as dose limiting toxicity.[34] In trials with purified urinary human M-CSF in patients undergoing BMT, thrombocytopenia was not observed and neutrophil recovery to 500/mm³ or 1000/mm³ was not altered.[119] Thirteen patients with lymphoma were given a single dose of purified urinary human M-CSF and monocyte respiratory burst activity, migration, phagocytosis and intracellular destruction of candida organisms were enhanced.[120] Thrombocytopenia was observed and was thought to have been related to enhanced phagocytic clearance of platelets by activated splenic macrophages.

RhM-CSF was given at doses ranging from 50 to 2000 µg/m²/day by 2 hour infusion for up to 30 days to 24 patients with either invasive fungal disease or with persistent fungemia in a phase I-II toxicity trial.[66] Twelve patients had Karnovsky scores ≤ 30% at the time of starting rhM-CSF. The primary site of tissue infection included the liver (8), lung (6), skin (3), blood (3), heart (1), sinus (1) and central nervous system (2). Hematopoietic cell responses to rhM-CSF are shown in Table 5. No changes in white blood cell, neutrophil, monocyte or lymphocyte count were detected, however, platelet counts consistently decreased in a dose-dependent manner. The average platelet count fell by 60 000/mm³ in patients given 2000 µg/m³/day of rhM-CSF. Thrombocytopenia was rapidly reversible after the rhM-CSF was discontinued. No patient suffered hemorrhagic complications. Further dose escalation of rhM-CSF was not attempted. The severity of GVHD was not affected in allografted patients. No other toxicities were noted.

The criteria for complete response of infection were histologic proof of resolution of infection or complete resolution of abnormalities on CT scan. Using these criteria, 6 patients responded, 6 did not and 12 were not evaluable. The patients were not evaluable either because the CT scan did not completely normalize when rhM-CSF was discontinued or they refused re-

Table 5. *Hematopoietic cell response to rhM-CSF (mean values ± standard deviation)*[66]

Cell Counts (×10³/mm³)	Pre	Post	P value
White blood cells	5.8 ± 4.7	7.8 ± 6.5	0.284
Absolute neutrophil count	3.3 ± 3.4	4.8 ± 4.8	0.218
Monocyte count	0.5 ± 0.5	0.4 ± 0.4	0.484
Lymphocyte count	0.7 ± 0.7	0.7 ± 0.7	0.741
Trough platelet count	95 ± 93	65 ± 67	0.011

biopsy. Ten patients (42%) survived 100 days after initiation of rhM-CSF and 14 died, 11 of non-fungal causes. This trial provided suggestive evidence for efficacy of rhM-CSF in the treatment of life-threatening fungal infections and defined thrombocytopenia as a dose limiting toxicity in BMT patients. Randomized, prospective trials to assess antifungal activity of rhM-CSF are ongoing.

Conclusions

Inflammatory mediators may be etiologic and certainly contribute to the morbidity of venoocclusive disease, diffuse idiopathic pneumonia and graft-versus-host disease. Tumor necrosis factor (TNF) is a potent inflammatory mediator and is felt to play an etiologic role in the disorders mentioned above. Approaches to suppressing the biologic effects of TNF, such as anti-TNF antibodies, soluble TNF receptors, and the methylxanthine derivative pentoxifylline, are currently being explored. Preliminary results with pentoxifylline (PTX) as a prophylactic agent in 30 BMT patients suggest this agent is well tolerated[121,122] and can partially reduce transplant-related morbidity. PTX suppressed circulating TNF levels compared to a control group of BMT patients. The PTX-treated patients had less mucositis (4 vs 19 days), less venoocclusive disease (10% vs 65%), less renal insufficiency (3% vs 65%) and less severe GVHD (35% vs 68%) compared to historical patients. Controlled clinical studies are ongoing to determine efficacy and risk of this therapy. Potential risks include an increased incidence of infection and an increase in relapse rate. If studies determine that pharmacologic inhibition of TNF-α is efficacious, studies combining this agent with hematopoietic growth factors will be of interest.

Despite reduced morbidity in patients receiving rhG-CSF and rhGM-CSF following autologous BMT, mortality was not decreased. Fewer than 15% of ABMT patients die from transplant associated complications.[69,70] The primary cause of death is relapse of their primary disease. Future trials need to evaluate strategies which utilize cytokines to assist in reducing the rate of relapse. Several approaches are possible. First, cytokines which hasten engraftment will permit earlier use of biologic anti-tumor agents, such as interferon,[123,124] IL-2,[125,126] TNF[124,126] and M-CSF.[12,67] This would allow use of these agents in patients while their tumor burden is minimal. Secondly, if the morbidity of the marrow transplant procedure can be sufficiently reduced, patients may be able to tolerate treatment above currently established maximum tolerated doses or sequential autologous BMTs. Pilot studies of double autografts in high risk patients without cytokines have been performed with mixed results.[127] Thirdly, it is possible to take clinical advantage of the ability of cytokines to stimulate proliferation of malignant hematopoietic cells. RhG-CSF, rhGM-CSF, rhIL-1 and rhIL-3 increase the rate of cell division of some AML blast cells. RhIL-1 and rhIL-6 may stimulate malignant plasma cells in multiple myeloma and neoplastic cells in B cell lymphoma. Cell cycle specific drugs may then be given with potentially greater efficacy.[128] Preliminary trials in patients with AML indicate that the administration of rhG-CSF and rhGM-CSF concurrently with cycle specific chemotherapy is tolerable and associated with a high rate of induction of complete remission.[129,130]

Cytokines used alone or in combination may be useful for expanding early progenitor cells in vitro before reinfusion. They also may be critical in enhancing the efficacy of gene transfer into hematopoietic stem cells.[131,132] ABMT with retrovirally marked stem cells has had limited success in mice, dogs, sheep and primates.[133–135] Two major problems limiting the use of gene therapy in ABMT are the lack of high efficiency insertion and low levels of gene expression. Insertion rate can be improved by increasing the percent of replicating cells at the time of insertion.[136] Both rhGM-CSF and IL-3 as single agents have been shown to do this. Combining IL-1 and GM-CSF, and IL-3 and IL-6 further increase efficiency of insertion.[133,137,138] Culture with other cytokines, such as c-kit ligand or additional combinations of cytokines coupled with selection of repopulating stem cells through use of differentiation antigens, such as CD34,[139,140] may also increase the efficiency of insertion. Such an advance may allow ABMT to be considered as an approach to genetic disorders and may enable genetic manipulation of hematopoietic cells allowing reinfusion of stem cells resistant to selected cytotoxic drugs (i.e. methotrexate resistance by transfer of dihydrofolate reductase gene).[134]

We are in an era that holds both excitement and promise for greatly increasing the utility of BMT by decreasing its toxicities with cytokines. A second generation of studies is in progress to further define the use of rhGM-CSF, rhG-CSF and rhM-CSF. Additional recombinant cytokines (rhIL-3, rhIL-1, rhIL-6, rhIL3-GMCSF fusion molecule, rhc-kit ligand) have also been cloned and produced in sufficient amounts for clinical use and will shortly enter clinical trials in BMT. Their initial use should be guided by in vitro and preclinical in vivo effects, and should address the residual problems in BMT.

Acknowledgements
Supported by PHS Grant Nos. CA 18029 and CA 26828, from the National Cancer Institute and DSHS.

References
(1) Thomas ED, Storb R, Clift RA et al. Bone marrow transplantation. *N Eng J Med* 1975; 292: 832–43, 895–902.
(2) Petersen FB, Appelbaum FR, Hill R et al. Autologous marrow transplantation for malignant lymphoma; a report of 101 cases from Seattle. *J Clin Oncol* 1990; 8: 638–47.

(3) Storb R, Prentice RL, Buckner CD. Graft-versus-host disease and survival in patients with aplastic anemia treated by marrow grafts from HLA-identical siblings. Beneficial effects of a protective environment. *N Eng J Med* 1983; 308: 302–7.

(4) Storb R, Deeg HJ, Whitehead J et al. Methotrexate and cyclosporine compared with cyclosporine alone for prophylaxsis of acute graft versus host disease after marrow transplantation for leukemia. *N Eng J Med* 1986; 314: 729–35.

(5) Moore MAS. Haemopoietic growth factor interactions: in vitro and in vivo preclinical evaluation. *Cancer Surveys* 1990; 9: 7–80.

(6) Metcalf D. The granulocyte-macrophage colony stimulating factors. *Science* 1985; 229: 16–22.

(7) Clark SC, Kamen R. The human hematopoietic colony-stimulating factors. *Science* 1987; 236: 1229–37.

(8) Cannistra SA, Griffin JD. Regulation of the production and function of granulocytes and monocytes. *Sem Hematol* 1988; 25: 173–88.

(9) Jacobs K, Shoemaker C, Rudersdorf R et al. Isolation and characterization of genomic and cDNA clones of human erythropoietin. *Nature* 1985; 313: 806–10.

(10) Souza LM, Boone TC, Gabrilowe J. Recombinant human granulocyte colony-stimulating factor: effects on normal and leukemic myeloid cells. *Science* 1986; 232: 61–5.

(11) Becker S, Warren MK, Haskill S. Colony-stimulating factor-induced monocyte survival and differentiation into macrophages in serum-free cultures. *J Immunol* 1987; 139: 3703–9.

(12) Ralph PWM. Biological properties and molecular biology of the human macrophage growth factor, CSF-1. *Immunobiol* 1986; 172: 194–204.

(13) Robinson BE, McGrath HE, Quesenberry PJ. Recombinant murine granulocyte-macrophage colony-stimulating factor has megakaryocyte colony-stimulating activity and augments megakaryocyte colony stimulation by interleukin-3. *J Clin Invest* 1987; 79: 1648–52.

(14) Li CL, Johnson GR. Stimulation of multipotential, erythroid, and other murine hematopoietic progenitor cells by adherent cell lines in the absence of detectable multi-CSF (IL-3). *Nature* 1985; 31: 633–5.

(15) Williams DE, Broxmeyer HE. Interleukin-1α enhances the in vitro survival of purified murine granulocyte-macrophage progenitor cells in the absence of colony-stimulating factors. Blood 1988; 72: 1608–15.

(16) Van Damme J, Cayphas S, Opdenakker G, Billiau A, Van Snick J. Interleukin 1 and poly (rI) poly (rC) induce production of a hybridoma growth factor by human fibroblasts. *Eur J Immunol* 1987; 17: 1–7.

(17) Sieff CA, Niemeyer CM, Metzer SJ, Faller DV. Interleukin-1 induces cultured human endothelial cell production of granulocyte-macrophage colony-stimulating factor. *J Clin Invest* 1987; 79: 48–51.

(18) Nemunaitis J, Andrews DF, Crittenden C, Kaushansky K, Singer JW. Response of simian virus 40 (SV40)-transformed, cultured human marrow stromal cells to hematopoietic growth factors. *J Clin Invest* 1989; 83: 593–601.

(19) Bartelmez SH, Bradley TR, Bertoncello I et al. Interleukin-1 plus Interleukin-3 plus colony-stimulating factor -1 are essential for clonal proliferation of primitive myeloid bone marrow cells. *Exp Hematol* 1989; 17: 240–5.

(20) Leary AG, Ikebuchi K, Yoshikatsu H et al. Synergism between interleukin-6 and interleukin-3 in supporting proliferation of human hematopoietic stem cells: Comparison with interleukin-1α. *Blood* 1988; 71: 1759–63.

(21) Stanley ER, Bartocci A, Patinkin D, Rosendaal M, Bradley TR. Regulation of very primitive, multipotent, hemopoietic cells by hemopoietin-1. *Cell* 1986; 45: 667–74.

(22) Neta R, Douches S, Oppenheim JJ. Interleukin-1 is a radioprotector. *J Immunol* 1986; 136: 2483–5.

(23) Cicco NA, Lindemann A, Content J et al. Inducible production of interleukin-6 by human polymorphonuclear neutrophils: Role of granulocyte-macrophage colony-stimulating factor and tumor necrosis factor-alpha. *Blood* 1990; 75: 2049–52.

(24) Nemunaitis J, Tompkins CK, Andrews DF, Singer JW. Transforming growth factor β expression in human marrow stromal cells. *Eur J Hematol* 1991; 46: 140–5.

(25) Sing GK, Keller JR, Ellingsworth LR, Ruscetti FW. Transforming growth factor β selectively inhibits normal and leukemic human bone marrow cell growth in vitro. *Blood* 1988; 72: 1504–11.

(26) Wing EJ, Magee DM, Whiteside TL, Kaplan SS, Shadduck RK. Recombinant human granulocyte/macrophage colony-stimulating factor enhances monocyte cytotoxicity and secretion of tumor necrosis factor α and interferon in cancer patients. *Blood* 1989; 73: 643–6.

(27) Bussolino F, Wang JM, Defilippi P et al. Granulocyte- and granulocyte-macrophage-colony stimulating factors induce human endothelial cells to migrate and proliferate. *Nature* 1989; 337: 471–3.

(28) Foulke RS, Marshall MH, Trotta PP, Von Hoff DD. In vitro assessment of the effects of granulocyte-macrophage colony-stimulating factor on primary human tumors and derived lines. *Cancer Research* 1990; 50: 6264–7.

(29) Hoang T, Haman A, Goncalves O, Wong GG, Clark SC. Interleukin-6 enhances growth factor-dependent proliferation of the blast cells of acute myeloblastic leukemia. *Blood* 1988; 72: 823–6.

(30) Hoang T, Nara N, Wong G, Clark S, Minden MD, McCulloch EA. Effects of recombinant GM-CSF on the blast cells of acute myeloblastic leukemia. *Blood* 1986; 68: 313.

(31) Park LS, Waldron PE, Friend D et al. Interleukin-3, GM-CSF, and G-CSF receptor expression on cell lines and primary leukemia cells: Receptor heterogeneity and relationship to growth factor responsiveness. *Blood* 1989; 74: 56–65.

(32) Van Damme J. Biochemical and biological properties of human HPGF/IL-6. *Ann NY Acad Sci* 1989; 557: 104–13.

(33) Klein B, Zhang X-G, Jourdan M et al. Paracrine rather than autocrine regulation of myeloma-cell growth and differentiation by interleukin-6. *Blood* 1989; 73: 517–26.

(34) Garnick MB, Stoudemire JB. Preclinical and clinical evaluation of recombinant human macrophage colony-stimulating factor (rhM-CSF). *Int J Cell Clon* 1990; 8(suppl 1): 356–73.

(35) Cohen AM, Zsebo KM, Inoue H et al. In vivo stimulation of granulopoiesis by recombinant human granulocyte colony-stimulating factor. *Proc Natl Acad Sci USA* 1991; 84: 2484–8.

(36) Welte K, Bonilla MA, Gilli AP et al. Recombinant human granulocyte colony-stimulating factor: effects on hematopoiesis in normal and cyclophosphamide-treated primates. *J Exp Med* 1987; 164: 941–8.

(37) Frenck RW, Sarman G, Harper TE, Buescher ES. The ability of recombinant murine granulocyte-macrophage colony-stimulating factor to protect neonatal rats from septic death due to *Staphylococcus aureus*. *J Infect Dis* 1990; 162: 109–14.

(38) Monroy RL, Skelly RR, MacVittie TJ et al. The effect of recombinant GM-CSF on the recovery of monkeys transplanted with autologous bone marrow. *Blood* 1987; 70: 1696–9.

(39) Blazar BR, Widmer MB, Soderling CB, Gillis S, Vallera DA. Enhanced survival but reduced engraftment in murine recipients of recombinant granulocyte/macrophage colony-stimulating factor following transplantation of T-cell depleted histoincompatible bone marrow. *Blood* 1988; 72: 1148–54.

(40) Nienhuis AW, Donahue RE, Karlsson S et al. Recombinant human granulocyte-macrophage colony-stimulating factor (GM-CSF) shortens the period of neutropenia after autologous bone marrow transplantation in a primate model. *J Clin Invest* 1987; 80: 572–7.

(41) Gillio AP, Gasparetto C, Laver J et al. Effects of interleukin-3 on hematopoietic recovery after 5-fluorouracil or cyclophosphamide treatment of cynomolgus primates. *J Clin Invest* 1990; 85: 1560–5.

(42) Oppenheim JJ, Neta R, Tiberghien P, Gress R, Kenny JJ, Longo DL. Interleukin-1 enhances survival of lethally irradiated mice treated with allogeneic bone marrow cells. *Blood* 1989; 74: 2257–63.

(43) Neta R, Sztein MB, Oppenheim JJ, Gillis S, Douches SD. The in vivo effects of interleukin-1. *J Immunol* 1987; 139: 1861–6.

(44) Castelli MP, Black PL, Schneider M, Pennington R, Abe F, Talmadge JE. Protective, restorative, and therapeutic properties of recombinant human IL-1 in rodent models. *J Immunol* 1988; 140: 3830–7.

(45) Donahue RE, Seehra J, Metzger M et al. Human IL-3 and GM-CSF act synergistically in stimulating hematopoiesis in primates. *Science* 1988; 241: 1820–3.

(46) Mayer P, Valent P, Schmidt G, Liehl E, Bettelheim P. The in vivo effects of recombinant human interleukin-3: demonstration of basophil differentiation factor, histamine-producing activity, and priming of GM-CSF-responsive progenitors in nonhuman primates. *Blood* 1989; 74: 613–21.

(47) Krumwieh D, Seiler FR. In vivo effects of recombinant colony stimulating factors on hematopoiesis in cynomolgus monkeys. *Transpl Proc* 1989; 21: 2964–7.

(48) Cenci E, Bartocci A, Puccetti P, Mocci S, Stanley ER, Bistoni F. Macrophage colony stimulating factor in murine candidiasis: Serum and tissue levels during infection and protective effect of exogenous administration. *Infect and Immunol* 1991; 59: 868–72.

(49) Van't Wout JW, Van der Meer JWM, Barza M, Dinarello CA. Protection of neutropenic mice from lethal *Candida albicans* infection by recombinant interleukin 1. *Eur J Immunol* 1988; 18: 1143–6.

(50) Smith PD, Lamerson CL, Banks SM et al. Granulocyte-macrophage colony-stimulating factor augments human monocyte fungicidal activity for *Candida albicans*. *J Infect Dis* 1990; 161: 999–1005.

(51) Mayer P, Schuetze E, Lam C, Kricek F, Liehl E. Recombinant murine granulocyte-macrophage colony stimulating factor augments neutrophil recovery and enhances resistance to infections in myelosuppressed mice. *J Infect Dis* 1990; 163: 584–90.

(52) Moore MAS. Hematopoietic growth factors in cancer. *Cancer* 1990; 65: 836–44.

(53) Robinson BE, Quesenberry PJ. Hematopoietic growth factors: overview and clinical applications, Part III. *Am J Med Sci* 1990; 300: 311–21.

(54) Glaspy JA, Golde DW. Clinical trials of myeloid growth factors. *Exp Hematol* 1990; 18: 1137–41.

(55) Brandt SJ, Peters WP, Atwate SK et al. Effect of recombinant human granulocyte- macrophage colony-stimulating factor on hematopoietic reconstitution after high-dose chemotherapy and autologous bone marrow transplantation. *N Eng J Med* 1988; 318: 869–76.

(56) Nemunaitis J, Singer JW, Buckner CD et al. Use of recombinant human granulocyte/macrophage colony stimulating factor in autologous bone marrow transplantation for lymphoid malignancies. *Blood* 1988; 72: 834–6.

(57) Nemunaitis J, Singer JW, Buckner CD et al. Use of recombinant human granulocyte-macrophage colony stimulating factor (rhGM-CSF) in autologous marrow transplantation for lymphoid malignancies. In: Dicke KA, ed. *Autologous bone marrow transplantation: Proceedings of the third international symposium.* Houston: University of Texas, 1989; 631–6.

(58) Devereaux S, Linch DC, Gribben JG, McMillan A, Patterson K, Goldstone AH. GM-CSF accelerates neutrophil recovery after autologous bone marrow transplantation for Hodgkin's disease. *Bone Marrow Transpl* 1989; 4: 49–54.

(59) Blazar BR, Kersey JH, McGlave PB et al. In vivo administration of recombinant human granulocyte/macrophage colony-stimulating factor in acute lymphoblastic leukemia patients receiving purged autografts. *Blood* 1989; 73: 849–57.

(60) Link H, Freund M, Kirchner H et al. Recombinant human granulocyte-macrophage colony-stimulating factor (rhGM-CSF) after bone marrow transplantation. *Behring Inst Mitt* 1988; 83: 313–19.

(61) Lazarus HM, Andersen J, Chen MG et al. Recombinant GM-CSF after autologous bone marrow transplantation for relapsed non-Hodgkin's lymphoma: Blood and bone marrow progenitor growth studies. A phase II Eastern Cooperative Oncology Group Trial. *Blood* 1991 (in press).

(62) Sheridan WP, Morstyn G, Wolf M et al. Granulocyte colony-stimulating factor and neutrophil recovery after high-dose chemotherapy and autologous bone marrow transplantation. *Lancet* 1989; ii: 891–5.

(63) Taylor KM, Jagannath S, Spitzer G et al. Recombinant human granulocyte colony-stimulating factor hastens granulocyte recovery after high-dose chemotherapy and autologous bone marrow transplantation in Hodgkin's disease. *J Clin Oncol* 1989; 7: 1791–9.

(64) Peters WP. The effect of recombinant human colony-stimulating factors on hematopoietic reconstitution following autologous bone marrow transplantation. *Sem Hematol* 1989; 26 (suppl. 2): 18–23.

(65) Auer I, Ribas A, Gale RP. What is the role of recombinant colony stimulating factors in bone marrow transplantation? *Bone Marrow Transpl* 1990; 6: 79–87.

(66) Nemunaitis J, Meyers J, Buckner CD et al. Phase I trial of recombinant human macrophage colony stimulating factor (rhM-CSF) in patients with invasive fungal infections. *Blood* 1991; 78 (4): 907–13.

(67) Nemunaitis J, Singer JW. Macrophage colony stimulating factor (M-CSF): Biology and clinical applications. In: *High dose cancer therapy: pharmacology, hematopoietics and stem cells*. Armitage JO, Antman KH (eds), in press.

(68) Nemunaitis J, Singer JW, Buckner CD et al. Long term follow-up of patients who receive recombinant human granulocyte macrophage-colony stimulating factor after autologous bone marrow transplantation for lymphoid malignancy. *Bone Marrow Transpl* 1991; 7: 49–52.

(69) Nemunaitis J, Rabinowe SN, Singer JW et al. Recombinant granulocyte-macrophage colony-stimulating factor after autologous bone marrow transplantation for lymphoid cancer. *N Eng J Med* 1991; 324: 1773–8.

(70) Rabinowe SN, Nemunaitis J, Armitage J, Nadler LM. The impact of myeloid growth factors on engraftment following autologous bone marrow transplantation for malignant lymphoma. *Sem Hematol* 1991; 28 (suppl. 2): 6–16.

(71) Gorin NC, Coiffier B, Pico J. Granulocyte-macrophage colony-stimulating factor (GM-CSF) shortens aplasia duration after autologous bone marrow transplantation (ABMT) in non-Hodgkin's lymphoma. A randomized placebo-controlled double-blind study. *Blood* 1990; 76: 542 (abstract).

(72) Link H, Boogaerts M, Carella A. Recombinant human granulocyte-macrophage colony-stimulating factor (RHGM-CSF) after autologous bone marrow transplantation for acute lymphoblastic leukemia and non-Hodgkin's lymphoma: A randomized double-blind multicenter trial in Europe. *Blood* 1990; 76 (suppl. 1): 152 (abstract).

(73) Gianni AM, Bregni M, Siena S et al. Rapid and complete hemopoietic reconstitution following combined transplantation of autologous blood and bone marrow cells. A changing role for high dose chemo-radiotherapy? *Hematological Oncology* 1989; 7: 139–48.

(74) Gianni AM, Bregni M, Stern AC, Siena S, Tarella C, Piler A, Bonnadonna G. Granulocyte-macrophage colony-stimulating factor to harvest circulating haemopoietic stem cells for autotransplantation. *Lancet* 1989; ii: 580–5.

(75) Peters WP, Kurtzberg J, Kirkpatrick G et al. GM-CSF primed peripheral blood progenitor cells (PBC) coupled with autologous bone marrow transplantation (ABMT) will eliminate absolute leukopenia following high dose chemotherapy (HDC). *Blood* 1989; 74: 50 (abstract).

(76) Kessinger A, Armitage JO, Landmark JD, Smith DM, Weisenburger DD. Autologous peripheral hematopoietic stem cell transplantation restores hematopoietic function following marrow ablative therapy. *Blood* 1988; 71: 723–7.

(77) Kessinger A, Armitage JO, Smith DM, Landmark JD, Bierman PJ,

J L Nemunaitis and J W Singer

Weisenburger DD. High-dose therapy and autologous peripheral blood stem cell transplantation for patients with lymphoma. *Blood* 1989; 74: 1260–5.

(78) Koerbling M, Holle R, Haas R et al. Autologous blood stem-cell transplantation in patients wth advanced Hodgkin's disease and prior radiation to the pelvic site. *J Clin Oncol* 1990; 8: 978–85.

(79) Hows J, Palmer S, Gordon-Smith EC. Successful haematopoietic reconstitution using autologous peripheral blood mononucleated cells in patients with acute promyelocytic leukemia. *Br J Hematol* 1986; 63: 209–11.

(80) Juttner CA, To LB, Haylock DN, Branford A, Kimber RJ. Circulating autologous stem cells collected in very early remission from acute non-lymphoblastic leukaemia produce prompt but incomplete haemopoietic reconstitution after high dose melphalan or supralethal chemoradiotherapy. *Br J Haematol* 1985; 61: 739–45.

(81) Juttner CA, To LB, Haylock DN et al. Autologous blood stem cell transplantation. *Transpl Proc* 1989; 21: 2929–31.

(82) Socinski MA, Cannistra SA, Elias A, Antman KH, Schnipper L, Griffin JD. Granulocyte-macrophage colony stimulating factor expands the circulating haemopoietic progenitor cell compartment in man. *Lancet* 1988; i: 1194–8.

(83) Molineux G, Pojda Z, Hampson IN, Lord B, Dexter TM. Transplantation potential of peripheral blood stem cells induced by granulocyte colony stimulating factor. *Blood* 1990: 2153–8.

(84) Haas R, Ho AD, Bredthauer U, Cayeux S, Egerer G, Knauf W et al. Successful autologous transplantation of blood stem cells mobilized with recombinant human granulocyte-macrophage colony-stimulating factor. *Exp Hematol* 1990; 18: 94–8.

(85) Moore MAS. The future of cytokine combination therapy. *Cancer* 1991; 67: 2718–26.

(86) Williams DE, Eisenman J, Baird A et al. Identification of a ligan for the c-kit proto-oncogene. *Cell* 1990; 63: 167–74.

(87) Zsebo CM, Wypych J, McNiece IK et al. Identification, purification and biological characterization of hematopoetic stem cell factor from Buffalo Rat liver-conditioned medium. *Cell* 1990; 63: 195–201.

(88) Anderson DM, Lyman SD, Baird A et al. Molecular cloning of mast cell growth factor, a hematopoietic that is active in both membrane board and soluble forms. *Cell* 1990; 63: 235–43.

(89) Williams DE, Park LS. Hematopoietic effects of a GM-CSF/IL3 fusion protein. *Cancer* 1991, in press.

(90) Metcalf D, Begley CG, Williamson DJ et al. Hemopoietic responses in mice injected with purified recombinant murine GM-CSF. *Exp Hematol* 1987; 15: 1–9.

(91) Wolfgang BE, Denhauser-Riedle S, Steinhouser G. Various human hematopoietic growth factors (IL-3, GM-CSF, G-CSF) stimulate clonal growth of non-hematopoietic tumor cells. *Blood* 1989; 73: 80–3.

(92) Nemunaitis J, Singer JW. The effect of recombinant human granulocyte macrophage colony stimulating factor (rhGM-CSF) and recombinant human interleukin 1 (rhIL-1) on proliferation of human tumor cell lines. *Cancer* 1989; 2(11): 369–71.

98

(93) Andreesen R, Scheibenbogen C, Brugger W et al. Adoptive transfer of tumor cytotoxic macrophages generated in vitro from circulating blood monocytes: A new approach to cancer immunotherapy. *Cancer Res* 1990; 50: 7450–6.

(94) Metcalf D. Hematopoietic effects in vivo of leukemia inhibitory factor (LIF). *Exp Hematol* 1990; 18(6): 597 (abstract).

(95) Champlin RE, Feig SA, Gale RP. Case problems in bone marrow transplantation. I. Graft failure in aplastic anemia: its biology and treatment. *Exp Hematol* 1984; 12: 728–33.

(96) Bolger GB, Sullivan KM, Storb R et al. Second marrow infusion for poor graft function after allogeneic marrow transplantation. *Bone Marrow Transpl* 1986; 1: 21–30.

(97) Nemunaitis J, Singer JW, Buckner CD et al. The use of recombinant human granulocyte-macrophage colony-stimulating factor in graft failure following bone marrow transplantation. *Blood* 1990; 76: 2450–530.

(98) Nemunaitis J, Singer JW. The use of rhGM-CSF in autologous bone marrow transplantation: Review. *LabMedica* 1991, in press.

(99) Brandwein JM, Nayar R, Baker MA et al. GM-CSF therapy for delayed engraftment after autologous bone marrow transplantation. *Exp Hematol* 1991; 19: 191–5.

(100) Moore RN, Oppenheim JJ, Farrar JJ, Carter CSJr, Waheed A, Shadduck RK. Production of lymphocyte-activating factor (Interleukin-1) by macrophages activated with colony-stimulating factors. *J Immunol* 1980; 125: 1302–5.

(101) Farrar WL, Mizel SB, Farrar JJ. Participation of lymphocyte activating factor (Interleukin-1) in the induction of cytotoxic T-cell responses. *J Immunol* 1980; 124: 1371–7.

(102) Shalaby MR, Fendly B, Sheehan KC, Schreiber RD, Ammann AJ. Prevention of the graft-versus-host reaction in newborn mice by antibodies to tumor necrosis factor. *Transplantation* 1989; 47: 1057–61.

(103) Piguet PF, Grau GE, Allet B, Vassalli P. Tumor necrosis factor/cachectin is an effector of skin and gut lesions of the acute phase of graft-versus-host disease. *J Exp Med* 1987; 1280: 9.

(104) Schmeiser Th, Kurrle E, Arnold R et al. Application of antimicrobial prophylactic treatment to the prevention of infection and graft-versus-host disease in allogeneic bone marrow transplantation (BMT). *Exp Hematol* 1984; 12: 105–6.

(105) Van Bekkum DW, Knaan S. Role of bacterial microflora in development of intestinal lesions from graft-versus-host-disease. *J Nat Cancer Inst* 1977; 58: 787–9.

(106) Van Bekkum DW, Roodenburg J, Heidt PJ, van der Waaij D. Mitigation of secondary disease of allogeneic radiation chimeras by modification of the intestinal microflora. *J Nat Cancer Inst* 1974; 52: 401–4.

(107) Blazar BR, Widmer MB, Soderling CRB et al. Augmentation of donor bone marrow engraftment in histoincompatible murine recipients by granulocyte-macrophage colony-stimulating factor. *Blood* 1988; 71: 320–8.

(108) Atkinson K, Matias C, Guiffre A et al. In vivo administration of G-CSF, GM-CSF, IL-1, IL-4, alone and in combination, after allogeneic murine hemopoietic stem cell transplantation. *Blood* 1991; 77: 1376–81.

(109) Ho AD, Haas R, Wulf G et al. Activation of lymphocytes induced by recom-

binant human granulocyte- macrophage colony-stimulating factor in patients with malignant lymphoma. *Blood* 1990; 75: 203–12.

(110) Hancock WW, Pleau ME, Kobzik L. Recombinant granulocyte-macrophage colony-stimulating factor down-regulates expression of IL-2 receptor on human mononuclear phagocytes by induction of prostaglandine. *J Immunol* 1988; 140: 3021–5.

(111) Nemunaitis J, Buckner CD, Appelbaum FR et al. Phase I/II trial of recombinant human granulocyte-macrophage colony-stimulating factor following allogeneic bone marrow transplantation. *Blood* 1991; 77: 2065–71.

(112) De Witte T, Gratwohl A, Van Del Lely N et al. A multicenter double blind randomized trial of recombinant human granulocyte-macrophage colony-stimulating factor (RhGM-CSF) in recipients of allogeneic T-cell depleted bone marrow. *Blood* 1990; (abstract).

(113) Powles R, Smith C, Milan S et al. Human recombinant GM-CSF in allogeneic bone-marrow transplantation for leukaemia: double-blind, placebo-controlled trial. *Lancet* 1990; 336: 1417–20.

(114) Nemunaitis J, Anasetti C, Storb R et al. Phase II trial of recombinant human granulocyte-macrophage colony-stimulating factor (rhGM-CSF) in patients undergoing allogeneic bone marrow transplantation from unrelated donors. *Blood* 1991 (submitted).

(115) Masaoka T, Takaku F, Kato S et al. Recombinant human granulocyte colony-stimulating factor in allogeneic bone marrow transplantation. *Exp Hematol* 1989; 17: 1047–50.

(116) Meyers JD. Infection in bone marrow transplant recipients. *Am J Med* 1986; 81: 27–38.

(117) Karbassi A, Becker JM, Foster JS, Moore RN. Enhanced killing of candida albicans by murine macrophages treated with macrophage colony-stimulating factor: evidence for augmented expression of mannose receptors. *J Immunol* 1987; 139: 417–21.

(118) Chong KT, Langlois L. Recombinant human macrophage colony stimulating factor (M-CSF): enhanced murine host defense against lethal *Candida albicans* infection. *ASM Annual Meeting* 1989; (abstract).

(119) Masoka T, Motoyoshi K, Takaku F et al. Administration of human urinary colony-stimulating factor after bone marrow transplantation. *Bone Marrow Transpl* 1988; 3: 121–7.

(120) Khwaja A, Johnson B, Addison IE et al. In vivo effects of macrophage colony-stimulating factor on human monocyte function. *Br J Haematol* 1991; 77: 25–31.

(121) Bianco JA, Appelbaum FR, Nemunaitis J et al. Phase I-II trial of pentoxifylline for the prevention of transplant related toxicities following bone marrow transplantation. *Blood* 1991 (in press).

(122) Bianco JA, Almgren J, Kern DL et al. Evidence that oral pentoxifylline reverses acute renal dysfunction in bone marrow transplant recipients receiving amphotericin B and cyclosporine. *Transplantation* 1991; 51: 925–7.

(123) Krown SE. Interferons and interferon inducers in cancer treatment. *Seminars in Oncol* 1986; 2: 207–17.

(124) Philip R, Epstein LB. Tumor necrosis factor as immunomodulator and

mediator of monocyte cytotoxicity induced by itself, τ-interferon and inter-leukin-1. *Nature* 1986; 323: 86–9.

(125) Nishimura T, Ohta S, Naoko S, Togashi Y, Goto M, Hashimoto Y. Combination tumor-immunotherapy with recombinant tumor necrosis factor and recombinant interleukin-2 in mice. *Int J Cancer* 1987; 40: 255–61.

(126) Rosenberg SA, Lotze MT, Muul LM et al. A progress report on the treatment of 157 patients with advanced cancer using lymphokine-activated killer cells and interleukin-2 or high-dose interleukin-2 alone. *N Eng J Med* 1987; 316: 889–942.

(127) Spitzer G, Huan S, Dunphy FR et al. Tandem high dose chemotherapy for metastatic breast cancer. In: Dicke KA, Armitage JO, Dicke-Evinger MJ (eds). *Autologous bone marrow transplantation. Proceedings of the Fifth International Symposium* 1990; V: 323–32.

(128) Cannistra SA, Groshek P, Griffin JD. Granulocyte-macrophage colony-stimulating factor enhances the cytotoxic effects of cytosine arabinoside in acute myeloblastic leukemia and in the myeloid blastic crisis phase of chronic myeloid leukemia. *Leukemia* 1989; 3: 328–34.

(129) Morishita Y, Kataoka T, Saito H. Granulocyte colony stimulating factor enhances cytosine arabinoside-mediated cytotoxicity in human myeloid leukemia cells. *Acta Haematol* JPN 1990; 53: 1526–32.

(130) Bettelheim P, Valent P, Andreeff M. Recombinant human granulocyte-macrophage colony stimulating factor in combination with standard induction chemotherapy in de novo acute myeloid leukemia. *Blood* 1991; 77: 700–11.

(131) Nienhuis AW, McDonagh KT, Bodine DM. Gene transfer into hematopoietic stem cells. *Cancer* 1991; 67: 2700–4.

(132) Anderson WF. Prospects of human gene therapy. *Science* 1984; 226: 401–9.

(133) Williams DA, Lemischka IR, Nathan DG, Mulligan RC. Introduction of new genetic material into pluripotent haematopoietic stem cells of the mouse. *Nature* 1984; 310: 476–80.

(134) Stead RB, Kwok WW, Storb R, Miller AD. Canine model for gene therapy: inefficient gene expression in dogs reconstituted with autologous marrow infected with retroviral vectors. *Blood* 1988; 71: 742–7.

(135) Bodine DM, McDonagh KT, Brandt SJ et al. Development of a high-titer retrovirus producer cell line capable of gene transfer into rhesus monkey hematopoietic stem cells. *Proc Natl Acad Sci USA* 1990; 87: 3738–42.

(136) Miller DG, Adam MA, Miller AD. Gene transfer by retrovirus vectors occurs only in cells that are actively replicating at the time of infection. *Mol and Cell Biol* 1990; 10: 4239–42.

(137) Bodine DM, Karlsson S, Nienhuis AW. Combination of interleukins 3 and 6 preserves stem cell function in culture and enhances retrovirus-mediated gene transfer into hematopoietic stem cells. *Proc Nat Acad Sci USA* 1989; 86: 8897–901.

(138) Hughes PFD, Eaves CJ, Hogge DE, Humphries RK. High-efficiency gene transfer to human hematopoietic cells maintained in long-term marrow culture. *Blood* 1989; 74: 1915–22.

(139) Andrews RG, Singer JW, Bernstein ID. Monoclonal antibody 12.8 recognizes a

115-kd molecule present on both unipotent and multipotent hematopoietic colony-forming cells and their precursors. *Blood* 1986; 67: 842–5.

(140) Berenson RJ, Andrews RG, Bensinger WI et al. Antigen CD34+ marrow cells engraft lethally irradiated baboons. *J Clin Invest* 1988; 81: 951–5.

Causes of leukemia

A BUTTURINI and R P GALE

Introduction

Leukemia accounts for about 10% of cancer deaths in humans.[1] In children, leukemia is the leading cause of death; its incidence is increasing.[2,3] The cause of most leukemia is unknown, as is the hematopoietic abnormality underlying its development. Here, data are reviewed from different clinical settings associated with increased leukemia risk, including children with congenital genetic disorders, persons exposed to radiation, chemicals or drugs and virus-associated leukemias.

These data offer insights on the etiology and pathogenesis of human leukemias. They suggest that leukemia is one of the several potential expressions of aberrant stem cell physiology whose range includes aplastic anemia and myelodysplasia.

Congenital genetic disorders

Several congenital disorders are associated with increased leukemia risk, including Fanconi anemia, Bloom syndrome, ataxia telangiectasia, Down's syndrome and other congenital syndromes.

Fanconi anemia is an autosomal recessive disorder characterized by progressive bone marrow failure.[4] The molecular defect is thought to be an inability to repair DNA crosslinks.[5] The precise abnormality is unknown and may differ in different cases.[6] Because the underlying genetic abnormality(ies) is undefined and the clinical phenotype is pleomorphic, the disease is best defined by increased chromosome strand breaks in lymphocytes following exposure to DNA crosslinkers.[7] The precise proportion of persons with Fanconi genotype developing bone marrow failure and leukemia is unknown.

Acute myelogenous leukemia (AML) is common in persons with Fanconi anemia surviving bone marrow failure; in recent studies actuarial incidence exceeds 50%.[8] Some persons develop AML directly or after antecedent

All correspondence to: Dr RP Gale, Division of Hematology and Oncology, Dept. of Medicine, UCLA School of Medicine, Los Angeles CA 90024, USA.

Cambridge Medical Reviews: Haematological Oncology Volume 2

myelodysplasia, without a clinically apparent aplastic phase. Different patterns of evolution to AML occur even within families, implying either variable phenotypic expression, a role for co-factors or both.

Bloom syndrome is a second autosomal recessive congenital disorder associated with increased leukemia risk.[9] The molecular basis is thought to be deficient DNA ligase I.[10] In contrast to Fanconi anemia, children with Bloom syndrome develop acute lymphoblastic leukemia (ALL) as well as AML. Also, there is no antecedent bone marrow failure.[11] Preliminary analyses suggest that the type of leukemia developing in Bloom syndrome is age related, mirroring leukemia in non-Bloom cases.[12]

Ataxia telangiectasia is an autosomal recessive disorder characterized by cerebral and vascular abnormalities.[13] The molecular basis may be a subtle abnormality in DNA repair.[14,15] Other abnormalities are also reported, such as impaired cysteine transport.[16] In ataxia telangiectasia, leukemia develops after the second decade of life; actuarial probability is about 10%.[17,18] In contrast to Fanconi anemia, where only AML develops, and Bloom syndrome, where both AML and ALL develop, leukemias in ataxia telangiectasia are exclusively lymphoid; most involve T-cells.[18]

Clones of T-cells with abnormalities of one or both chromosomes 14, typically involving the beta T-cell receptor locus, are common in persons with ataxia telangiectasia, only few of them ultimately develop leukemia.[19,20] Some abnormal clones expand with time, others disappear spontaneously. Leukemia may develop within a previously detected clone or in a new clone, however, chromosome 14 abnormalities are always present. One conclusion is that abnormalities of chromosome 14 are a necessary prelude of leukemia, but other (genetic?) changes are required.

Children with Down's syndrome also have an increased risk of developing ALL and AML.[21,22] The actuarial risk is reported to be about 1.5%. The age-related pattern of ALL development in children with Down's syndrome is similar to children without Down's syndrome.[12] In contrast, the pattern of AML shows a considerable excess of cases in children less than 2 years old. Most of these cases are acute megakaryocytic leukemia (AML M7).[23]

Myelodysplasia, including bone marrow fibrosis, uncommon before leukemia in normal children, is a frequent antecedent of AML in Down's syndrome.[23] Also, children with Down's syndrome have an increased risk of transient leukemoid reactions postnatally. This is a clonal disorder that in Down's mosaic develops only in trisomic cells and in some (but not all) cases is followed by leukemia in the next 1–2 years.[24]

Leukemia developing in Down's children is also clonal and in Down's mosaic develops only in trisomic cells.[25] In contrast to transient leukemoid reactions, leukemia cells often contain additional acquired cytogenetical abnormalities.[26] These data suggest that trisomy 21 is a necessary, but insufficient cause of leukemia in Down's syndrome and are conceptually similar to those discussed in ataxia–telangiectasia. Interestingly, trisomy 21 is a common acquired genetical abnormality in AML and ALL unassociated with Down's syndrome.[27]

Other congenital disorders associated with leukemia include Schwachman-–Diamond syndrome, N and Poland syndromes, and others.[28-32] Because these disorders are rare, and prospective studies are lacking, the actuarial probability of progression to leukemia and the relationship between age and type of leukemia that develops are uncertain.

Radiation, chemicals and drugs
Exposure to radiation, chemicals and drugs is a rare cause of leukemia. The best studied model is radiation-related leukemogenesis in persons exposed to atomic bomb radiation, persons receiving radiation therapy for malignant or nonmalignant diseases and children exposed to diagnostic X-ray in utero.

Persons exposed to atomic bomb radiation had a substantial increase in leukemia, with a relative risk of about fivefold. An increased risk was first detected about 3 years after exposure, peaked between 5 and 10 years and declined slowly thereafter. Increased leukemia risk showed a linear or a linear–quadratic relationship to radiation dose, with a threshold at 0.5 to 2.0 Gy.[33-35] Risk correlated with age and was greatest in younger persons. Because the estimated 50% lethal dose of the atomic bomb explosions was about 2 Gy, the actuarial risk of leukemia in heavily exposed persons is unknown.

Several forms of leukemia were increased after atomic bomb exposure, including AML, ALL and chronic myelogenous leukemia (CML).[36] There was no correlation between age at exposure and the type of leukemia developing.[12] For example, children were as likely to develop CML as ALL. Interestingly, chronic lymphocytic leukemia (CLL) was not increased.[36] Whether this is because CLL is not a radiogenic cancer or because of host factors (CLL is exceedingly rare in Japan) is unknown.

Several studies of persons receiving radiation therapy for cancer, including breast, cervical and endometrial cancers and lymphomas, show an increased risk of leukemia, mostly AML and rarely CML.[37-41] However, defining the precise role of radiation therapy in leukemogenesis is difficult. In most studies, chemotherapy was combined with radiation; synergy between radiation and alkylating drugs in leukemia induction is described.[42] In cancer patients, radiotherapy alone causes no detectable increased leukemia risk.[39-43] In contrast, persons receiving radiotherapy alone for non-malignant diseases such as ankylosing spondylitis and tinea capitis are at increased risk of AML and CML.[44-46] Whether the different risk is associated with radiation dose or statistical biases due to different survival in malignant and non-malignant diseases is unknown.

Children exposed to diagnostic X-ray in utero are also at increased risk of leukemia. Most cases develop within 2 years and appear to be ALL.[47–49] In contrast, children exposed in utero to the atomic bomb radiations have an increased incidence of solid tumors but not leukemia.[50] This difference is ascribed to the different radiation dose and dose rate.

There is considerable controversy whether radiation causes leukemia in other settings. For example, some studies report that children living near nuclear facilities, such as weapon plants, atmospheric test sites, fuel reprocessing plants and commercial power stations, have an increased risk of developing ALL.[51,52] Other studies fail to report this association.[53] Also, a study in the United Kingdom reports increased ALL in children living in sites selected for nuclear facilities that were never constructed.[54] This has led to the notion that geographic or epidemiologic features of these sites, rather than radiation, may explain the increased incidence of leukemia. A viral etiology has been proposed.[55,56] Although the cause of this ALL excess is unknown, radiation doses received by persons living near these facilities are substantially below those presumed to cause leukemia in humans. Similarly, a recent study reported increased leukemia in children of fathers working at nuclear power stations who were exposed to radiation doses of >10 mSV in the 6 months before conception.[57] These data confirm a preceding study showing increased leukemia in children of fathers who received diagnostic X-ray preconceptionally,[58] but are at variance with studies in progeny of persons exposed to atomic bomb radiation.[59]

Other controversial data are those regarding increased incidence of leukemia in other settings, such as radium watch dial painters, persons receiving diagnostic X-ray or thorotrast and radiology personnel.[60] Also, the role of α-radiation in leukemogenesis remains unclear, although some studies report increased leukemia risk in persons exposed to radon.[61–63] Again, variation in radiation doses and exposure, additional risk factors and statistical biases can account for discrepancies in the studies.

The possible role of non-ionizing radiation in leukemogenesis is also undefined. Several reports describe an increase in leukemias in children living near high-voltage electrical transmission wires, amateur radio operators and electrical industry workers.[64] These data are controversial and are the subject of prospective studies. Presently, there is little data suggesting how electromagnetic radiation might permanently alter hematopoietic cells.

The evidence that chemicals and drugs cause leukemia mostly derive from studies showing an increased incidence of leukemia in persons who received cytotoxic drugs for cancers. As discussed before, many of these studies show a synergy between radiation and drugs in causing leukemia, however increased incidence is shown also in persons receiving drugs alone, especially alkylans and epydophyllins.[39–41,65,66] Treatment-related leukemias are mostly AML in both children and adults.

Exposure to benzene, chloramphenicol and phenylbutazone is also reported to increase leukemia risk.[67,68] Here, leukemia is often preceded by bone marrow aplasia and/or myelodysplasia. Prospective epidemiologic studies are not reported, and the actuarial risk of developing preleukemia and leukemia is unknown.

Virus-related leukemias

Viruses are a common cause of leukemia in animals, including primates. However, the search for a viral etiology of most human leukemias has been unsuccessful. Although considerable epidemiologic data suggest that ALL in children reflects an uncommon response to a common infection,[55,56,69,70] no specific virus has been detected. There are, however, some well documented virus-related types of lymphoid malignancies: adult T-cell leukemia and human T-cell lymphotropic virus 1 (HTLV-1) and Burkitt lymphoma–leukemia and Epstein Barr virus (EBV).

Adult T cell leukemia (ATL), endemic in Japan, the Caribbean and West Africa, is characterized by monoclonal proliferation of CD4-, CD25-positive T cells.[71] Although the precise mechanism of virus-induced transformation is unclear, epidemiologic and experimental data suggest a role of HTLV-1 in leukemogenesis.

HTLV-1 is a human retrovirus[72] transmitted via maternal–fetal infection and from breast feeding.[73] Infections via blood products are also reported in nonendemic areas.[74,75]

Considerable data indicate that HTLV-1 causes T cell proliferation by inducing expression of the IL-2 receptor and possibly activating paracrine or autocrine mechanisms.[76–80] Also, expression of the HTLV-1-related TAT gene results in mesenchimal tumors in transgenic mice.[81] Data in humans suggest that HTLV-1 is necessary but insufficient to cause leukemia; additional factors likely contribute. For example, leukemia develops after a long latent period, up to 20–30 years and occurs in less than 0.1% of infected persons.[71] Monoclonal or oligogoclonal integration of HTLV-1 sequences is detected in the leukemia cells, but cells have no detectable expression of viral encoded RNA or proteins.[82–84] These observations also suggest that HTLV-1 may initiate the process that ultimately leads to leukemia, but that viral gene expression is not required to maintain the transformed phenotype.

Burkitt lymphoma–leukemia is a B-lymphocyte malignancy endemic in Central Africa and sporadic elsewhere. Tumor cells contain specific chromosome translocations, t(8;14), t(2;8) or t(8;22) involving the MYC protooncogene on chromosome 8 and immunoglobulin heavy or light chain loci on chromosomes 2, 14 or 22. These translocations appear to deregulate MYC expression likely by loss or mutation of MYC regulatory sequences and the juxtaposition to immunoglobulin regulatory sequences.[85]

EBV, a DNA virus, causes infectious mononucleosis. A lifelong latent infection is established after an acute EBV infection. Latency reflects a balance between viral replication and host immunity.[86] A role of EBV in the pathogenesis of Burkitt lymphoma–leukemia is suggested by the detection of monoclonal virus integration in the genome of almost all endemic and 10–20% of sporadic lymphoma.[87] Also, EBV immortalizes human B lymphoblasts in vitro and causes poli-, oligo- or monoclonal lymphoproliferative diseases in immune deficient persons.[88–91]

These data suggest that EBV infection precedes and possibly causes clonal expansion of B cells in Burkitt lymphoma. The relation between EBV infection and MYC translocation is controversial. EBV might result in expansion of immortalized B cells, thereby increasing the target cell population for additional events like MYC translocation.[92] Other data suggest that EBV infection causes clonal expansion of cells containing an altered MYC.[93]

Discussion

The data reviewed indicate that different situations associated with increased risk of leukemia share common features. Often, they cause or are associated with genetic alterations. Examples are congenital genetic disorders, where spontaneous or inducible chromosome abnormalities are reported,[94] and radiation and alkylating drugs, which cause chromosomal or subchromosomal aberrations.[42] Also, considerable data indicate that viruses cause leukemia in animals by transducing oncogenes or activating cellular oncogenes via viral insertion.[95,96] Mechanisms of viral leukemogenesis in humans are unknown.

The incidence and significance of chromosome and gene abnormalities in 'spontaneous' leukemias is discussed elsewhere.[96,97] It is however important to note that leukemia developing in individuals 'at risk' for underlying congenital syndromes, radiations, chemicals or viruses have similar alterations to those reported in 'spontaneous' leukemias. For example, trisomy 21 and chromosome 14 translocations typical of leukemias in persons with Down's syndrome and ataxia telangiectasia are common in 'spontaneous' leukemias.[27] Also, the authors and others report that atomic bomb induced CML has similar molecular rearrangement of BCR and ABL genes as CML unrelated to radiation.[98] A possible exception is EBV-related endemic Burkitt lymphoma, where the locus of MYC breakpoint differs from the one present in the sporadic non-EBV-related forms.[99]

A second common characteristic is that not all persons with these risk features develop leukemia. This issue is discussed in relation to congenital genetic disorders and virus induced leukemia. A similar concept applies in other settings. For example, some persons exposed to atomic bomb radiation have stable chromosome abnormalities in hematopoietic progenitor cells for many years without evolution to leukemia.[100] Whether similar antecedent abnormalities were present in exposed persons ultimately developing leukemia is unknown.

Also, in most of the situations we review, leukemia is often preceded by one or more preleukemia phases, including clonal expansion, bone marrow hypoplasia or myelodysplasia. This is reported in Fanconi anemia, ataxia telangiectasia, Down's syndrome, radiation and drug-induced leukemia. This mode of leukemia development also occurs in 'spontaneous' leukemias.

Another common feature is immune deficiency. Impaired immune function is described in persons with Bloom or Down's syndromes, ataxia telangiectasia or in those exposed to radiation.[13,101-103] The role of the immune system in regulating leukemia is controversial. However, some data suggest that cellular or humoral mechanisms influence leukemia development.[104,105] Also, EBV-induced lymphomas are described in immune deficient persons.[89-91]

These observations suggest that in the situations reviewed and possibly also in 'spontaneous' leukemias, the pathogenesis of leukemia is likely to be multistep. A single agent or situation may initiate the process but additional events are needed for leukemia development. These additional events may be random or the consequence of other agents. This model is well described in experimental carcinogenesis.[106,107]

In some cases, the first detectable event is abnormal cell proliferation. The role of poly-, pauci- or clonal cell expansion in leukemogenesis is unclear. In man, both HTLV-1 and EBV result in expansion of T- and B-cells, respectively.[76,77,88-91] Cell proliferation might cause leukemia by increasing the number of cells at risk for transformation. Malaria and possibly HTLV-1 infections are reported to influence the likelihood of developing CLL and Burkitt lymphoma by a similar mechanism.[108-110] However, other data indicate that policlonal or clonal expansion do not always eventuate in leukemia. For example, studies in experimental animals constitutively expressing myeloid growth factors, such as IL-3, GM-CSF and erythropoietin, show no relationship between hematopoietic cell growth and leukemia.[111-113] Also, pauci- or clonal B-cell proliferation is described in persons with immune thrombocytopenia and other autoimmune diseases or with hyperactive malarial splenomegaly who did not develop leukemia.[114,115]

The role of promoting agents in progression of human leukemia is unproven. However, several data indicate that interaction of different agents is necessary in leukemogenesis. For example, a role for milkbush has been postulated to be important in the development of EBV-related Burkitt lymphoma.[116] Also, synergy between radiation and viruses or chemicals in leukemia induction is reported.[42,117]

To date, it is also impossible to identify cells where leukemogenesis begins. In 'spontaneous' leukemias, it is commonly thought that CML begins in a stem cell and acute leukemias in committed cells. Here, stem cells are defined as cells capable of self-renewal, including totipotent hematopoietic stem cells and most lymphoid cells, while committed cells are differentiating cells lacking self-renewal capability. Considerable data, however, suggest that stem cells are always the site of transformation in leukemia. For example, most acute leukemias developing in persons 'at risk' and some 'spontaneous' acute leukemia are preceded by preleukemia. Notably, clonal hematopoiesis, aplastic anemia and myelodysplastic syndromes are considered hematopoietic stem cell disorders.[118]

There are additional reasons why leukemia transformation should typically occur in stem cells rather than in more mature cells. In dividing stem cells, DNA replication is conservative. When the cell divides to form one new stem cell and one more differentiated progeny, the DNA in the stem cell is more likely to be the original strand. Since this DNA is 'older', it is more likely to undergo additional alterations than the 'new' DNA in differentiated progeny.[119,120] Also, because the long timescale of multistep leukemogenesis, long-lived stem cells, rather than their shorter-lived progeny, are a more likely site of transformation.

The authors envision a model of leukemogenesis which begins with a genetic change in a hematopoietic cell. This may occur spontaneously or because of leukemogens. The extent of the damage varies from subtle to lethal. Genetic changes in committed cells may result in cell death or abnormal cell functions. However, the corresponding disorders are likely to be transient, since the altered cells are replaced by new cells. When the genetic alterations affect cells capable of self-renewal, consequences are different. Lethal abnormalities in a stem cell cause clonal extinction. Subtle abnormalities may start a process leading to neoplastic transformation through one or more preleukemia phases. For example, it is possible that in Down's syndrome, transient leukemoid reactions represent a disorder of committed hematopoietic cells, whereas leukemia arises from stem cell abnormalities.

Conclusions

Most cases of leukemia reflect a stem cell disorder. The pathogenesis is often multistep. Etiology is usually unknown, but may result from the interaction of endogenous or exogenous factors. Among the former are inherent chromosome instability, abnormal DNA repair and altered immune function. Among the latter are radiation, chemicals and viruses. Despite the increased incidence of leukemia in congenital syndromes, most leukemia are likely acquired. Data indicating increased leukemia in children of fathers who received radiation before conception need confirmation.[121]

References

(1) Linet MS. *The leukemias.* Oxford University Press. New York 1985: 20.
(2) Court-Brown WM, Doll R. Leukemia in childhood and young adult life. Trend in mortality in relation to etiology. *Br Med J* 26: 981, 1961.
(3) van Hoff J, Schymura MJ, McCrea Curnam MG. Trends in the incidence of childhood and adolescent cancer in Connecticut 1935–79. *Med Ped Oncol* 1988; 16: 78.

(4) Auerbach A. *Fanconi syndrome*. Springer Verlag. Berlin 1989.
(5) Sasaki MS. Is Fanconi's anaemia defective in a process essential to repair DNA cross links? *Nature* 1975; 257: 501.
(6) Gordon-Smith EC, Rutherford TR. Fanconi anemia: constitutional aplastic anemia. *Sem Hematol* 1991; 28: 104.
(7) Auerbach AD, Rogatko A, Schroeder-Kurt TM. International Fanconi Anemia Registry: relation of clinical symptoms to diepoxybutane sensivity. *Blood* 1989; 73: 391.
(8) Auerbach A, Allen RC. Leukemia and preleukemia in Fanconi anemia patients. *Cancer Genet Cytogenet* 1991; 51: 1.
(9) Miller RW. Persons with exceptionally high risk of leukemia. *Cancer Res.* 1967; 27: 2420.
(10) Willis AE, Lindahl T. DNA ligase I deficiency in Bloom syndrome. *Nature* 1987; 325: 355.
(11) German J, Gardin C. Bloom's syndrome. XV. The instances of acute myelogenous leukemia in the Bloom's syndrome registry. In: Gale RP, ed. *Acute myelogenous leukemia: progress and controversies*. New York, Wiley-Liss Inc., 1990: 35.
(12) Butturini A, Gale RP. Age onset and type of leukemia. *Lancet* 1989; ii: 798.
(13) Waldmann TA, Misiti J, Nelson DI, Kzamer KH. Ataxia telangienctasia: a multisystem hereditary disease with immunodeficiency, impaired organ maturation, X-ray hypersensivity and a high incidence of neoplasia. *Ann Int Med* 1983; 99: 367.
(14) Cox R, Debenham PG, Masson WK et al. Ataxia telangiectasia: a human mutation giving high frequency misrepair of DNA double-stranded scission. *Mol Biol Med* 1986; 3: 220.
(15) Cunliffe PM, Mann JR, Cameron AH. Radiosensivity in ataxia telangiectasia. *Br J Radiol* 1975; 48: 37.
(16) Meredith HJ, Dudson ML. Impaired glutathione biosynthesis in cultured human ataxia telangiectasia cells. *Cancer Res* 1987; 47: 4576.
(17) Kersey JH, Spector BD, Good RA. Primary immunodeficiency diseases and cancer: the immunodeficiency cancer registry. *Int J Cancer* 1973; 12: 333.
(18) Duhrsen U, Uppenkamp M, Uppenkamp I et al. Chronic T cell leukemia with unusual characteristics in ataxia telangiectasia. *Blood* 1986; 68: 577.
(19) Sparkes RS, Como R, Golde DW. Cytogenetic abnormalities in ataxia telangiectasia with T cell chronic lymphocytic leukemia. *Cancer Genet Cytogenet* 1980; 1: 329.
(20) Stern MH, Theodorou I, Aurias A et al. T-cell non-malignant clonal proliferation in ataxia–telangiectasia: a cytological, immunological and molecular characterization. *Blood* 1989; 73: 1285.
(21) Fabia J, Drolette M. Malformations and leukemia in children with Down's syndrome. *Pediatrics* 1970; 45: 60.
(22) Fong C, Brodeur GM. Down's syndrome and leukemia: epidemiology, genetics, cytogenetics and mechanisms of leukemogenesis. *Cancer Genet Cytogenet* 1987; 28: 55.
(23) Zipursky A, Peeters M, Poon A. Megakaryoblastic leukemia and Down syn-

drome – a review. In: McCoy EE, Epstein CJ, eds. *Ongolocy and immunology of Down's syndrome*. New York: Alan Liss, 1987: 19.

(24) Kurahashi H, Hara J, Yumura-Yagi K et al. Monoclonal nature of transient abnormal myelopoiesis in Down's syndrome. *Blood* 1991; 77: 1161.

(25) Rowley JD. Down's syndrome and acute leukemia: increased risk may be due to trisomy 21. *Lancet* 1981; ii: 1020.

(26) Hayashi Y, Eguchi M, Sugita K et al. Cytogenetic findings and proliferative features in acute leukemia and transient myeloproliferative disorder in Down's syndrome. *Blood* 1988; 72: 15.

(27) Mittleman F. Catalog of chromosome aberrations in cancer. In: Sandberg A, ed. *Topics in cytogenetics*. New York: Alan Liss, 1985: 5.

(28) Woods WG, Roloff JS, Lukens JN, Krivit W. The occurrence of leukemia in patients with the Shwachman syndrome. *J Pediatr* 1981; 99: 425.

(29) Hess RO, Hafez GR, Meisner LF. Updating the N syndrome: occurrence of lymphoid malignancy and possible association with an increased rate of chromosome breakage. *Am J Med Genet* 1987; Suppl. 3: 383.

(30) Miller RA, Miller DR. Congenital absence of the pectoralis major muscle with acute lymphoblastic leukemia and genitourinary anomalies. J. Pediatr 1975; 87: 146.

(31) Jonas DM, Heilbron DC, Ablin AR. Rubinstein–Taybi syndrome and acute leukemia. *J Pediatr* 1978; 92: 851.

(32) Mulvihill JJ. Genetic repertory of human neoplasia. In: Mulvihill JJ, Miller RW. *Genetics of human cancer*. New York: Raven Press, 1977: 137.

(33) Bizzozzero OJ, Johnson KG, Ciocco A, Kawasaki S, Toyoda S. Radiation-related leukemia in Hiroshima and Nagasaki 1946–64. *Ann Int Med* 1967; 66: 522.

(34) Ishimaru T, Otake M, Ichimaru M. Dose–response relationship of neutrons and gamma ray to leukemia incidence among atomic bomb survivors in Hiroshima and Nagasaki by type of leukemia 1950–71. *Radiation Res* 1979; 77: 377.

(35) Lambert BE. Radiation-induced cancer risks. *Lancet* 1988; i: 1045.

(36) Moloney WC. Radiogenic leukemia revisited. *Blood* 1987; 70: 905.

(37) Pedersen-Bjergaard J, Larsen SO, Struck J et al. Risk of therapy-related leukemia and preleukemia after Hodgkin's disease. *Lancet* 1987; ii: 830.

(38) Wagoner JK. Leukemia and other malignancies following radiation therapy for gynecological disorders. In: Boice JD, Fraumeni JF, eds. *Radiation carcinogenesis: epidemiology and biological significance*. New York: Raven Press, 1984: 153.

(39) Pui CH, Hancock ML, Raimondi SC et al. Myeloid leukemia in children treated for solid tumours. *Lancet* 1990; 336: 417.

(40) Kaldor JM, Day NE, Clarke EA et al. Leukemia following Hodgkin's disease. *N Eng J Med* 1990; 322: 7.

(41) Kaldor JM, Day NE, Petterson F et al. Leukemia following chemotherapy for ovarian cancer. *N Eng J Med* 1990; 322: 1.

(42) Wald N, Connor MK. Induced chromosome damage after irradiation and cytotoxic drugs. In: Testa N, Gale RP, eds. *Hematopoiesis. Long-term effects of chemotherapy and radiation*. New York: Dekker, 1988: 159.

(43) Curtis RE, Boice JM, Stovall M, Flannery JT, Moloney WC. Leukemia risk following radiotherapy for breast cancer. *J Clin Oncol* 1989; 7: 21.

(44) Court-Brown WM, Doll R. Mortality from cancer and other causes after radiotherapy for ankylosising spondylitis. *Br Med J* 1965; 2: 1327.

(45) Smith PG. Late effects of X-ray treatment of ankylosing spondylitis. In Boice JD, Fraumeni JF, eds. *Radiation carcinogenesis: epidemiology and biological significance*. New York: Raven Press, 1984: 107.

(46) Kohn HI, Fry RJM. Radiation carcinogenesis. *N Eng J Med* 1984; 301: 504.

(47) Gibson RW, Bross IDJ, Graham S et al. Leukemia in children exposed to multiple risk factors. *N Eng J Med* 1968; 279: 906.

(48) MacMahon B. Prenatal X ray exposure and childhood cancer. *J Nat Cancer Inst* 1962; 28: 1173.

(49) Bithell J, Stewart A. Prenatal irradiation and childhood malignancy: a review of British data from Oxford survey. *Br J Cancer* 1975; 31: 271.

(50) Yoshimoto Y, Kato H, Schull WJ. Risk of cancer among children exposed in utero to A-bomb radiations, 1950–84. *Lancet* 1988; ii: 665.

(51) Committee on Medical Aspects of Radiation in the Environment (COMARE). First report: the implications of the new data on the releases from Sellafield in the 1950s for the conclusions of the report of the investigation of the possible increased incidence of cancer in West Cumbria. Chairman: Prof. M. Bobrow, London, HM Stationery Office. 1986.

(52) Committee on Medical Aspects of Radiation in the Environment (COMARE). Second report: investigation of the possible increased incidence of leukaemia in young people near the Dounreay nuclear establishment, Caithness, Scotland. Chairman: Prof. M. Bobrow, London, HM Stationery Office. 1988.

(53) Clapp RW, Cobb S, Chen CK, Walter B. Leukemia near Massachusetts nuclear power plant. *Lancet* 1987; i: 1324.

(54) Cook-Mozzafarri P, Darby S, Doll R. Cancer near potential sites of nuclear installations. *Lancet* 1989; ii: 145.

(55) Kinlen L. Evidence for an infective cause of childhood leukemia: comparison of a Scottish new town with nuclear reprocessing sites in Britain. *Lancet* 1988; i: 1323.

(56) Kinlen LJ, Clarke K, Hudson C. Evidence from population mixing in British new towns 1946–85 of an infective basis for childhood leukemia. *Lancet* 1990; 336: 577.

(57) Editorial. Childhood leukemia, radiation and the paternal germ cell. *Lancet* 1990; 335: 447.

(58) Shu XO, Gao YT, Bruton LA et al. A population-based cased-control study of childhood leukemia in Shangai. *Cancer* 1988; 62: 635.

(59) Ishimura T, Ichimaru M, Mihauni M. Leukemia incidence among individuals exposed in vitro, children of atomic bomb survivers and their controls. Hiroshima and Nagasaki 1945–1979. (RERF Tech. Rep. 11–18) Hiroshima. Radiation Effect Research Foundation 1981.

(60) Boice JD, Fraumeni JF. *Radiation carcinogenesis: epidemiology and biological significance*. New York: Raven Press, 1984.

(61) Breckon G, Cox R. Alpha particle leukemogenesis. *Lancet* 1990; 335: 656–7.

(62) Lucia NP. Radon exposure and leukemia. *Lancet* 1989; ii: 99.

(63) Henshaw DL, Elatough JP, Richardson RB. Radon as a causative factor in induction of myeloid leukemia and other cancers. *Lancet* 1990; 335: 1008.

(64) Byus CV. Possible relationship of exposure to low energy electromagnetic fields and cancer. In: Gale RP, ed. *Acute myelogenous leukemia: progress and controversies*. New York: Wiley-Liss Inc., 1990: 51.

(65) Tucker MA, Meadows AT, Boice JD. Leukemia after therapy with alkylating agents for childhood cancer. *J Nat Cancer Inst* 1987; 78: 459.

(66) Pui CH, Behm FG, Raimondi SC et al. Secondary acute myeloid in children treated for acute lymphoid leukemia. *N Eng J Med* 1989; 321: 136.

(67) Rinsky RA, Smith AB, Horning R et al. Benzene and leukemia: an epidemiologic risk assessment. *N Eng J Med* 1987; 316: 1037.

(68) Chemicals, industrial processes and industries associated with cancer in humans. *IARC Monogr* (suppl. 4) 1982.

(69) Greaves MF. Speculations on the cause of childhood acute lymphoblastic leukemia. *Leukemia* 1988; 2: 120.

(70) Editorial. Childhood leukemia: an infectious disease? *Lancet* 1990; 336: 1477.

(71) Kuefler PR, Bunn PA. Adult T-cell leukemia-lymphoma. *Clin Hematol* 1986; 15: 695.

(72) Wong-Staal F, Gallo RC. Human T-lymphotrophic retroviruses. *Nature* 1984; 317: 395.

(73) Kajiyama W, Kashiwagi S, Iketmashu H, Hayashi J, Nomura H, Okochi K. Intrafamiliar transmission of adult T-cell leukemia virus. *J Infect Dis* 1986; 154: 851.

(74) Mueller N, Tachibana N, Stuver S et al. Epidemiologic perspective of HTLV-1. In Blattner WA, ed. *Human retrovirology: HTLV*. New York: Raven Press, 1990: 281.

(75) Anderson DW, Epstein JS, Lee TH et al. Serological confirmation of human T lymphotropic virus type 1 infection in healthy blood and plasma donors. *Blood* 1989; 74: 2585.

(76) Popovich M, Sarin PS, Robert-Guroff M et al. Isolation and transmission of human retrovirus (human T-cell leukemia virus). *Science* 1983; 219: 856.

(77) Kinoshita K, Amagasaki T, Ikeda S et al. Preleukemic state of adult T-cell leukemia: abnormal T-lymphocytosis induced by human adult T-cell leukemia lymphoma virus. *Blood* 1985; 66: 120.

(78) Duc Dodon M, Gazzolo L. Loss of interleukin-2 requirement for the generation of T-colonies defines an early event of human T-lymphotropic virus type 1 infection. *Blood* 1987; 69: 12.

(79) Siekevitz M, Feinberg MB, Holbrook N, Wong Staal F, Greene WC. Activation of interleukin 2 and interleukin 2 receptor (TAC) promoter expression by the transactivator (TAT) gene product of human T cell leukemia virus, type 1. *Proc Natl Acad Sci USA* 1987; 84: 5389.

(80) Ruben S, Poteat H, Tan TH et al. Cellular transcription factors and regulation of IL2 receptor gene expression by HTLV 1 TAX gene product. *Science* 1988; 241: 89.

(81) Neremberg M, Hinrichs SH, Reynolds RK, Khoury G, Jay G. The TAT gene of human T-lymphotropic virus type 1 induces mesenchimal tumors in transgenic mice. *Science* 1987; 237: 1325.

(82) Yamaguchi K, Seiki M, Yoshida M, Nishimura H, Kawano F, Takatsuki K. The detection of human T cell leukemia virus proviral DNA and its application for classification and diagnosis of T-cell malignancy. *Blood* 1984; 63: 1235.

(83) Yoshida M, Seiki M, Yamaguchi K, Takatsuki K. Monoclonal integration of human T-cell leukemia provirus in all primary tumors of adult T-cell leukemia suggests a causative role of human T-cell leukemia virus in the disease. *Proc Natl Acad Sci USA* 1984; 81: 2534.

(84) Franceschini G, Wong-Staal F, Gallo R. Human T-cell leukemia virus (HTLV-1) transcripts in fresh and cultured cells of patients with adult T-cell leukemia. *Proc Natl Acad Sci USA* 1984; 81: 6207.

(85) Croce CM, Nowell PC. Molecular basis of human B cell neoplasia. *Blood* 1985; 65: 1.

(86) Thorley-Lawson DA. Basic virologic aspects of Ebstein Barr virus infection. *Sem Hematol* 1988; 25: 247.

(87) Neri A, Barriga F, Inghirami G et al. Epstein Barr virus infection precedes clonal expansion in Burkitt's and acquired immunodeficiency syndrome associated lymphoma. *Blood* 1991; 77: 1092.

(88) Henle W, Diehl V, Kohn G, zur Hausen H, Henle G. Herpes-type virus and chromosome marker in normal lymphocytes after growth with irradiated Burkitt cells. *Science* 1967; 1578: 1064.

(89) Shapiro RS, Mc Clani K, Frizzera G et al. Epstein Barr virus associated B cell lymphoproliferative disorders following bone marrow transplantation. *Blood* 1988; 71: 1234.

(90) Borzy MS, Hong R, Horowitz SD et al. Fatal lymphoma after transplantation of cultured thymus in children with combined immunodeficiency disease. *N Eng J Med* 1979; 301: 565.

(91) Cleary ML, Nalesnik MA, Shearer W, Sklar J. Clonal analysis of transplant associated lymphoproliferation based on the structure of the genomic termini of the Epstein Barr virus. *Blood* 1988; 72: 349.

(92) Lombardi L, Newcomb EW, Dalla Favera R. Pathogenesis of Burkitt Lymphoma: expression of an activated c-myc oncogene causes the tumorigenic conversion of EBV infected lymphoblasts. *Cell* 1987; 49: 161.

(93) Bornkamm GW, Polack A, Eick D, Berger R, Lenoir GM. Chromosome translocation and Epstein Barr virus in Burkitt's lymphoma. *Onkologie* 1987; 10: 196.

(94) Schroeder TM, Kuth R. Spontaneous chromosomal breakage and high incidence of leukemia in inheredited disease. *Blood* 1971; 37: 96.

(95) Wyke J. Principles of viral leukemogenesis. *Sem Hematol* 1986; 23: 198.

(96) Butturini A, Gale RP. Oncogenes and leukemias. *Leukemia* 1990; 4: 138.

(97) Sandberg AA. The chromosomes in human leukemia. *Sem Hematol* 1986; 23: 201.

(98) Aurer I, Junbashi T, Sekine I, Tomonaga M, Gale RP. Analysis of high molecular weight DNA and RNA from old formalin-fixed and paraffin-embedded specimens. *Am J Clin Path* (in press).

(99) Shiramizu B, Barriga F, Neequaye J et al. Patterns of chromosomal breakpoint locations in Burkitt's lymphoma: relevance to geography and Epstein Barr virus association. *Blood* 1991; 77: 1516.

(100) Tanaka K, Kamada N. Leukemogenesis and chromosome aberrations: de novo leukemia in humans with special reference to atomic bomb survivers. *Acta Haematol.* JPN. 1985; 48: 1830.

(101) Hutteroth TH, Litwin SD, German J. Abnormal immune responses of Bloom's syndrome lymphocytes in vitro. *J Clin Invest* 1975; 56: 1.

(102) McCoy EE, Epstein CJ, eds. *Oncology and immunology of Down's syndrome.* New York: Alan Liss, 1987.

(103) Naparstek E, Slavin S. Long term damage to the immune system after irradiation. In Testa NG, Gale RP, eds. *Hematopoiesis - long term effects of chemotherapy and radiation.* New York: Dekker, 1988: 217.

(104) Butturini A, Gale RP. Graft versus leukemia. *Immunol Res* (in press).

(105) Truitt RL, Gale RP, Bortin MM. *Cellular immunotherapy of cancer.* New York: Alan Liss, 1987.

(106) Rous P, Kidd JG. Conditional neoplasms and subthreshold neoplastic states. *J Exp Med* 1941; 73: 365.

(107) Pivot HC, Sirica AE. The stages of initiation and promotion in hepatocarcinogenesis. *Biochim Biophys Acta* 1980; 605: 191.

(108) Fakunle Y. Tropical splenomegaly. Part 1. Tropical Africa. *Clin Haematol* 1981; 10: 963.

(109) Rosenblatt JD, Wachsman W, Chen ISY. Retroviruses and leukemia. Recent developments. In: Gale RP, Rai K, eds. *Chronic lymphocytic leukemia: recent progress and future direction.* New York: Alan Liss, 1987: 11.

(110) Sugden B. Synthesis for a complex role. *Nature* 1989; 339: 179.

(111) Chang JM, Metcalf D, Lang RA, Gonda TJ, Johnson GR. Non-neoplastic hematopoietic myeloproliferative syndrome induced by dysregulated multi CSF (IL-3) expression. *Blood* 1989; 73: 1487.

(112) Lang RA, Metcalf D, Cuthbertson S et al. Transgenic mice expressing a hematopoietic growth factor gene (GM-CSF) develop accumulations of macrophages, blindness, and a fatal syndrome of tissue damage. *Cell* 1987; 51: 675.

(113) Semenza GL, Traystman MD, Gearhart JD, Antonarakis SE. Polycythemia in transgenic mice expressing the human erythropoietin gene. *Proc Natl Acad Sci USA* 1989; 86: 2301.

(114) van der Harst D, de Jong D et al. Clonal B-cell populations in patients with idiopathic trombocytopenia purpura. *Blood* 1990; 76: 2321.

(115) Bates I, Bedu-Addo G, Beran DH, Rutherford TR. Use of immunoglobulin gene rearrangements to show clonal lymphoproliferation in hyper-reactive malaria spenomegaly. *Lancet* 1991; 337: 505.

(116) Aya T, Kinoshita T, Imai S et al. Chromosome translocation and c-MYC activation by Epstein–Barr virus and *Euphorbia tirucalli* in B lymphocytes. *Lancet* 1991; 337: 1190.

(117) Henderson EE, Ribecky R. Transformation of human leukocytes with Epstein Barr virus after cellular exposure to chemical or physical mutagens. *J Natl Cancer Inst* 1980; 64: 33.

(118) Butturini A, Gale RP. New concepts in leukemia development and cure. *N Eng J Med* submitted.

(119) Cairns J. Mutation selection and natural history of cancer. *Nature* 1975; 255: 197.
(120) Hall PA, Watt FM. Stem cells and generation of cellular diversity. *Development* (in press).
(121) Editorial: Childhood leukemia, radiation and the paternal germ cell. *Lancet* 1990; 335: 447.

Chronic lymphocytic leukemia: biology and therapeutic options

A POLLIACK

Introduction

Chronic lymphocytic leukemia (CLL) was first described in 1845 and distinguished from other forms of leukemia in 1903.[1-3] Since then CLL has been recognized as the most common type of leukemia in man.[4] During the past two decades, advances and developments in immunology, cytogenetics and molecular biology have contributed much to the basic understanding of the disease. Nevertheless, the molecular etiology of the disease still remains elusive and basically unknown.

Some progress, however, has been made in the therapy of CLL thanks to a better understanding of the prognostic factors, which determine the patient's outcome at the time of diagnosis and during the course of the disease. Furthermore, the development of more accurate staging systems with a better definition of progressive disease has enabled the indications for initiating therapy in patients with CLL to be defined more clearly. Some therapeutic advances have also been made in patients with progressive disease and recent studies have identified a subgroup of patients with early disease who should not be treated because they have the same survival and lifespan as normal age and sex matched controls in the general population who lack CLL.[5] These advances in the understanding of the disease and its biology are reflected in the vast literature accumulated in recent years, by the number of symposia and workshops organized and by the books on CLL published recently. These basically reflect the growing and renewed interest of clinicians, investigators and basic researchers, in this disease. Since 1987, publications have included the proceedings of the International Workshops on CLL[6,7] and at least two books on CLL in 1988 and 1990 respectively.[8,9] In this chapter, the current 'state of the art' for this disease will be presented and details of new

All correspondence to: Professor A Polliack, Lymphoma-Leukemia Unit, Department of Hematology, Hadassah University Hospital, Jerusalem, Israel.

Cambridge Medical Reviews: Haematological Oncology Volume 2

data relating to its biology provided and current views expressed on the therapy of CLL.

Incidence, geographic distribution and age

B-CLL is recognized as the most common form of leukemia in man. According to Linet and Blattner[10] it comprises 0.9% of all malignancies in whites and 0.7% in blacks. B-CLL also has an obvious ethnic and geographic distribution, for it constitutes 26–29% of all leukemias in the USA[11] and 38% of all leukemias in Denmark.[12] In contrast, in Japan and China it only represents 2.5–5% of all leukemias and also has a low incidence in Japanese immigrants living in the USA.[10,13] Of further interest is the increased incidence of CLL amongst Jews with a much higher frequency in Jews of Eastern European origin, particularly from countries like Russia, Poland, Rumania and Hungary[14] compared to a lower incidence in Jews from Oriental and Arab geographical origin. Furthermore, the disease is rare in black Africans; however in West Africa both Williams et al[15] and Fleming[16] have reported two groups of CLL patients: one under the age of 45 years which is likely to occur twice as frequently in females and another group over the age of 45 years in which the sex ratio is reversed. It has been suggested that younger women of lower socioeconomic class in West Africa, may develop CLL because of a relative decrease in their immune status due to multiple pregnancies. However, data from Kenya do not support these observations[17] and there seems to be no doubt that some of the geographic and racial variations are probably due to genetic factors. They have no relation to HTLV-1 antibody status of the patients concerned.

In the USA, rates of CLL have increased markedly with increasing age in males. In general, the disease is most frequent in elderly patients and only about 5% of cases are seen under the age of 50 years,[4,10] while very few are even evident under the age of 40.[18,19] Experienced physicians have seldom seen the disease occurring in patients less than 30 years of age, and in this respect cases of low grade lymphocytic or intermediate type lymphoma in leukemic phase, must be distinguished from CLL. However, today, these cases may easily be distinguished on the basis of cytology and immunophenotyping. Recently, 3 young males under the age of 30 with CLL have been described (29, 27 and 25 years old respectively).[18] All had typical CLL morphologically, with relatively rapidly progressive disease requiring chemotherapy within 1 to 3 years. All 3 developed bulky disease and 2 had night sweats. All of the patients responded dramatically to therapy, returning to stage 0–1 disease. In one case, the disease remained quiescent for over 4 years, and the patient is currently in Stage O(A) after 9 years.

In a larger series of cases with a mean age of 46, the Italian Co-operative Group has shown that younger patients seem to have a higher incidence of hepatosplenomegaly,[20] lower mean levels of peripheral blood lymphocytes and higher median values for hemoglobin and platelets. Multivariate analysis of the data seem to suggest that the extent and pattern of bone marrow lymphocytosis may be the most important variable in this respect. Bennett et al. have also described 22 cases under the age of 50, the youngest being 35 years of age. Of the 22 cases, 21 were males who appeared to present with more advanced disease but responded well to therapy.[19]

It is, indeed, possible that younger patients with CLL should be treated differently, particularly in the light of the predicted life expectancy of 10–12 years, which could be considered inadequate in this age group. Newer strategies of therapy could be designed for this group of patients who may require a more radical approach for their disease, using chemotherapy earlier and perhaps considering the option of bone marrow transplantation at an earlier stage, if a donor is available.[21] It is obvious that more factors which determine the correct therapeutic approach still need to be defined for this group and in this respect the data accumulating in Europe from the IWCLL and collected by Pangalis et al.[22] will be of great importance.

Familial aggregation; occupational exposure and second malignancies
Familial aggregation of CLL has been described with a 2–7-fold increased incidence in first degree relatives of patients with CLL.[10,23,24] Several reports of familial CLL affecting siblings in 1 or even 2 generations have been recorded. However, because of the adult distribution of the disease, carefully planned studies of this nature are very difficult to perform. In these instances, there are obviously common genetic and environmental factors involved in the pathogenesis of the disease. Familial cases have included the report of an unusual family prone to B-CLL and, in this instance, 4 siblings and a parent who had CLL were followed for a period of 18–20 years. One of the siblings had a rare spontaneous remission, while another unaffected sibling had a persistent absolute CD4+ lymphocytosis. In this report, Marti and colleagues[25] suggest that, in the early stages of CLL, there may be a monoclonal CD4+ CD5+ lymphocytosis, followed later on by the development of a more pleomorphic monoclonal lymphocytosis.

Some occupational exposures have been recorded for CLL and these include the occurrence in workers involved with soya bean production, cattle raising, dairy production and herbicides.[10,26,27] In addition, other exposures such as rubber manufacturing, solvents including benzene but not radiation, have also been reported in CLL.[28–30] However, these observations should still be viewed with caution in terms of etiology. Second malignancies are prevalent in CLL and there is up to a 2–4-fold excess of skin cancers including melanoma, and other skin neoplasias[31] as well as lung carcinoma and rectal cancer in patients with CLL.

CLL as a clonal disease – cell derivation, immunophenotype

In the vast majority of cases, CLL is a clonal disease of neoplastic B lymphocytes, while only a small proportion are of T-cell origin. CLL cells are
morphologically difficult to distinguish from normal lymphocytes by almost
all methods, however, they are not the neoplastic counterparts of the normal
circulating B cells in the blood. They probably derive from a minor subpopulation of 'activated' B cells, which lack some of the antigens normally
present on resting B cells. This subpopulation of B-cells is found at the
periphery of the germinal centers of adult lymph nodes or tonsils. Some may
be found in the peripheral blood but they are not present in the marrow.
These CD5+ lymphocytes are found in fetal tissues and are increased in
patients with auto-immune disorders, such as rheumatoid arthritis or SLE.
Recently these monoclonal CD5+ B-CLL subpopulations have been shown
to be able to produce auto-antibodies after short-term culture in vitro with or
without mitogenic stimulation.[32,33] In these instances autoantibodies dis-
played monotypic L-chains identical to those expressed on B-CLL cells'
surface. In over half of the cases studied the autoantibodies were reactive with
either IgG, ssDNA or dsDNA; reactivity often seen in association with autoimmune disorders. Thus B-CLL appears to represent a clonal overexpansion
of a putative autoantibody producing B-lymphocyte, perhaps explaining why
the sera of CLL patients often contain auto-antibodies and why autoimmune
phenomena are so frequently encountered in this disease.[33]

B-CLL cells express monoclonal surface membrane immunoglobulin (Ig),
have clonally rearranged Ig genes and bear B-cell restricted antigens. In
contrast to normal B cells, CLL cells generally display surface IgM/D which
has a weaker staining pattern than normal cells. They may also express C3d
receptors (EBV receptor = CD21) but not C3b receptors (which are the
complement cleavage fragments) frequently seen in normal B cells. In addition, cells are invariably CD5+ and a high proportion form spontaneous
MRBC rosettes. Other B-cell restricted antigens like CD19+ and CD20 are
also commonly expressed, as is CD24[34] while CD23 also gives a high number
of positive reactions in a large proportion of patients with CLL and in a recent
series 68% of cases were positive.[35] This spectrum of reactivity with different
monoclonal antibodies may well help to distinguish CLL from other B-cell
neoplasias. In general cells are CALLA negative and CD25 (IL-2r) are usually
absent in most cases.

However, some subpopulations of CLL cells have a different phenotype
showing CD11c+ CD5+ and CD20+. In these cases, cells are reported to be
larger in size with lower nuclear-cytoplasmic ratios than the small B-CLL.
These cells resemble hairy cells but the clinical features are different from
those seen in HCL.[36]

Further evidence to support the hypothesis that B-CLL cells may in fact be
derived from a clone of lymphocytes which have undergone activation is

122

provided by the fact that faintly staining surface membrane Ig is frequently seen after lymphocyte activation when normal B cells lose their surface Ig. Furthermore, the relative lack of CD21+ and CD22+ in CLL in the presence of CD23+ positivity may also be regarded as evidence of an 'activated' B cell state particularly when CD71, CD25, CD30 and CD40 are also expressed on some cells.[37] Some recent studies have, in fact, shown[38,40] that a significantly higher percentage of B-CLL cells expressed activation antigens than normal healthy B-lymphocytes. Furthermore, their in vitro responses to growth factors including IL-2, interferon and IL-4 and their own production of other growth factors such as IL-1, IL-6 and TNF also support the hypothesis that they are not strictly mature resting cells.[37]

B-CLL activation in vitro

In CLL there is an heterogeneous response to activation in vitro; in some cases there is little in vitro response and while some respond to EBV, others react even better to PWM or LPS.[41-44] These studies suggest that a high response to B cell mitogens may be associated with a more aggressive course of the disease, whereas unresponsive cells are a reflection of indolent and more benign disease with a longer survival.[43-45] In their elegant serial in vitro studies Tötterman and colleagues confirmed these observations using different stimulatory agents.[46] Higher cellular responses to phorbol esters (TPA) appeared to reflect progressive disease and may even provide more information than the clinical staging system. It appears that B-CLL cells are already activated and receptors are induced in vitro, which enable the cells to respond to a variety of growth factors including interferon and IL-2, which may mediate differentiation. Cells now take on plasmacytic, prolymphocytic or immunoblastic appearance[47,48] and may even show some features of hairy cell leukemia (HCL) cells.[49,50] These changes seem to occur only in clones with enhanced levels of 2'5'-oligo adenylate synthetase.

The phenotypic differentiation towards plasmacytic–immunoblastic maturation and IgM secretion appears to be transcriptional, translational and posttranslational. C-myc proto-oncogene expression is rapidly increased and sustained after TPA induction of maturation, while C-fos is only transiently elevated.[51] DNA and RNA measurements show that adult B-CLL cells appear to be arrested in the G0-G1 phase of the cell cycle and only about 0.1% of cells are Ki67+.[52] However, there seem to be more proliferating Ki67+ cells in the splenic white pulp in CLL, and it is indeed possible that these cells represent the microenvironmental inducer for CD21+ expression on B-CLL cells when they reach the spleen, thereby enabling them to bind B cell growth factors produced locally by CD4+ T cells present in the spleen. The presence of CD21+ B-CLL cells in the white pulp of the spleen may imply proliferation and may also correlate with the severity of the disease.[53] It appears that the induction of maturation and differentiation of B-CLL cells is regulated and augmented by the presence of a small number of T-helper cells (CD4+) and by some other factors.

Recently, TNF receptors have been found on B-CLL cells and TNF itself has been shown to serve as a growth factor[54-56] in CLL, inducing cell proliferation, transcription of TNF-mRNA and eventually synthesis of TNF protein. This occurs particularly in the early stages of CLL, suggesting that it plays a regulatory role in CLL. In vitro treatment of B-CLL cells with TNF induces the transcription of some proto-oncogenes such as c-fos, c-jun and c-myc, the products of which may be involved in signal transmission initiated via the phospho-inositol lipid and protein kinase C (PKC) signal transduction pathway. The induction of proto-oncogene expression by TNF is delayed, when compared to the effects of TPA alone or TPA in combination with the calcium ionophore A23187 which directly activates PKC.[57] The mechanism for this delayed induction still remains to be elucidated. Once again the fact that these B-CLL cells may still respond in vitro to growth factors, including IL-1, IL-6, BCGF and TNF, further supports the hypothesis that in B-CLL, the cells are not regular resting phase B-cells.

Clonogenic cell growth in CLL
Recently, clonogenic B-CLL cells have been grown in fluid agar or methylcellulose. B-CLL colony growth formation has been induced after coculture with irradiated cells, a variety of conditioned media (CM), mitogens or IL-2 in combination with either TPA or PHA.[58] These cells have been shown to be clonogenic bearing the B-cell phenotype seen on the same cells prior to culture. In this recent report the phenotype and growth requirements of clonogenic cells from 28 patients with CLL were determined using the same techniques. Different clinical risk groups were studied and colonies were obtained in 25 of 28 patients. The number of colonies and the colony size were high in patients with low risk CLL. Irradiated activated T cells or irradiated unstimulated T cells with or without culture medium were essential for successful colony formation. On the other hand clonogenic cells from intermediate or high risk CLL patients formed less and smaller sized colonies and both irradiated cells and CM were required for growth in all instances. These results indicate that, with progression of the disease, there is a loss of clonogenic ability in the circulating pool in CLL. In addition, it seems that factors provided by activated T cells and CM are required for clonogenic activity to take place. Further studies in this field will be awaited with great interest.

Membrane abnormalities and metabolic function in B-CLL
CLL cells show abnormal membrane fluidity and decreased cap formation in the presence of anti-Ig antibodies[59] and Concanavalin A.[60] Cellular ecto-ATPase, 5-nucleotidase and amino acid transport systems are also abnormal

and markedly reduced.[61,62] Furthermore, cells have altered motility, changes in the cholesterol/tocopherol content[63] and decreased actin content and vimentin abnormalities have also been reported.[64,65] B-CLL cells have many surface microvilli which can be easily visualized by scanning electron microscopy but they appear to be less densely distributed on the surface than in normal or activated B cells,[66] however, this has not been carefully studied using morphometric techniques.

Oestrogen receptors (OR) have been shown to be present on CLL cells but are infrequently encountered. Using a new monoclonal antibody and immunocytochemistry to detect the OR, we have recently shown that OR are rarely found on B-CLL cells and when present may be indicative of progressive disease or transformation to Richter's syndrome as described in some earlier clinical studies.[67] The higher incidence of OR on CLL cells, encountered in earlier studies, may be related to the methodology used at the time and the advent of highly specific monoclonal antibodies may explain why these are so infrequently seen now.

Immune function of CLL cells
As described earlier, B-CLL cells have abnormal cell membrane fluidity shown by low concanavalin A-induced capping.[59,60] Although responses are very heterogeneous, B-CLL cells frequently have decreased in vitro response to B-cell mitogens including EBV, lipopolysacharides, and pokeweed mitogen. Despite the fact that they do have Ia antigens they frequently display no stimulatory effect in autologous and allogeneic MLC, and decreased activity in antibody dependent cytotoxicity.[68] Low levels of immunoglobulin are present in the serum and about half the patients have hypogammaglobulinemia. As a result, infections are a common cause of death and morbidity.[69] This defect is in part due to primary B-cell failure and possibly also to T-helper cell deficiency or increased CD8+ T-cell suppressor activity.

T-cells in B-CLL
In most cases of CLL there is an absolute increase in the number of T-cells[70-72] with an inversion of the CD4:CD8 ratio and a decrease in the number of circulating CD4+ cells in the peripheral blood but not in the bone marrow. In addition there appears to be an increase in CD8+ T-suppressor cells which may explain why hypogammaglobulinemia is so frequently encountered.[73,74]

Usually T-cells in CLL have normal in vitro function and respond normally to T-cell mitogens in most cases.[75,76] NK-cell (LGL) function, however, may be abnormal.[77,78] Part of the problem relates to the fact that the results from studies of T-helper and suppressor cells in CLL have been difficult to interpret and at times are even contradictory.[41,79,80] Nevertheless, it seems that helper function may be depressed while suppressor function may be marginally increased.[73,74,81,82] It is indeed possible that some of these contradictory results may relate to the fact that some patients received chemoradiotherapy at the time these studies were performed while others did not. Some of the T-cell abnormalities and NK function may improve after splenectomy, splenic irradiation or after interferon.[41,74,83,84] Most recently Crockard et al.[85] have shown that CD4+ Leu8+ lymphocytes are reduced in CLL with a decrease in the CD4+ Leu8+/CD4+ Leu8-cell ratio. This decrease appears to be associated with disease activity while other CD4+ subpopulations, including CD45RA+ CD45RO+ and CD29+ cells are unaltered.

Examples of the abnormal immunoregulation seen in CLL are the presence of autoimmune hemolytic anemia in 10–25% of patients, most of which are of IgG type, while a smaller proportion of cases develop autoimmune thrombocytopenic purpura, or neutropenia and autoimmune pure red cell aplasia. The former conditions are probably due to the production of autoantibodies by B-cells and the latter to T-cell factors.[86–89] The etiology of these phenomena is still unclear but may well relate to the predominance of CD5+ CLL cells in this disease as described earlier. In this respect, other autoimmune stigmata including the presence of ANF+, SLE like manifestations, positive rheumatoid arthritis serology, cold urticaria and Raynaud's phenomenon may also be seen in CLL and other lymphocytic lymphomas.[90–93] Cases of SLE in association with B-CLL have been reported,[90–93] while an increased risk of autoimmune disorders in family relatives has also been recorded in CLL.[25,94]

Chromosomal aberrations in B-CLL

Malignancies of the B-cell lineage frequently exhibit chromosomal abnormalities such as t(14;18) and t(11;14).[95,96] Specific genes are involved in these translocations, particularly Bcl 1 and Bcl 2 which are localized to the site of the IgH chain locus on chromosome 14. After it was evident that B-CLL cells could proliferate in vitro after stimulation with mitogenic agents,[97] it was possible to show that chromosomal aberrations were also frequently present in CLL. Initially,[44,45,98–104] trisomy 12 was described as the most frequent chromosomal aberration, however t(11;14) was also present but was less common. Until now, no consistent abnormalities at specific breakpoints have been found and it has not yet been possible to identify specific genes of pathogenetic significance in CLL.

Until quite recently one could well have asked what the significance of trisomy 12 was. Did its presence significantly affect the evolution of the disease? Is there a correlation between karyotypic abnormalities, immunophenotype, clinical features and stage of disease? Some of these questions have already been answered in recent studies.[105,106] Firstly it does seem that patients with chromosomal changes have a worse prognosis than those who lack these aberrations. About one-third of the CLL patients with chromosomal aberrations (i.e. 1 in 6–8 CLL patients) have trisomy 12 and using RLFP analysis it seems that this consists of a duplication of one of the chromosomes no. 12,[107–109] while triplication of one chromosome 12 with loss of mitosis and nondisjunction of chromosome no. 12 are not usually found.[109] The high incidence of this abnormality suggests some role for trisomy 12 in the pathogenesis of CLL, however until now there is no evidence for the presence of a consistent specific CLL gene comparable to the BCL1 and BCL2 found in B-NHL, although they may be involved in CLL. Of the known defined oncogenes, 2 are present on chromosome 12, k-ras-2[110] and int-1.[111] However there are not enough data yet to support a role for these oncogenes in CLL. Other pathogenetic mechanisms must be involved as many CLL patients do not show any changes of chromosome 12.[96,112]

Initially, results concerning chromosomal aberrations in CLL were quite controversial[98–104] but a multicenter collaborative study published recently by Juliusson et al.[106] seems to have settled some of these issues. Earlier studies by Juliusson and Gahrton[105] only obtained metaphases in 85 of 102 CLL patients, while only 58 of these had chromosomal aberrations. Trisomy 12 was found in only 26 patients and represented a single aberrant in only 9 of these. Other relatively frequent abnormalities recorded then included 14 q and deletions of the long arm of chromosomes 6, 11 or 13. From this initial study it seemed that Rai stage 1 or more advanced cases had more frequent clonal aberrations than patients with Rai stage 0 and that they had a poorer survival than those with a normal karyotype. Those with a higher proportion of abnormal metaphases also appeared to have a slightly poorer prognosis than patients with an admixture of normal metaphases. Patients who had 14 q abnormalities and trisomy 12 also seemed to have a poorer prognosis than cases with 6 q – while those with abnormalities of chromosome 13 tended to have a better prognosis. Clonal evolution was rare but the presence of a complex karyotype tended to be an adverse prognostic sign. Furthermore signal karyotypic abnormalities were more common in Rai stages 1 and 2 while complex karyotypes were more frequent in Rai stages 3 and 4. There did not seem to be any correlation of karyotypic abnormalities with peripheral blood lymphocyte counts, surface markers or the number of T-cells present. Therapeutic responses in patients with a normal karyotype were higher in CLL than in those with multiple chromosomal abnormalities, while the chances of developing Richter's syndrome were also higher in patients with multiple chromosomal aberrations than in those who had trisomy 12 alone or normal karyotypes. Other studies[98–105] showed quite similar results in many respects but also suggested that Rai stage 0–2 CLL with trisomy 12 appeared to have a significantly poorer survival than those with other aberrations irrespective of whether they had additional aberrations or not; while 14q + CLL seemed to have a more aggressive course. Some of the conflicting views concerning chromosomal abnormalities reported at the time could have been due to inadequate numbers of cases with insignificant statistical significance.

Most recently, Juliusson et al.[106] have attempted to answer many of these questions via a larger multicenter collaborative European study which included and reviewed data from almost half of the cases of CLL with reported karyotypes in Europe. Of the 391 patients collected, 218 had chromosomal changes, the most frequent of which were trisomy 12 (67 patients), structural abnormalities of chromosome 13 (50 patients), involving the site of the retinoblastoma gene, and abnormalities of chromosome 14 (41 patients). Cases with a normal karyotype had a median survival of more than 15 years compared with 7.7 years for those with chromosomal changes. Patients with a single abnormality did significantly better than those with complex karyotypes and patients with 14 q abnormalities had a poorer survival than those with aberrations of 13 q. Among the patients with a single abnormality those with trisomy 12 had a poorer prognosis than those with a single aberration of chromosome 13 q who were shown to have the same survival as those with normal karyotypes.

The cytogenetic measurement with the most prognostic importance appeared to be the presence of a high percentage of cells in metaphase which was indicative of a more proliferative type of CLL and a poorer survival. Cox type analysis identified age, sex, the percentage of cells in metaphase and the clinical stage of the disease as independent prognostic variables. Thus it is evident that chromosomal analysis provides additional prognostic information concerning survival in addition to other clinical parameters. Another important fact to be considered is that when restriction fragment length polymorphism (RFLP) is studied in cells from patients with trisomy 12, using probes for polymorphic genes on chromosome 12, it seems that almost all cells in the sample have trisomy 12 despite the fact that some may appear cytogenetically normal.[109] Thus patients with cells that divide more readily on mitogenic stimulation fare worse clinically than those who are unresponsive to mitogens in vitro. The karyotypic abnormalities recorded seem to be similar in different institutes, despite the fact that different in vitro methods are used. Thus cytogenetic examination provides an additional tool for the identification of poor or good prognosis subgroups at the time of diagnosis.

Clinical features, staging systems, prognostic factors and differential diagnosis

The clinical course of CLL is often variable and unpredictable, however since the introduction of the different staging systems, both the clinical course and indications for therapy are better understood. In recent years a number of prognostic factors have been established as prognostic signs in this disease and their presence at the time of diagnosis or during the course of the disease may predict the outcome in many instances. Different studies have shown that bone marrow histopathology,[113,114] cytogenetic findings,[104–106] peripheral blood lymphocyte doubling time[30,115] and size and morphology of the individual circulating lymphoid cells,[34,116-118] all determine the survival and are important factors governing the prognosis of the disease.[20,115,116] Some of these will be discussed further.

Convincing data have been proposed to indicate that the number of larger prolymphocytes (PL) present in the peripheral blood are predictive of survival. The more prolymphocytic cells present, the worse the prognosis appears to be.[4,34] From these studies, it is evident that there are cases of typical CLL which show a slow but progressive increase in the percentage of prolymphocytes during the course of their disease and evolve into what has been termed CLL/PL. In these cases, 11–55% prolymphocytes are seen and patients tend to remain more stable as opposed to others who present with a mixture of cells (> 55% prolymphocytes) at the time of diagnosis. The latter seem to represent a more aggressive form of CLL which probably had more than 10% prolymphocytes present from the beginning of the disease.

In these instances CLL must be distinguished from other chronic lymphoid leukemias which have also been more clearly defined in recent years[34,119-124] and include prolymphocytic leukemia (PLL), hairy cell leukemia (HCL), HCL-variant (HCL-V), splenic lymphoma with villous lymphocytes (SLVL) and non-Hodgkin's lymphoma (NHL) in leukemic phase, mostly follicular type and intermediate lymphoma. It is indeed possible that some of the earlier studies predating immunophenotyping with monoclonal antibodies, may have included up to 10% of cases which were not truly CLL.

Criteria for the diagnosis of the different chronic lymphoid neoplasias have been more clearly defined most recently by the FAB group[124] who have outlined morphological and immunophenotypic characteristics for each group and stressed what is relevant in terms of the differential diagnosis. Although there is obviously some heterogeneity within the different groups the combination of a certain immunophenotype, morphology and clinical features make it possible to recognize the different entities quite easily. Typical HCL is seldom if ever misdiagnosed as CLL and the principal forms of B-type leukemia to be distinguished from B-CLL are B-PLL, HCL-variant and SLVL. The HCL-v may have features which are intermediate between PLL and SLVL and is also important to recognize and distinguish from classical HCL.

Thus the typical immunophenotype for CLL would read as follows:

SmIg, weakly + (usually IgM/D; about 20% may in fact lack detectable SmIg).

CD5+	(over half the cells)
CD23+	(over half the cells)
HLA DR+	(most of the cells)
MRBC	rosettes (usually more than 30%)

FMC7+	less than 30% of the cells
CD21+	some cells; many negative
CD19+	most cells
CD20+	most cells
CD22−	most cells
CD25−	most cells
CD38−	all
CD10−	all
PCAI−	all
CD24+	most cells

As mentioned earlier, some workers have found the presence of 'activation antigens' on B-CLL cells and there are obviously subtypes of B-CLL with varying surface marker patterns but the combination of the above immunophenotypic pattern is the most typical for CLL. When CLL progresses to CLL/PL the surface markers may change with more than 30% of the cells being positive for FMC7, accompanied by some changes in the expression of the SmIg.

PLL is a very different disease with distinct clinical and hematological features, constituting about 1–2% of all lymphoid neoplasias. There is progressive splenic enlargement without significant lymphadenopathy and the disease is more frequent in males than females. It occurs in the elderly with a mean age of 70 years. The WBC is usually very high with a mean count of 176 × 10⁹/l, but can reach 500–1000 × 10⁹/l. Cells are larger than in CLL, have a characteristic morphology with a large centrally placed vesicular nucleolus and abundant cytoplasm and are TRAP negative. The disease is usually relentlessly progressive with increasing splenomegaly and WBC counts associated with progressive bone marrow failure. The spleen usually shows mostly white pulp involvement and t(11;14) is the most characteristic karyotype encountered. Monoclonal IgM bands may be found in about 30% of the cases. In contrast to CLL, cells have more brightly staining SmIg and are usually FMC7 positive. MRBC are lower than in CLL while cells may still be CD5+ positive.

In *SLVL*, the cells are also larger than in CLL and many are elongated in shape, with plasmacytoid features. The cytoplasmic membrane is villous and cells often show polarized villi. The disease also occurs in elderly patients (mean age about 70 years) and is also more frequent in males than females (1.9:1). The mean WBC count is 17 × 10⁹/l and splenomegaly is very prominent. Lymphadenopathy may be present in about 20% of cases but is not significant, while a monoclonal IgM peak is present in over 60% of patients. The spleen shows both white and red pulp involvement and patients will benefit from splenectomy. Cells are TRAP negative, have strongly staining surface Ig, and low MRBC rosette qualities. CD5 is not strongly expressed while FMC7 is strongly positive. $t^{14;18}$ is the most common karyotype encountered.

In the *HCL-variant*, the cells are larger than in CLL having a prominent nucleolus and resemble PLL more than CLL. This is also a disease affecting males more than females (4:1) and the median age is similar but slightly less than PLL (60 years). The mean WBC count is close to $90 \times 10^9/l$ and splenomegaly is prominent but unaccompanied by lymphadenopathy (approaching 0%). No monoclonal IgM bands are found. Cells are, in contrast to HCL, TRAP negative but do express surface membrane Ig strongly. They are however CD5 negative, FMC7 negative and have very low MRBC rosetting qualities. They are also negative for other typical HCL markers such as CD25 (TAC) and HC2. Splenic histology shows mainly red pulp involvement. Patients may well be resistant to interferon and responsive to splenectomy.

Thus although there are similarities and some overlap amongst these entities a combination of clinical, morphological and immunophenotypic qualities enables ready distinction in most cases.

Richter's Syndrome

In some cases of CLL the morphology may alter in the peripheral nodes and this is frequently associated with a rapidly progressive lymphomatous type of clinical picture.[125–127] The cells are very much larger and more irregular than in CLL and display more cytoplasmic basophilia. The disease is frequently bulky in nature and often associated with gross abdominal node enlargement and a precipitous drop in WBC counts. This entity represents a 'switch' in B cell distribution and maturation with cells migrating to solid organs and lymph nodes often associated with a drop in the number of circulating cells. The immunophenotype is also altered and cells are now almost immunoblastic in nature, CD5− but with strongly staining surface membrane Ig, and CALLA +. These immunophenotypic changes are usually associated with the development of refractory and less stable disease. Studies of the homing receptors LFA-1, LFA-3 and ICAM will be of great interest in these cases in the future.

Recently molecular biology studies have shown that about two-thirds of the cases with Richter's are in fact derived from the original B-cell clone and bear the same H and L chains of Ig, while others represent the development of another additional lymphoma.[128,129] Thus the immunological, molecular genetic and cytogenetic features of Richter's syndrome are more variable than originally thought and display more heterogeneity.[128,129]

Staging in CLL and prognostic features

The introduction of a variety of staging systems has advanced the concept of evolution of CLL as a disease with a gradual increase in the total mass of lymphocytes which leads to a sequence of developments involving the bone marrow, peripheral blood, lymph nodes, spleen and liver with eventual bone marrow failure, reprsenting distinct landmarks in the disease process.

Rai et al.[130] first proposed a staging system for CLL in 1975 which was in fact based on Dameshek's initial definition of the original pathophysiology of CLL.[131] The Rai system is simple to use and gave an idea of the progression of the disease and its prognosis. Despite the fact that not all CLL patients can easily be plotted into the scheme, it provided the first means by which results and prognosis could be compared on an International scale.

The original Rai stages 0–4 were based on measurable disease. Earlier stages (0–2) reflected minimal disease without widespread involvement, while more advanced disease reflected the development of bone marrow insufficiency in particular anemia (stage 3) and thrombocytopenia (stage 4). Stage 0 implies absolute lymphocytosis alone, stage 1 represents lymphocytosis and lymphadenopathy and stage 2 lymphocytosis and splenomegaly. Medial survival according to the Rai scheme was >150 months (stage 0), >100 months (stage 1), 71 months (stage 2) and 19 months (for stages 3 and 4). When survival was calculated according to stage 0, 1 and 2, and 3–4 as 3 groups only, further differences are also evident. In fact, in 1975 Rai had already indicated that the suggested 5 categories could be merged into 3 groups (stage 0, stages 1 and 2 and stages 3 and 4) which could be classified as low, intermediate and high risk respectively with over 60% survival for at least 12 years in the low risk group, more than 50% survival at 6–9 years for the intermediate group and a survival of 2 years for the high risk group.

Subsequent modifications to this system have been made and in fact these offer obvious additional advantages.[132] The Binet system provided further information dividing cases into those with anemia (less than 100g/l) and thrombocytopenia (less than 100×10 /l) as stage C disease and others within the category A or B according to the number of lymphoid areas involved (more than 3, (B) and less than 3 (A)). Binet C includes Rai stages 3 and 4 while A and B broke down the Rai stages 1 and 2 more clearly in terms of bulk of the disease. There is no doubt that this is a valid method and stage A patients have a survival of 40–120 months (median 60), stage B, 40–84 months (median 54) and stage C 8–24 months (median 20). However other workers have shown different results using this scheme, particularly for stage A.

During the past decade, there has been a tendency to compromise and to incorporate this into one system proposed initially in 1981 by the IWCLL,[133] however, this too has not been widely used. Other staging systems have also been proposed and are of interest, particularly the one described by Jaksic and Vitale[134] who estimated the total mass in CLL using a scoring system which included (1) square root of the number of peripheral blood lymphocytes/nanoliter (2) the diameter of the largest palpable node and (3) the perpendicular diameter of the spleen. Patients with a score above 9 had a median survival of 39 months while those with a score of less than 9 had a median survival of 101 months.

However, despite the fact that both the major staging systems define the extent of the disease well they have not related effectively to the major issue in CLL, which is to identify, as early as possible, cases that will become progressive and require therapy and those that will remain stable and will not need treatment. Recently, some national studies in Europe have attempted to address these issues, to define what is meant by progressive disease and to outline criteria for the onset of therapy in individual cases. In this respect it is worthwhile referring to a report by Tura et al.[135] who studied 52 cases of stage 0 Rai CLL over a period of 13 years. Only 27 of these cases progressed to a higher stage while the remaining 25 remained at stage 0. The probability of changing to a different stage was 65% at 14 years and 53% at 8 years respectively, however the survival curves for both groups were basically the same. There were no CLL related deaths in the stable Rai stage 0 CLL group as opposed to 7 leukemia-associated deaths in the progressive group. In this study it appeared that doubling time of the PBL (less than 24 months) was a significant factor in the prognosis, however no factors could predict at the onset which patients would progress more rapidly although it seemed that this occurred more frequently in males and in patients with higher peripheral blood lymphocyte counts and lower serum immunoglobulin levels.

The importance of bone marrow histopathology as a guide to prognosis

The pattern of bone marrow involvement has recently been shown to be a very good guide to the eventual prognosis in CLL.[113,114,135] Patients with a diffuse pattern of involvement are associated with more advanced disease and a poorer prognosis, while all other patterns (including nodular, interstitial and mixed) had a better prognosis.[113,136] These findings were readily reproducible and based upon more than 300 cases. In these studies, the bone marrow biopsy patterns emerged as the most reliable criteria compared to other single variables which included age over 60, more than 2 areas of lymphadenopathy, hepatosplenomegaly, anemia (<10g%), absolute/lymphocytic count of more than $30 \times 10^9/l$, thrombocytopenia (<$100 \times 10^9/l$) or Rai/Binet staging. The median survival of diffuse bone marrow involvement was about 20 months compared with non-diffuse patterns which were close to 80 months. Stage A diffuse pattern was 40 months as opposed to 90 months for A with non-diffuse pattern, 35 months for B, with diffuse pattern compared to 65 months with a non-diffuse pattern while in stage C there were no differences and the survival was 15 months for both groups.

Similar findings were described by Pangalis et al.[114] in a study of 120 patients. From the latter, it was obvious that the diffuse pattern was more frequently encountered in advanced (stage C) disease and 64% of cases with diffuse bone marrow pattern of involvement had stage C disease. Survival appeared to correlate with the pattern of bone marrow involvement and in addition prediction of progression also correlated well with the type of marrow involvement; 66–80% of stage A and B patients with diffuse involvement progressed, compared with 8.6–33% of patients with non-diffuse patterns. Thus this parameter appears to be an independent significant prognostic value in CLL. For this to be used reliably, bone marrow biopsies would have to be performed quite frequently, in order to attempt to predict progression during the course of the disease. Some may validly argue that this may limit its practical utility as a guide to progression in CLL.

Other prognostic factors

The absolute peripheral blood lymphocyte count and its doubling time are no doubt of great importance as a predicting prognosis in CLL[20,113,115] and a number of recent studies have stressed that a doubling time of less than 12 months in untreated patients is a reliable indicator of progression. In addition, the number of larger circulating cells and the degree of prolymphocytic change is also a significant prognostic variable in CLL.[34,116–118] Cytogenetic findings are of great significance in this respect and these have already been discussed in the sections dealing with cytogenetics and CLL. In the last UK MRC trial involving 600 patients, Catovsky et al.[137] showed that age, sex and response to treatment were of great importance in terms of survival. Stratified and multivariate analysis indicated that age and response to treatment were the major prognostic factors after the stage, while women always fared better than men, independent of age or stage of disease. The significant influence of treatment response on survival also suggests that the search for better therapy for CLL is valid and may well be rewarding in the future. In this study, at least half of the deaths in patients with stage A disease appeared to be unrelated to CLL, while close to 33% of all CLL deaths were not leukemia-associated.

In 1989, data relating to early stage CLL were collected from several large randomized multicenter European trials and presented at a meeting of the IWELL held in the United Kingdom.[5] These studies attempted to define which cases of CLL may be progressive in nature and require therapy and which were better left untreated. Attempts were also made to define the concept of progression of CLL and to suggest this as a possible indication for therapy. From these studies it was evident that the overall survival for stage A was very good and more than half of the deaths in these cases were unrelated to CLL. It is apparent that these cases, if asymptomatic, do not require any therapy. The likelihood of progression in this group related once again to the WBC count, the peripheral blood lymphocyte doubling time and to the type of karyotypic aberration encountered.

From the above data it was possible to identify a subgroup of patients with stage A with less than $30 \times 10^9/l$ lymphocytes and a hemoglobin of more than 120g/l with an extremely favorable prognosis. This group termed stage A^1 had the same 5-year median survival rate and life expectancy as an age and sex-matched patient group without CLL (87% vs 69%). Similar data were obtained from France, UK, Barcelona (Spain) and Athens (Greece). If Rai substages of Binet stage A were compared A_0 and A_1 had 82% and 79%, 5-year survival rates, and A2 and A3 had 66% and 50% five year survival rates respectively. There was very little variation from center to center in this respect. Of the Binet stage A', 25% progressed to a higher stage in 5 years while in stage A" (Hb < 120g/liter and WBC $> 30 \times 10^9/l$), 54% progressed to a higher stage. Progression in these cases was best defined by the development of B symptoms, enlargement of lymph nodes, advancing splenomegaly, a change in karyotype and in particular by a doubling time of less than 12 months. The Barcelona group were able to define what they termed as 'smouldering CLL', cases with Hb > 130g/l, WBC $< 30 \times 10^9/l$ and a doubling time of > 12 months. Of this group only 5% progressed, as opposed to 52% of cases without the above features. The criteria proposed for progression could well serve as an indication for therapy in CLL. This group will have to be studied carefully in the future in order to determine whether therapy will, in fact, influence long-term survival.

Therapy of chronic lymphocytic leukemia
Before reviewing therapy in CLL, it is perhaps worthwhile stressing a number of facts which may directly relate to the future planning of the therapeutic strategy for this disease and which has influenced the choice of treatment given during the past 20 years. These include the fact that uniform response criteria have not been used until quite recently in therapeutic trials for CLL. Earlier studies did not always attempt to achieve complete remission (CR) or even to define accurately what was meant by CR or partial remission (PR). This makes it extremely difficult to compare the results of a number of studies reported by different authors from various centers throughout the world. Some of these studies were also reported prior to the use of the current staging systems defined by Rai or Binet. In recent years, CR and PR and the concept of progression of CLL have been more clearly defined and Rai and Binet staging systems have been used. As a result, present and future comparative studies will be easier to perform and consequently the results of these trials may be more meaningful.

In CLL, as in other chronic indolent lymphoproliferative disorders, increasingly, more aggressive therapeutic approaches employed in other hematooncological disorders with success particularly in younger patients, are not applicable, since the majority of patients are over the age of 60 years. Furthermore the general principle of early (aggressive) therapy for early stage disease, which applies well in most cancers is also not acceptable for CLL, particularly since single agent chemotherapy has not been shown to be effective when given in the early stages of the disease. Some of the principles outlined by Kempin[138] are relevant for CLL and include: (a) life expectancy of elderly patients with CLL is probably comparable to that of the same population of individuals without CLL. Therefore, any chemotherapy given may not only decrease survival but also the quality of life for this particular group of elderly patients. The above however does not hold for younger patients under the age of 60 and particularly for the small group 40–60 years of age, who may respond well to therapy and achieve CR or PR if treated at the first indication of progression of the disease; (b) the natural history of CLL appears to be one of inevitable recurrence despite therapy and as a result, achieving PR or CR may not be important. However, from recent studies it seems that CR can be achieved after chemotherapy and median survival improved in advanced disease. Accordingly, this concept could be challenged. Until recently single oral alkylating agents have been the basis for most treatment schedules in CLL, mainly because most physicians wanted to treat but not eradicate the CLL. This concept may also be incorrect and the recent entry of effective alternative single intravenous agents and newer combination schedules may result in improved survival for patients with progressive disease. The price to be paid for these successes includes increased morbidity or mortality due to myelosuppression and subsequent infection. However not all of the newer agents cause severe myelosuppression and results of these ongoing studies are eagerly awaited.

Definition of progression in CLL, complete remission (CR) and partial remission (PR)

Criteria for progression, CR and PR have been more clearly identified and defined in recent years. Clinical and laboratory criteria are used to establish CR or PR while immunophenotypic, cytogenetic or molecular genetic techniques have until now not been routinely used in order to define remission status. Recently Keating et al.[139] used the following criteria for CR and PR, which are no doubt acceptable for this disease.

CR: Hemoglobin > 110g/liter and platelets $> 100 \times 10^9$/l, $< 4 \times 10^9$/l peripheral blood lymphocytes, $< 30\%$ lymphocytic infiltrate in the bone marrow with no nodules on biopsy, liver and spleen not palpable and no palpable lymph nodes.

PR: Hemoglobin > 110g/liter, platelets $> 100 \times 10^9$/l; $> 4 \times 10^9$ total peripheral blood lymphocytes, > 1 log reduction of peripheral blood cells $> 40\%$ decrease in the size of the spleen or liver, $> 50\%$ decrease in the product of the perpendicular diameters of lymph nodes, 50% decrease in bone marrow infiltrate with $> 30\%$ lymphocytes or nodules on biopsy.

From most recent studies[5,140,141] it is evident that patients who have stage A CLL have similar lifespans to age and sex matched individuals in the general population without CLL. In this particular group of patients it certainly is not justified to administer chemotherapy. However, when patients with the above stage show signs of progression they should probably receive therapy. Patients with more advanced disease such as Binet B stages or C (stages 3 and 4 Rai) should receive chemotherapy. The criteria for 'progression' have been more clearly defined recently and are described earlier in this review. However one could suggest the following parameters: a doubling time of < 12 months, doubling of the peripheral blood lymphocyte count to a total of more than $20 \times 10^9/l$, $> 50\%$ increase in the size of liver, spleen or lymph nodes or $> 0\%$ increase in the extent of the disease in the bone marrow over a period of 3–4 months; increasing neutropenia ($< 1\cdot0 \times 10^9$ neutrophils/l) with evidence of infection, bulky disease with signs of pressure, development of B symptoms including fever, loss of weight or night sweats, increasing percentage ($> 20\%$) of prolymphocytes in the peripheral blood, the development of a diffuse pattern of infiltration on bone marrow biopsy and the development of certain cytogenetic chromosomal aberrations as outlined earlier.

Ongoing multicenter trials will probably provide answers to some of the questions relating to therapy posed earlier in this review.

Single agent chemotherapy, immunotherapy or radiotherapy

Radiotherapy

This was first used to treat CLL but was abandoned in the mid-1940s.[142,143] Later during the 1960s, Johnson in particular[144-146] used TBI, 50–100 cGy, 3–5 times a week to a total dose of 10–40 Gy, with very good response rates, approximating 80%, including the achievement of CR and improved survival. However since then these results have not been obtained by others and have remained controversial.[147-149] In retrospect, the response rates were no better than with chlorambucil and prednisone. Based upon Johnson's original data, Kempin et al.[138] treated patients with TBI, cyclophosphamide and prednisone. The median follow-up at 4 years showed no major differences compared with chlorambucil and prednisone and cyclophosphamide alone. Remissions were achieved in both groups.[150]

Low dose splenic irradiation has also been used, particularly in cases with huge or painful splenomegaly with some effective responses.[150] The dose used may be extremely small (10–15 rads/day) and a total dose of 140–200 rads has been recommended. The author has seen a number of patients who have obtained significant responses with alterations of the total WBC count, after very small amounts of splenic irradiation. It certainly can provide symptomatic relief.

Thymic irradiation first proposed by Richards et al.[151] was shown to be effective in their patients. However, other groups recorded severe toxicity with no beneficial effects,[152] and subsequently this therapy was discontinued. In 2 cases the author found that this showed no benefit and the disease remained unaffected by the dose given but no untoward toxicity was encountered. The described effect probably relates to the fact that the large blood vessels and thoracic duct may receive radiation with lysis of circulating lymphocytes in these vessels.

Chemotherapy – single agents

Chlorambucil (with or without prednisone) has been the backbone of treatment for most cases of CLL in the past and has remained so until now. Different schedules for administering chlorambucil have been described. One may start with a loading dose of 0.1 – 0.2 mg/kg and once the disease is under control or toxicity is achieved, the dose may be lowered.[153–160] Higher doses (0.4 – 0.6 mg/kg) may also be given every 3–4 weeks as pulse therapy, while other schedules using 10 mg/m^2 (15–25 mg/day) for 5–6 days every 28 days have also been employed. Responses using cyclic therapy appear to be comparable to those obtained by continuous daily doses.[154] In general, about 60% of patients respond and 8–20% may even achieve CR[17,18,25] using conventional criteria or CR. In 1973 Han et al.,[161] comparing chlorambucil alone and chlorambucil with prednisone showed that 3 of 15 obtained CR with the combined approach and 1 of 11, with the single agent. Similar results were described by Sawitzky et al.[162] who also were unable to show any significant differences comparing intermittent and continuous administration of both agents. In general, CR or PR was obtained in 40–77% of previously untreated patients while responses are lower in previously treated cases, in the order of 30% with a median survival of about 15 months. In the later stages of disease (Rai stages 3 and 4) 37–43% response rates were recorded while responding patients appeared to survive longer than non responders in all groups. Prednisone is useful for the therapy of autoimmune hemolytic anemia and thrombocytopenia in CLL and should always be given in these conditions.

Cyclophosphamide may be given as a single agent either orally or intravenously, usually at 2–3 mg/kg/day or 20 mg/kg every 3 weeks[163] and may be just as effective as chlorambucil. Some have even used escalating high doses (3–5 – 7.0 g/m^2) in 6 cycles.[164] In this somewhat unorthodox regimen the drug was certainly effective in tumor lysis, but only short-term benefits were achieved with substantial morbidity.[28] Cyclophosphamide has also been used in combination with Oncovin and prednisone and similar results have been obtained as with chlorambucil alone.[165,166] Other regimens also employ cyclophosphamide in combination with anthracyclines, however, those have not been shown to improve the response rate or survival of CLL beyond that achieved by chlorambucil and steroids.[137,165–172] These regimens will be discussed briefly later.

In recent years, new single-agent drugs have also been used in the treatment of CLL, including α-interferon, Fludarabine phosphate, 2 chloro-deoxyadenosine and mitozantrone, all of which look promising for the future and will have to be compared with chlorambucil in randomized trials, particularly for patients who have progressive or stage C (Binet) disease. Some of these agents are already currently in use in phase 2 trials.

Interferon: (IFN) Crude alpha IFN extracts were first shown to be active in the treatment of lymphoma and CLL in 1980–1982[173, 174] and some PR were initially recorded.[175] Early data by Montserrat et al. showed that untreated patients with relatively early disease may respond to IFN[176,177] while others have shown a lack of response when IFN is given to patients with refractory disease who have failed earlier conventional chemotherapy.[175] There seems to be no doubt that the drug is active in CLL, however it appears from other data[178–180] that the addition of IFN to chlorambucil does not change the rate or degree of response in the initial induction phase of treatment. However it may best be used as maintenance therapy for disease already controlled by earlier chemotherapy. Pangalis using different regimens[178–179] was initially able to obtain responses in 65% of patients within 3 months and of these about one half were still responding after 12 months' therapy. IFN may have a role in the maintenance of response initially obtained with other agents. Its efficacy is now being tested in several studies.

Fludarabine phosphate This relatively new drug, a fluorinated analogue of adenine (9β-D-arabinofuranosyl-2-fluoro-adenine monophosphate) resistant to deamination, has been used in the treatment of advanced CLL since 1986.[181] In very early studies 9 out of 26 (35%) refractory cases of CLL responded to therapy, while only one achieved CR.[181,182] Later data[182–185] showed the drug to be effective cytoreductive therapy in more than half (56%) of the patients who had previously untreated disease. The response was quite rapid and 36 of 39 cases achieved at least a PR after the first 3 cycles, and the drug was very well tolerated. Comparison of these results with other regimens is difficult for a number of reasons, but mostly because the criteria for response to chemotherapy, entry of patients into the study and the extent of previous therapy, have not been accurately defined in many of the earlier studies. At first glance, the results with Fludarabine look better than using other schedules such as POACH,[170] COP[165,166] and the M-2 protocol[168] which achieve about a 25–30% PR in previously treated patients. However, in terms of median survival, the end results do not appear to be any different.

CR was achieved in about 13% of patients and this is an improvement on other results. If one added to this group all the patients with PR with a residual nodular infiltrate in the marrow after therapy, the figures appear to be even better reaching a total response rate of 57% (13% CR, 28% PR and

16% PR with residual nodules in the bone marrow). The median survival of the entire group was 16 months while all PR patients with residual nodules in the marrow and CR patients were still alive 4–37 months after treatment. Seven of the PR patients had died.

The drug is usually given in 5-day cycles every 4 weeks at 25–30 mg/m^2 for a minimum period of 3 cycles. Major side effects included myelosuppression with 56% developing neutropenia, 25% minor thrombocytopenia, 9% major infections, and FUO and minor infections. Other toxicities were mild and no major pulmonary or central nervous system toxicity was seen at all. Of the Rai stage 43% 1–3 patients and 19% of the Rai stage 4 patients returned to Rai stage 0 after therapy. Thus these initial results are indeed encouraging and the drug is currently being studied both in refractory patients at the NIH and in a phase 2 study together with interferon.[186] The current MRC trial in the UK uses Fludarabine in patients who have become resistant to chlorambucil or chlorambucil and epirubicin. Dose scheduling seems to be important for the drug as a different schedule used in the New York area, employing a loading dose of 20 mg/m^2 (IV bolus) followed by continuous infusion of 30 mg/m^2 daily for 2 days every 28 days,[186,187] did not achieve the same results as those described from the MD Anderson Institute.[185] No CR was obtained but 52% achieved a PR while 36% progressed while still on therapy. Of the 22 responders 15 improved their Rai stage to 0 and these patients appeared to have an improved survival. More myelosuppression and an increased rate of infection associated with mortality was noted than in earlier studies. The new trial from this group using Fludarabine and interferon will be awaited with interest.

Recently the author has seen some dramatic responses in a few cases, particularly those with very high WBC counts and bulky disease. A tumor lysis syndrome may occur in the wake of these responses. This complication should be recognized and can be prevented and adequately treated with good supportive care.

Mitoxantrone Hansen and the Danish CLL groups[188] have utilized Mitoxantrone alone in CLL. Initially 21 patients were treated with 5 mg/m^2 IV/day for 3 days every 4 weeks as a single agent. Ten of these were previously untreated patients while 11 had received prior therapy and were regarded as failures. Most patients had advanced disease. Four patients achieved CR, 4 PR, 5 improved on therapy, while 5 had no response at all. The duration of response was up to 18 months and no major toxicity was observed. This agent appears to be effective in CLL and in low grade lymphomas[189,190] and is currently being used in combination with chlorambucil and prednisone in a randomized national study in Israel.

2-chlorodeoxyadenosine (2-CDA) Recently 2-CDA, an adenosine deaminase resistant purine analogue, which selectively accumulates as a $5'$ triphosphate derivative in cells rich in deoxycytidine kinase has been used successfully in CLL.[191] This agent which appears to have few side effects, appears to be effective in low grade lymphomas and particularly in hairy cell leukemia.[192] This drug will have to be compared to other active agents currently used in randomized CLL trials, but undoubtedly 2-CDA will be most useful in the treatment of CLL in the future.

Leukapheresis
The routine use of leukapheresis in CLL does not seem to be justified but can be used in selected patients with significant leukocytosis, who are unable to tolerate chemotherapy. It seems to be a safe procedure for cytoreduction but provides only temporary benefits.[193–195]

Splenectomy
This is not a curative procedure but can be used successfully when there is hypersplenism, auto-immune thrombocytopenia and hemolytic anemia and for the removal of bulky disease. Some studies, which are not randomized, suggest that patients who had splenectomy had a better survival than those not splenectomized.[196,197]

Combination chemotherapy
The role of combination chemotherapy has been somewhat controversial until now. Of previously untreated patients 40–80% will respond, however. From a number of studies it is evident that they do not improve the PR or CR rate when compared to results obtained with chlorambucil and prednisone.[163–171] When given to patients who have failed other regimens, PR and CR rates are consistently inferior to those obtained in previously untreated patients yielding only about 30% responses and median survivals in the range of 15 months.

COP regimen
This combination has been used in CLL and overall response rates range from 44–72% with an increase in the median survival for responding patients of 38 months as opposed to 5 months for patients not responding to COP. This regimen has not been more successful than the conventional oral combination of chlorambucil and prednisone given in advanced disease[158,165–167,171] and it appears to have no advantage over single or dual agent therapy with chlorambucil as a base.[198,199]

CHOP

In the more intense CHOP regimens given and developed primarily by the French Cooperative Study group, adriamycin is given at a low dose (25 mg/m^2). Earlier randomized studies comparing CVP and CHOP suggested a beneficial effect of the adriamycin bearing regimen. However despite differences in survival between COP and CHOP which appeared to be obvious in 1986 and in later studies[140,141,169,200-202] the patient groups are basically not very large and results still require further confirmation. The Danish CLL study group also obtained high responses with CHOP (82% response rate) but survival advantage compared to dual therapy with chlorambucil has not yet become apparent.[203]

From these studies it seems that the anthracycline appears to be the active agent in the CHOP combination and as a result a number of new trials have been started to study the effect of anthracycline derivatives or anthracycline-like compounds such as epirubicin or mitoxantrone. These may well be as effective as adriamycin with less cardiotoxicity.

M-2 regimen (cyclophosphamide, BCNU, vincristine, prednisone, melphalan)

This combination was initially used for progressive Rai stage 2 and advanced stage 3–4 CLL by the Memorial Sloan Kettering Cancer Center group[168] and was shown to be effective in early studies with very few side effects. Overall responses were 62% (with 18% PR and 44% PR) and a median survival of 76 months for patients who achieved CR, 40 months for PR patients and 14 months for non responders. However longer follow-up on this group of patients showed no significant advantages for patients in terms of survival.[138,204] In 40 cases of CLL, the author has found this an easy regimen to use with very few side effects. Three patients had remarkably good responses after receiving the M-2 regimen for progressive disease, two achieving stable PR while one is in CR 14 years after the therapy. The two PR had responses lasting up to 4 years.

POACH regimen

Cytosine arabinoside has been used alone in CLL with little survival advantage while low doses of 5–20 mg/m^2 have also been employed in a few patients with significant but very short responses.[159] When combined in high doses with dexamethasone and cisplatinum[205] there appears to be quite significant activity. Ara C may well be useful in combination regimens in the future. Recently results with the POACH regimen for CLL have been reported.[170] This regimen employs prednisone (100 mg/per os days 1–7), cyclophosphamide (50 mg IV, day 1). Vincristine (2 mg/m^2 IV on day 1), adriamycin (15 mg/m^2 IV days 1,8,15) and Ara C (25 mg/m^2 IV q 12 hours, days 1–5). 65 patients were treated and of these 34 were previously untreated cases. Of the latter 19 responded with 21% obtaining CR. Of the 31 previously treated patients only 8 responded (25% response rate) and of these 2 had a CR and 6 a

PR. All patients who achieved CR or PR had a significantly longer survival than those with no response, 47% returning to stage 0 in the previously untreated group and 29% returned to stage 0 in the previously treated group. The latter had a median survival of 15 months compared with 58 months in the former group.

Overall, mortality was higher in previously treated patients. However when results of the group treated with POACH were compared with those patients who had in other studies received chlorambucil and prednisone, the CR-PR rate was the same, as was median survival (59–72 months). Thus POACH may be used in elderly patients but mostly in previously treated patients as it is not more effective than oral therapy when given to previously untreated patients.

CAP regimen

In 1990 Keating et al.[139] reported long-term results with the CAP regimen used in 47 previously untreated patients with CLL. All patients had advanced stage 3 or 4 disease or progressive stage 0–2 disease. CAP included 750 mg/m^2 cyclophosphamide IV and 50 mg/m^2 IV Adriamycin on day 1 and 100 mg prednisone on days 1–5, given every 21 days until CR or PR was achieved. Maintenance with 750 mg/m^2 IV cyclophosphamide on day 1 and 100 mg prednisone (on days 1–5) were then given every 3 weeks as maintenance for 18 months.

Twenty patients (43%) achieved a CR and 11 (23%) had a PR while the remainder (34%) had no response. Patients were followed for 10 years and CR/PR status was established by bone marrow biopsy using strict criteria for the definition of CR. Median survival for the entire group was 259 weeks, but no patient remained in CR and no impact on survival has been noted. However, the response rate and survival appear to be higher and longer for patients with more advanced disease or bulky tumor mass with a predicted 10% survival at 5 years. The median survival for Rai stage 4 and Binet stage C disease is 93 and 83 months respectively. Thus the regimen which is well tolerated with about a 5% incidence of congestive failure (all in patients who had previous cardiac risk factors), shows some promise for patients with advanced disease.

Conclusion

It is evident that combination chemotherapy is effective in advanced CLL or in progressive early stage CLL and that anthracyclines can be well tolerated in the elderly. However no real impact on survival has been noted and results do not appear better than those obtained with single or dual agents. The results of a number of ongoing (multi)national randomized studies employing chlorambucil, 2-CDA, interferon, epirubicin and mitoxantrone are awaited with interest.

A Polliack

Acknowledgement
The author wishes to thank the following for their constant support and collaboration. Rachel Leizerowitz, Hannah Ben-Bassat and Michael Schlesinger, Hadassah University Hospital, and Hebrew University Medical School, Jerusalem, Israel. This study was supported by the Paul Ehrlich Center for the Study of Leukemic and Normal White Blood Cells.

References

(1) Craigie D. Case of disease of the spleen in which death took place in consequence of the presence of purulent matter in the blood. *Edinburgh Med Surg J* 1845; 64: 400.

(2) Bennett JH. Cases of hypertrophy of spleen and liver in which death took place from suppuration of blood. *Edinburgh Med Surg J* 1845; 64: 413.

(3) Turk W. Ein system der lymphomatosem. *Wien Klin Wochenschr* 1903; 16: 1073.

(4) Galton DAG. B-chronic lymphocytic leukemia: Some diagnostic and clinical aspects. In: Polliack A, Catovsky D, eds. *Chronic lymphocytic leukemia.* Harwood Academic Publishers, 1988: p. 33.

(5) Binet JL, Catovsky D, Chastang C et al. Prognostic features of early chronic lymphocytic leukaemia. *Lancet* 1989; 21: 968–9.

(6) Fourth International Workshop on Chronic Lymphocytic Leukemia. Paris 1988. *Nouv Rev Franc Hematol* 1988; vol. 30.

(7) Gale RP, Rai KR, eds. *UCLA Symposium on molecular and cellular biology,* vol. 59. Allan R. Liss, Inc., New York 1987.

(8) Polliack A, Catovsky D, eds. *Chronic lymphocytic leukemia.* Harwood Academic Publishers, London, 1988.

(9) Catovsky D, Foa R. *Chronic lymphoid leukemias.* Butterworths, UK, 1990.

(10) Linet MS, Blattner WA. The epidemiology of chronic lymphcytic leukemia. In: Polliack A, Catovsky D, eds. *Chronic lymphocytic leukemia.* Harwood Academic Publishers, 1988: pp. 11–32.

(11) Young JL, Percy CL, Asire AJ. Cancer incidence and mortality in the United States. *NCI Monograph* 1981; 57: 1–187.

(12) Brincker H. Population-based age- and sex-specific incidence rates in specific incidence rates in the 4 main types of leukaemia. *Scand J Haematol* 1982; 29: 241–9.

(13) Wakisaka G, Uchino H, Nakamura T et al. Present status of leukemia in Japan with special reference to epidemiology and studies on the effect of chemotherapy. *Acta Haematol (Basel)* 1964; 31: 214–24.

(14) Graham S, Gibson R, Lilienfeld AM et al. Religious and ethnicity in leukemia. *Am J Pub Health* 1970; 60: 266–74.

(15) Williams CKO, Essien EM, Bamgboye EA. In: Magrath I, O'Connor GT, Ramot B, eds. *Pathogenesis of leukemias and lymphomas: environmental influence.* New York, Raven Press, 1984: pp. 17–27.

(16) Fleming AF. The epidemiology of lymphomas and leukemias in Africa – An Overview. *Leuk Res* 1985; 9: 735–40.

(17) Oloo AJ, Ogada TA. Chronic lymphocytic leukemia (CLL): clinical study at Kenyatta National Hospital (KNH). *E Afr Med J* 1984; 61: 797–801.
(18) Lugassy G, Bouissiotos VA, Ruchlemer R, Pangalis GA, Berrebi A, Polliack A. Chronic lymphocytic leukemia in younger adults: report of 6 cases under the age of 30 years. Proceedings 5th International Workshop on CLL, Barcelona 1991. *Leukemia and Lymphoma* 1991; 5(suppl): 179–82.
(19) Bennett JM, Raphael B, Oken MM et al. The prognosis and therapy of chronic lymphocytic leukemia under age 50 years. *Nouv Res Fr Hematol* 1988; 30: 411–12.
(20) DeRossi G, Mandelli F, Covelli A et al. In: Gale RP, Rai KR, eds. *Chronic lymphocytic leukemia. Recent progress and future direction.* Allan R. Liss Inc., New York, 1987: pp. 289–306.
(21) Michaellet M, Corront B, Hollard D. Allogeneic bone marrow transplantation in chronic lymphocytic leukemia: Report from the European Cooperative Group for Bone Marrow Transplantation (8 Cases). *Nouv Rev Franc Hematol* 1988; 30: 467–70.
(22) Pangalis GA (personal communication) 1990.
(23) Gunz FW, Veale AMO. Leukemia in close relatives – accident or predisposition? *J Natl Cancer Inst* 1969; 42: 517–24.
(24) Gunz FW, Gunz JP, Veale AMO. Familial leukaemia: A study of 909 families. *Scand J Haematol* 1975; 15: 117–31.
(25) Caporaso NE, Whitehouse J, Bertin P et al. A 20 year old clinical and laboratory study of familial B-CLL in a single kindred. *Leukemia and Lymphoma* 1991; 3(5&6): 331–42.
(26) Bernard SM, Cartwright RA, Bird CC et al. Aetologic factors in lymphoid malignancies: A case-control epidemiological study. *Leuk Res* 1984; 8: 681–9.
(27) Burmeister LF, van Lier SF, Isacson P. Leukemia and farm practices in Iowa. *Am J Epidemiol* 1982; 115: 720–8.
(28) McMichael AJ, Spirtas R, Kapper LL, Gamble JF. Solvent exposure and leukemia among rubber workers: an epidemiologic study. *J Occup Med* 1975; 17: 234–9.
(29) Arp EW, Wolfe PH, Checkoway ZH. Lymphocytic Leukemia and Exposures to Benzene and Other Solvents in the Rubber Industry. *J Occup Med* 1989; 25: 598–602.
(30) Monson RR, Fine LJ. Cancer mortality and morbidity among rubber workers. *J Natl Cancer Inst* 1978; 61: 1047–53.
(31) Videbaek A. Chronic lymphocytic leukemia associated with other malignancies. In: Polliack A, Catovsky D, eds. *Chronic lymphocytic leukemia.* Harwood Academic Publishers, 1988: pp. 219–30.
(32) Sthoeger Zm, Wakai M, Tse DB. Production of autoantibodies by CD5-expressing B lymphocytes from patients with chronic lymphocytic leukemia. *J Exp Med* 1989; 169: 255–68.
(33) Borche L, Lim A, Binet JL, Dighiero G. Evidence that chronic lymphocytic leukemia B lymphocytes are frequently committed to production of natural autoantibodies. *Blood* 1990; 76: 562–9.
(34) Melo JV, Robinson DSF, Catovsky D. The differential diagnosis between chronic lymphocytic leukemia and other B-cell lymphoproliferative disorder:

Morphological and Immunological Studies. In: Polliack A, Catovsky D, eds. *Chronic lymphocytic leukemia*. Harwood Academic Publishers, 1988: pp. 85–103.

(35) Bain B, Morilla R, Monard S et al. Spectrum of reactivity with three monoclonal antibodies – MHM6 (CD23), L30 (CD24) and UCHB1 – in B-cell leukaemias. *Leukemia and Lymphoma* 1990; 3: 97–103.

(36) Wormsley SB, Baird SM, Gadol N. Characteristics of CD11c+ CD5+ chronic B-cell leukemias and the identification of novel peripheral blood B-cell subsets with chronic lymphoid leukemia immunophenotypes. *Blood* 1990; 76: 123–30.

(37) Freedman AS, Nadler LM. The relationship of chronic lymphocytic leukemia to normal activated B cells. *Leukemia and Lymphoma* 1990; 1: 293–300.

(38) Paloczi K, Pocsik E, Mihalik R et al. Detection of activation antigens on chronic lymphocytic leukaemia cells. *Leukemia and Lymphoma* 1990; 3: 31–6.

(39) Freedman AS, Boyd A, Bieber W et al. Normal cellular counterparts of B cell chronic lymphocytic leukemia. *Blood* 1987; 70: 418–27.

(40) Dorken B, Moldenhauer G, Pezzuto A et al. HD39(B3), a B lineage-restricted antigen whose cell surface expression is limited to resting and activated human B lymphocytes. *J Immunol* 1986; 136: 4470–9.

(41) Fu SM, Chiorazzi N, Kunkel HG et al. Induction of in vitro differentiation and immunoglobulin synthesis of human leukemic B lymphocytes. *J Exp Med* 1978; 148: 1570–8.

(42) Nowell P, Shankey TV, Finan J et al. Proliferation, differentiation, and cytogenetics of chronic leukemic B lymphocytes cultured with mitomycin-treated normal cells. *Blood* 1981; 57: 444–51.

(43) Juliusson G, Robert KH, Nilsson B et al. Prognostic value of B-cell mitogen-induced and spontaneous thymidine uptake in vitro in chronic B-lymphocytic leukaemia cells. *Brit J Haematol* 1985; 60: 429–36.

(44) Robert KH, Juliusson J, Gahrton G. Activation of malignant B-lymphocytes in the clinical evaluation of chronic lymphocytic leukemia (B-CLL). In: Polliack A, Catovsky D, eds. *Chronic lymphocytic leukemia*. Harwood Academic Publishers, 1988: pp. 315–23.

(45) Juliusson G. Immunologic and cytogenetic studies improve prognosis prediction in chronic B-lymphocytic leukemia. *Cancer* 1986; 58: 688–92.

(46) Totterman TH, Carlsson M, Larsson LG et al. Chronic lymphocytic leukemia as a model of B-cell differentiation. In: Gale RP, Rai KR, eds. *Chronic lymphocytic leukemias: recent progress and future direction*. UCLA Symposium on Molecular and Cell Biology, New Series vol. 59. Allan Liss Inc, NY, 1987; pp. 29–39.

(47) Ostlund L, Einhorn S, Robert KH et al. Chronic B-lymphocytic leukemia cells proliferate and differentiate following exposure to interferon in vitro. *Blood* 1986; 67: 152–9.

(48) Robert KH, Einhorn S, Juliusson G et al. Interferon induces proliferation in leukemic and normal B-cell subsets. *Hematol Oncol* 1986; 4: 113–18.

(49) Caligaris-Cappio F, Pizzolo G, Chilosi M et al. Phorbol ester induces abnormal chronic lymphocytic leukemia cells to express features of hairy cell leukemia. *Blood* 1985; 66: 1035–42.

(50) Gazitt Y, Leizerowitz R, Polliack A. Effect of the differentiating agents, TPA

and retinoic Acid, in B-lymphocytic leukemias. In: Polliack A, Catovsky D, eds. *Chronic lymphocytic leukemia*. Harwood Academic Publishers, 1988: pp. 325–51.

(51) Totterman TH, Nilsson K. Differentiation of B-chronic lymphocytic leukemia Cells in vitro. In: Polliack A, Catovsky D, eds. *Chronic lymphocytic leukemia*. Harwood Academic Publishers, 1988: pp. 353–68.

(52) Caligaris-Cappio F Schena M, Bergui L et al. C3b receptors mediate the growth factor-induced proliferation of malignant B-chronic lymphocytic leukemia lymphocytes. *Leukemia* 1987; 1: 746–52.

(53) Lampert IA, Hegde U, Van Noorden S. The splenic white pulp in chronic lymphocytic leukaemia: A microenvironmental association with CR2 (CD21) expression, cell transformation and proliferation. *Leukemia and Lymphoma* 1990; 1: 319–26.

(54) Cordingley FT, Bianchi A, Hoffbrand AV et al. Tumour necrosis factor as an autocrine tumour growth factor for chronic B-cell malignancies. *Lancet* 1988; ii: 969–71.

(55) Foa R, Massaia M, Cardona S et al. Production of tumor necrosis factor-alpha by B-cell chronic lymphocytic leukemia cells: A possible regulatory role of TNF in the progression of the disease. *Blood* 1990; 76: 393–400.

(56) Hahn T, Shylman L, Karov Y, Vorst E, Berrcbi A. Involvement of interleukin-6 in the autocrine stimulation of CLL B cells by tumor necrosis factor. Proceedings of 5th International Workshop on CLL, Barcelona 1991. *Leukemia and Lymphoma* 1991; 5(Suppl): 65–70.

(57) Gignac SM, Buschle M, Heslop HE et al. Delayed induction of proto-oncogene expression in B-CLL cells by tumor necrosis factors. *Leukemia and Lymphoma* 1990; 3: 37–43.

(58) Dadmarz R, Rabinowe SN, Cannistra SA et al. Association between clonogenic cell growth and clinical risk group in B-cell chronic lymphocytic leukemia. *Blood* 1990; 76: 142–9.

(59) Ben-Bassat H, Polliack A, Penchas S et al. Changes in the con-A-induced redistribution patterns of lymphocytes: A possible aid in the differential diagnosis between malignant lymphoma and other diseases. *Blood* 1980; 55: 205–9.

(60) Cohen HJ. B-Cell Lymphosarcoma cell leukemia: dynamics of surface-membrane immunoglobulin (value differentiation from chronic lymphocytic leukemia). *Ann Int Med* 1978; 88: 317–22.

(61) Conklyn MJ, Silber R. Properties of lymphocyte 5′ nucleotidase in normal subjects and patients with chronic lymphocytic leukemia. *Leuk Res* 1982; 6: 203–10.

(62) Gutmann HR, Chow YM, Vesella RL et al. The kinetic properties of the ecto-AT pase of Human peripheral blood lymphocytes and of chronic lymphocytic leukemia cells. *Blood* 1983; 62: 1041–6.

(63) Kajden HJ, Hatam L, Traber MG et al. Anomalous function of vimentia in chronic lymphocytic leukemia lymphocytes. *Blood* 1984; 63: 213–15.

(64) Stark RS, Liebes LF, Shelanski ML, Silber R. Anomalous function of vimentin in chronic lymphocytic leukemia lymphocytes. *Blood* 1984; 63: 415–30.

(65) Stark R, Liebes LF, Nevrla D, Conklyn M, Silber R. Decreased actin content

of lymphocytes from patients with chronic lymphocytic leukemia. *Blood* 1982; 59: 536–41.

(66) Polliack A. Normal, transformed and leukemic leukocytes. *A scanning electron microscopy atlas.* Springer Verlag, New York, 1978.

(67) Melo N, Hobday C, Catovsky D, Matutes E, Morillo R, Polliack A. Oestrogen receptors in chronic lymphocytic leukemia. *Leuk Res* 1990; 14: 949–52.

(68) Gale RP, Foon KA. Biology of chronic lymphocytic leukemia. In: Polliack A, Catovsky D, eds. *Chronic lymphocytic Leukemia.* Harwood Academic Publishers, 1988: pp. 263–87.

(69) Ultmann JE, Fish W, Osserman E et al. The clinical implications of hypogammaglobulinemia in patients wth chronic lymphocytic leukemia and lymphocytic lymphosarcoma. *Ann Intern Med* 1959; 51: 501–16.

(70) Catovsky D, Miliani E, Okos A, Galton DA. Clinical significance of T-cells in chronic lymphocytic leukaemia. *Lancet* 1974; ii: 751–2.

(71) Kay NE, Johnson JD, Stanek R, Douglas SD. T-cell subpopulations in chronic lymphocyic leukemia: abnormalities in distribution and in in vitro receptor maturation. *Blood* 1979; 54: 540–4.

(72) Foa R, Catovsky D, Brozovic M et al. Clinical staging and immunological findings in chronic lymphocytic leukemia. *Cancer* 1979; 44: 483–7.

(73) Chirazzi N, Fu SM, Moutazen G et al. T cell helper defect in patients with chronic lymphocytic leukemia. *J Immunol* 1979; 122: 1097–1090.

(74) Lauria F, Foa R, Catovsky D et al. Increase in T$_\gamma$ lymphocytes in B-cell chronic lymphocytic leukaemia. *Scand J Haematol* 1980; 24: 187–90.

(75) Han T, Bloom ML, Dadey B et al. Lack of autologous mixed lymphocyte reaction in patients with chronic lymphocytic leukemia: evidence for autoreactive T-cell dysfunction not correlated with phenotype, karyotype or clinical status. *Blood* 1982; 60: 1075–81.

(76) Smith JB, Knowlton RP, Koons LS. Immunologic studies in chronic lymphocytic leukemia: defective stimulation of T-cell proliferation in autologous mixed lymphocyte culture. *J Natl Cancer Inst* 1977; 58: 579–85.

(77) Platsoucas CD, Fernandez G, Gupta SL et al. Defective spontaneous and antibody dependent cytotoxicity mediated by E-rosette positive and rosette-negative cells in untreated patients with chronic lymphocytic leukemia: augmentation by in vitro treatment with interferon. *J Immunol* 1980; 125: 1216–23.

(78) Zieler HW, Kay NE, Zorling JM. Deficiency of natural killer cell activity in patients with chronic lymphocytic leukemia. *Int J Cancer* 1981; 27: 321–7.

(79) Kay NE. Abnormal T-cell subpopulation function in CLL: excessive (T$_\gamma$) and deficient helper (T$_\mu$) activity with respect to B-cell proliferation. *Blood* 1981; 57: 418–20.

(80) Lauria F, Foa R, Mantovani B et al. T-Cell functional abnormality in B-chronic lymphocytic leukaemia: evidence of a defect of the T-helper subset. *Br J Haematol* 1983; 54: 277–84.

(81) Kay NE, Oken MM, Perri RT. The influential T-cell in B-cell neoplasms. *J Clin Oncol* 1983; 1: 810–16.

(82) Catovsky D, Lauria F, Matutes E et al. Increase in T$_\gamma$ lymphocytes in B-cell chronic lymphocytic leukaemia. *Br J Haematol* 1981; 47: 539–44.

(83) Izaquirre ZA, Minden MD, Howatson AF et al. Colony formation by normal and malignant human B-lymphocytes. *Br J Cancer* 1980; 42: 430–7.

(84) Lauria F, Raspadore D, Tura D. Effect of a thymic factor on T lymphocytes in B cell chronic lymphocytic leukemia: in vitro and in vivo studies. *Blood* 1984; 64: 667–71.

(85) Crockard AD, Alexander HD, Stephenson CF et al. An analysis of circulating CD4 lymphocyte subpopulations in B-cell chronic lymphocytic leukaemia. *Leukemia and Lymphoma* 1990; 3: 127–34.

(86) Bergsagel DE. The chronic leukemias CA review of disease manifestations and the aims of therapy. *Can Med Assoc J* 1967; 96: 1615–20.

(87) Carey RW, McGinnis A, Jacobson BM et al. Idiopathic thrombocytopenic purpura complicating chronic lymphocytic leukemia. *Arch Intern Med* 1976; 136: 62–6.

(88) Rustagi P, Han T, Ziolkowski L et al. Antigranulocyte antibodies in chronic lymphocytic leukemia and other chronic lymphoproliferative diseases. *Blood* 1983; 62(suppl 1): 106.

(89) Mangan KF, Chikkappa G, Farley PC. T gamma (T_γ) cells suppress growth of erythroid colony forming units in the pure-red cell aplastic of B-cell chronic lymphocytic leukemia. *J Clin Invest* 1982; 70: 1148–56.

(90) Andreev VC, Zlatkov NB. Systemic lupus erythematosus and neoplasia of the lymphoreticular system. *Br J Dermatol* 1968; 80: 503–8.

(91) Lishner M, Hawkee G, Amato D. Chronic lymphocytic leukemia in patients with systemic lupus erythematosus. *Acta Haematol* 1990; 84: 38–9.

(92) Green JA, Dawson AA, Walker W. Systemic lupus erythematosus and lymphoma. *Lancet* 1978; ii: 753–56.

(93) Michaeli J, Lugassy G, Polliack A. Chronic lymphocytic leukemia, lymphoma and autoimmunity. In: Polliack A, Catovsky D, eds. *Chronic lymphocytic leukemia.* Harwood Academic Publishers, 1988: pp. 231–47.

(94) Tibebu M, Polliack A. Familial lymphomas – a review of the literature with report of cases in Jerusalem. *Leukemia and Lymphoma* 1990; 1: 195–202.

(95) Yunis JJ, Oken MM, Kaplan ME et al. Distinctive chromosomal abnormalities in histologic subtypes of non-Hodgkin's lymphoma. *N Engl J Med* 1982; 307: 1231–6.

(96) Tsujimoto Y, Finger LR, Yunis J et al. Cloning of the chromosome breakpoint of neoplastic B cells with the t(14;18) chromsome translocation. *Science* 1984; 226: 1097–9.

(97) Robert KH, Moller E, Gahrton G, Eriksson H, Nilsson B. B-cell activation of peripheral blood lymphocytes from patients with chronic lymphatic leukaemia. *Clin Exp Immunol* 1978; 33: 302–8.

(98) Gahrton G, Zech L, Robert KH, Bird AG. Mitogenic stimulation of leukemia cells by Epstein-Barr virus (letter). *N Engl J Med* 1979; 301: 438–9.

(99) Morita M, Minowada J, Sandberg AA. Chromosomes and causation of human cancer and leukemia XLV chromosome patterns in stimulated lymphocytes of chronic lymphocytic leukemia. *Cancer Genet Cytogenet* 1981; 3: 293–306.

(100) Han T, Ozer H, Sandamori N et al. Prognostic importance of cytogenetic abnormalities in patients with chronic lymphocytic leukemia. *N Engl J Med* 1984; 310: 288–92.

(101) Juliusson G, Robert KH, Ost A et al. Prognostic information from cytogenetic analysis in chronic B-lymphocytic leukemia and leukemic immunocytoma. *Blood* 1985; 65: 1341–41.

(102) Pittman and Catovsky D. Prognostic significance of chromosome abnormalities in chronic lymphocytic leukemia. *Br J Haematol* 1984; 58: 649–60.

(103) Han T, Emrich LJ, Ozer H, Sandberg AA. Prognostic implication of trisomy 12 and non-trisomy 12 karyotypes in B cell chronic lymphocytic leukemia (letter). *Blood* 1985; 66: 470–2.

(104) Han T, Sadamori N, Block AMW et al. Cytogenetic studies in chronic lymphocytic leukemia, prolymphocytic leukemia and hairy cell leukemia: a progress report. *Nouv Rev Tranc Hematol* 1988; 30: 393–5.

(105) Juliusson G, Gahrton G. Chromosome aberrations in B-cell chronic lymphocytic leukemia. Pathogenetic and clinical implications. *Cancer Genet Cytogenet* 1990; 45: 143–60.

(106) Juliusson G, Oscier DG, Fitchett M et al. Prognostic subgroups in B-cell chronic lymphocytic leukemia defined by specific chromosomal abnormalities. *N Engl J Med* 1990; 323: 720–4.

(107) Han T, Henderson ES, Emrich LJ, Sandberg AA. Cytogenetic studies with clinical correlations in 102 patients with chronic lymphocytic leukemia: a progress report. In: Gale RP, Rai KR, eds. *Chronic lymphocytic leukemias: recent progress and future direction.* UCLA Symposium on Molecular and Cell Biology, New Series vol. 59. Allan Liss, Inc, NY: 1987; pp. 177–86.

(108) Crossen PE, Horn HL. Origin of trisomy 12 in B-cell chronic lymphocytic leukemia (letter). *Cancer Genet Cytogenet* 1987; 28: 185–6.

(109) Einhorn S, Burvall K, Juliusson G et al. Molecular analyses of chromosomes 12 in chronic lymphocytic leukemia. *Leukemia* 1989; 3(12): 871–4.

(110) Jhanwar SC, Neel BG, Hayward WS, Chaganti RS. Localization of c-ras oncogene family on human germ-line chromosomes. *Proc Soc Natl Acad Sci USA* 1983; 80: 4794–7.

(111) Van't Veer LJ, Van Kessel AG, Van Heerikhuizen et al. Molecular cloning and chromosomal assignment of the human homolog of int-1, a mouse gene implicated in mammary tumorigenesis. *Mol Cell Biol* 1984; 4: 2532–4.

(112) Bakshi A, Jensen JP, Coldman P et al. Cloning the chromosomal breakpoints of T(14;19) human lymphomas: clustering around JH on chromosome 19 and near a transcriptional unit on 18. *Cell* 1985; 41: 899–906.

(113) Rozman C, Montserrat E. Bone marrow biopsy in chronic lymphocytic leukemia. In: Polliack A, Catovsky D, eds. *Chronic lymphocytic leukemia.* Harwood Academic Publishers, 1988: pp. 183–91.

(114) Pangalis GA. Bone marrow involvement in chronic lymphocytic leukemia, small lymphocytic (well-differentiated) and lymphoplasmacytic (macroglobulinemia of Waldenstrom) non-Hodgkin's lymphoma. In: Polliack A, Catovsky D, eds. *Chronic lymphocytic leukemia.* Harwood Academic Publishers, 1988: pp. 173–81.

(115) Montserrat E, Sanchez-Bisono J, Vinolos et al. Lymphocyte doubling time to chronic lymphocytic leukaemia: Analysis of its prognostic significant. *Br J Haematol* 1986; 62: 567–70.

(116) Vallespi T, Torrabadella M, Julia A et al. In: Gale RP, Rai K, eds. *Chronic lymphocytic leukemia: recent progress and future direction.* UCLA Symposia, Vol. 59, Alan R. Liss Inc., New York, 1987: pp. 277–88.

(117) Rozman C, Montserrat E, Fulfu E et al. Lymphocyte size and survival of patients with chronic lymphocytic leukaemia (B-Type). *Scand J Haematol* 1980; 24: 315–18.

(118) Dubner HN, Crowley JJ, Schilling RF et al. Prognosis value of nucleoli and cell size in chronic lymphocytic leukemia. *Am J Hematol* 1978; 4: 337–40.

(119) Melo JV, Hegde A, Parreira et al. Splenic B cell lymphoma with circulating villous lymphocytes: differential diagnosis of B cell leukaemias with large spleens. *J Clin Pathol* 1987; 40: 642–6.

(120) Cawley JC, Burns GF, Hayhoe FGJ. A chronic lymphoproliferative disorder with distinctive features: A distinct variant of hairy-cell leukemia. *Leuk Res* 1980; 4: 547–51.

(121) Catovsky D, O'Brien M, Melo JV et al. Hairy cell leukaemia (HCL) variant: an intermediate disease between HCL and B prolymphocytic leukemia. *Semin Oncol* 1984; 11: 362–6.

(122) Sainati L, Matutes E, Mulligan S et al. A variant form of hairy cell leukemia resistant to α-interferon: clinical and phenotypic characteristics of 17 patients. *Blood* 1990; 76: 157–62.

(123) Galton DAG, Goldman JM, Wiltshaw E et al. Prolymphocytic leukaemia. *Br J Haematol* 1974; 27: 7–12.

(124) Bennett JM, Catovsky D, Daniel MT et al. Proposals for the classification of chronic (mature) B and T lymphoid leukaemias. *J Clin Pathol* 1989; 42: 567–84.

(125) Dumont J, Flandrin G, Basch A et al. Le syndrome de Richter. *Nouv Rev Fr Hematol* 1971; 11: 496–502.

(126) Foucar K, Rydell RE. Richter's syndrome in chronic lymphocytic leukemia. *Cancer* 1980; 46: 118–34.

(127) Flandrin G. Richter's Syndrome. In: Polliack A, Catovsky D, eds. *Chronic lymphocytic leukemia.* Harwood Academic Publishers, 1988: pp. 209–18.

(128) Michiels J, Van Dongen JJM, Hagemeijer A et al. Richter's syndrome with identical immunoglobulin gene rearrangements in the chronic lymphocytic leukemia and the supervening non-Hodgkin lymphoma. *Leukemia* 1989; 3: 819–24.

(129) Flandrin G. Richter's syndrome in chronic lymphocytic leukemia. Polliack A, Catovsky D, eds. *Chronic lymphocytic leukemia.* Harwood Academic Publishers, 1988: pp. 209–18.

(130) Rai KR, Sawitsky A, Cronkite EP, Chanana AD, Levy RN, Pasternack BS. Clinical staging of chronic lymphocytic leukemia. *Blood* 1975; 46: 219–34.

(131) Dameshek W. Chronic lymphocytic leukemia – an accumulative disease of immunologically incompetent lymphocytes. *Blood* 1967; 29: 566–84.

(132) Binet JL, Auguierz A, Dighiero G et al. A new prognosis classification of chronic lymphocytic leukemia derived from a multivariate survival analysis. *Cancer* 1981; 48: 198–206.

(133) International Workshop on CLL. Chronic lymphocytic leukaemia: proposals for a revised prognostic staging system. *Br J Haematol* 1981; 48: 365.

(134) Jaksic B, Vitale B. Total tumour mass score (TTM): A new parameter in chronic lymphocytic leukaemia. *Br J Haematol* 1981; 49: 405–13.

(135) Tura S, Cavo M, Baccarani M. In: Gale RP and Rai K, eds. *Chronic lymphocytic leukemia: recent progress and future direction.* Allan R. Liss Inc., 1987: pp. 2665–75.

(136) Rozman C, Montserrat, Rodriguez-Fernandez JM et al. Bone marrow histologic pattern – the best single prognostic parameter in chronic lymphocytic leukemia: a multivariate survival analysis of 329 cases. *Blood* 1984; 64: 642–6.

(137) Catovsky D, Fooks J, Richards S. Prognostic factors in chronic lymphocytic leukaemia: the importance of age, sex and response to treatment in survival. *Br J Haematol* 1989; 72: 141–9.

(138) Kempin SJ. Treatment strategy in chronic lymphocytic leukemia. In: Polliack A, Catovsky D, eds. *Chronic Lymphocytic Leukemia.* Harwood Academic Publishers, 1988: pp. 159–72.

(139) Keating MJ, Hester JP, McCredie KB et al. The long-term results of CAP therapy in chronic lymphocytic leukemia. *Leukemia and Lymphoma* 1990; 2: 391–9.

(140) French Cooperative Group on CLL. Natural history of stage in a chronic lymphocytic leukemia untreated patients. *Br J Haematol* 1990; 76: 45–57.

(141) French Cooperative Group on CLL. Effects of chlorambucil and therapeutic decision in initial forms of chronic lymphocytic leukemia (stage A): results of a randomized clinical trial on 612 patients. *Blood* 1990; 75: 1414–21.

(142) Osgood EE. Titrated, regularly spaced radioactive phosphorus or spray roentgen therapy of leukemia. *Arch Intern Med* 1951; 87: 329–48.

(143) Osgood EE, Seanan AJ, Tivey H. Comparative survival times of x-ray treated versus P^{32} treated patients with chronic lymphocytic leukemia under the program of titrated regularly spaced total body irradiation. *Radiology* 1955; 64: 373–82.

(144) Johnson RE. Treatment of chronic lymphocytic leukemia by total body irradiation alone and combined with chemotherapy. *Int J Radiat Oncol Biol Phys* 1979; 5: 159.

(145) Johnson RE. Evaluating of fractionated total-body irradiation in patients with leukemia and disseminated lymphomas. *Radiology* 1966; 86: 1085.

(146) Johnson RE. Total body irradiation of chronic lymphocytic leukemia. *Cancer* 1976; 37: 2691–6.

(147) Byhardt RW, Brace KC, Wiernik PH. The role of splenic irradiation in chronic lymphocytic leukemia. *Cancer* 1975; 35: 1621–5.

(148) Rubin P, Bennett JM, Begg C et al. The comparison of total body irradiation vs chlorambucil and prednisone for remission induction of active chronic lymphocytic leukemia: an ECOG study part I: total body irradiation – response and toxicity. *Int J Radiat Oncol Biol Phys* 1981; 7: 1623–32.

(149) Jacobs P, King HS, Dent DM et al. 2nd Int Conf on Malignant Lymphoma, Lugano, Switzerland, 1988. In: RP Gale and KA Foon, eds. *Chronic lymphocytic leukemia.* Harwood Academic Publishers, 1988; pp. 145–6.

(150) Al-Mondhiry H, Stryker J, Kempin SJ. Splenic irradiation (SI) in chronic

lymphocytic leukemia (CLL). *Proc Am Soc Clin Oncol* 1984; 3: 192, #C746 (abstract).

(151) Richards F Jr, Spurr CL, Ferree C et al. The control of chronic lymphocytic leukemia with mediastinal irradiation. *Am J Med* 1978; 64: 947–54.

(152) Sawitsky A, Rai KR, Aral I et al. Mediastinal irradiation for chronic lymphocytic leukemia. *Am J Med* 1976; 61: 892–6.

(153) Huguley CM Jr. Long-term study of chronic lymphocytic leukemia: interim report after 45 months. *Cancer Chemotherapy Reports* 1962; 16: 241–4.

(154) Knospe WH, Loeb V Jr, Huguley Jr. Bi-weekly chlorambucil treatment of chronic lymphocytic leukemia. *Cancer* 1974; 33: 555–62.

(155) Galton DA, Wiltshaw E, Szur L, Dacie JV. The use of chlorambucil and steroids in treatment of chronic lymphocytic leukaemia. *Br J Haematol* 1961; 7: 73–98.

(156) Rundles RW, Grizzle J, Bell WN et al. Comparison of chlorambucil and myleran in chronic lymphocytic and granulocytic leukemia. *Am J Med* 1959; 27: 424–32.

(157) Yunis AA, Harrington WJ. Clinical use of methyl prednisolone in certain hematologic disorders. *Metabolism* 1958; 7: 543–68.

(158) Ezdinli E, Pocock S, Berard CW et al. Comparison of intensive versus moderate chemotherapy of lymphocytic lymphomas. *Cancer* 1976; 38: 1060.

(159) Keller JW, Knospe WH, Raney M et al. Treatment of chronic lymphocytic leukemia using chlorambucil and prednisone with or without cycle-active consolidation chemotherapy. *Cancer* 1986; 58: 1185.

(160) Idestrom K, Kimby E, Bjorkholm et al. Treatment of chronic lymphocytic leukemia and well-differentiated lymphoma with continuous low -or intermittent high dose prednisone vs chlorambucil/prednisone. *Eur J Cancer* 1982; 18: 1117.

(161) Han T, Ezdinli EZ, Shimaoka K et al. Chlorambucil vs combined chlorambucil-corticosteroid therapy in chronic lymphocytic leukemia. *Cancer* 1973; 31: 502.

(162) Sawitsky A, Rai KR, Glidewell O, Silver RT. Comparison of daily versus intermittent chlorambucil and prednisone therapy in the treatment of patients with chronic lymphocytic leukemia. *Blood* 1977; 50: 1049–59.

(163) Huguley CM Jr. Treatment of chronic lymphocytic leukemia. *Cancer Treat Rev* 1977; 4: 261–73.

(164) Jacobs P, Wood L. High dose cyclophosphamide in patients with chronic lymphocytic leukemia. A feasibility study. *10th Congress of the International Society of Haematology*, Jerusalem, Israel, 1989; p. 32 (abstract).

(165) Montserrat F, Alcala A, Parody R et al. Treatment of chronic lymphocytic leukemia in advanced stages. A randomized trial comparing chlorambucil plus prednisone versus cyclophosphamide, vincristine, and prednisone. *Cancer* 1985; 56: 2369–75.

(166) Oken MM, Kaplan ME. Usefulness of cyclophosphamide, vincristine and prednisone therapy in refractory chronic lymphocytic leukemia. *Blood* 1977; 50: 202–9.

(167) Liepman M, Votaw ML. The treatment of chronic lymphocytic leukemia with COP chemotherapy. *Cancer* 1978; 41: 1664.

A Polliack

(168) Kempin SJ, Lee BJ, Thaler HT et al. Combination chemotherapy of advanced chronic lymphocytic leukemia: the M-2 protocol (vincristine, BCNU, cyclophosphamide, melphalan, and prednisone). *Blood* 1982; 60: 1110.
(169) French-Cooperative Group on CLL. Effectiveness of 'CHOP' regimen in advanced untreated chronic lymphocytic leukaemia. *Lancet* 1986; i: 1346–9.
(170) Keating MJ, Scouros M, Murphy S et al. Multiple agent chemotherapy (POACH) in previously treated and untreated patients with chronic lymphocytic leukemia. *Leukemia* 1988; 2: 157–64.
(171) Oken MM, Kaplan ME. Combination chemotherapy with cyclophosphamide, vincristine and prednisone on the treatment of refractory chronic lymphocytic leukemia. *Cancer Treat Rep* 1979; 63: 441–7.
(172) Catovsky D, Fooks, Richards S. The UK Medical Research Council CLL trials 1 and 2. *Nouv Rev Fr Hematol* 1988; 30: 423–7.
(173) Gutterman JU, Blumenschein G, Alexanian R et al. Leukocyte interferon-induced tumor regression in human metastatic breast cancer, multiple myeloma, and malignant lymphoma. *Ann Intern Med* 1980; 93: 399–406.
(174) Huang A, Laszlo J, Brenckman W. Lymphoblastoid interferon (Wellferon) trial in chronic lymphocytic leukemia in progressive phase. *Proc Am Assoc Cancer Res* 1982; 23: 441 (abstract).
(175) Foon KA, Boltino GC, Abrams PG et al. Phase II trial of recombinant leukocyte a interferon in patients with advanced chronic lymphocytic leukemia. *Am J Med* 1985; 78: 216–20.
(176) Montserrat E, Vinolas N, Urbano-Ispizua A et al. Treatment of B-CLL in early stages with alfa 2 recombinant interferon: a pilot study. *Blood* 1986; 68: 227a.
(177) Rozman C, Montserrat E et al. Recombinant α_2-interferon in the treatment of B chronic lymphocytic leukemia in early stages. *Blood* 1988; 5: 1295–8.
(178) Pangalis GA, Griva E. Recombinant alfa-2b-inteferon therapy in untreated, stages A and B chronic lymphocytic leukemia. *Cancer* 1988; 61: 869.
(179) Boussiotis VA, Pangalis GA. Randomized clinical trial with α 2b-interferon in 26 stage A untreated B-chronic lymphocytic leukemia patients. *Nouv Rev Trans Hematol* 1988; 30: 471–3.
(180) Pini M, Foa R. Combined use of alpha 2B interferon and chlorambucil in the management of previously treated B-cell chronic lymphocytic leukemia. *Leukemia and Lymphoma* 1991; 5(suppl): 143–8.
(181) Grever MR, Coltman CA, Files JC et al. Fludarabine monophosphate in chronic lymphocytic leukemia. *Blood* 1986; 68: 223a.
(182) Grever MR, Kopecky KJ, Coltman CA. Fludarabine monophosphate: A potentially useful agent in chronic lymphocytic leukemia. *Nouv Rev Fr Hematol* 1988; 30: 457–9.
(183) Keating MJ, Kantarjian H, O'Brien S, Robertson L, Huh Y. New agents and strategies in CLL treatment. *Proceedings 5th International Workshop on Chronic Lymphocytic Leukemia*, Barcelona 1991. Leukemia and Lymphoma 1991; 5(suppl): 139–42.
(184) Keating MJ, Kantarjian H, Talpaz M et al. Fludarabine therapy in chronic lymphocytic leukemia (CLL). *Nouv Rev Fr Hematol* 1988; 30: 461–8.
(185) Keating MJ, Kantarjian H, Talpaz M et al. Fludarabine: a new agent with major activity against chronic lymphocytic leukemia. *Blood* 1989; 74: 19–25.

(186) Mittelman A, Lichtman SM. Personal Communication 1990.

(187) Mittelman A, Lichtman SM, Silver R et al. Therapy of CLL with fludarabine phosphate (FAMP). *10th Congress of the International Society of Haematology*, Jerusalem, Israel, September 1989: p. 31.

(188) Hansen MM. Mitoxantrone in the treatment of chronic lymphocytic leukemia. *10th Congress of the International Society of Haematology*, Jerusalem, Israel, September 1989, p. 32.

(189) Hansen SW, Nissen NI, Hansen MM et al. High activity of mitoxantrone in previously untreated low grade lymphomas. *Cancer Chemother and Pharmacol* 1988; 22: 77–9.

(190) Hansen MM, Hansen SW, Pedersen-Bjergaard, Nissen NI. Mitoxantrone in the treatment of chronic lymphocytic leukemia. *Leukemia and Lymphoma* 1992; 17: (in press).

(191) Piro LD, Carrera CJ, Beutler E, Carson DA. 2-Chlorodeoxyadenosine: an effective new agent for the treatment of chronic lymphocytic leukemia. *Blood* 1988; 72: 1069–73.

(192) Piro LD, Carrera CJ, Carson D, Beutler E. Lasting remission in hairy-cell leukemia induced by a single infusion of 2-chlorodeoxyadenosine. *N Engl J Med* 1990; 322: 1117–21.

(193) Cooper IA, Ding JC, Adams PB et al. Intensive leukapheresis in the management of cytopenias in patients with chronic lymphocytic lymphoma. *Am J Hematol* 1979; 6: 387–98.

(194) Goldfinger D, Capostagno V, Lowe C et al. Use of long-term leukapheresis in the treatment of chronic lymphocytic leukemia. *Transfusion* 1980; 20: 450–4.

(195) Marti GE, Folks T, Lingo DL et al. Therapeutic cytapheresis in chronic lymphocytic leukemia. *J Clin Apheresis* 1983; 1: 243–8.

(196) Adler S, Stutzman L, Sokal JE et al. Splenectomy for hematologic depression in lymphocytic lymphoma and leukemia. *Cancer* 1975; 35: 521–8.

(197) Meryl SA, Theodorakis ME, Goldberg J et al. Splenectomy for thrombocytopenia in chronic lymphocytic leukemia. *Am J Hematol* 1983; 15: 253–9.

(198) Montserrat E, Rosman C. Combination chemotherapy in chronic lymphocytic leukemia: a brief review. *Nouv Rev Franc Hematol* 1984; 26: 87–93.

(199) Raphael B, Silber R, Moore DF, Oken MM, Glick J. Survival duration and complete remission (CR) incidence in advanced chronic lymphocytic leukemia: a randomized ECOG study. *Blood* 1986; 68(Suppl 1): 229a.

(200) French Cooperative Group on CLL. A randomized comparison of chlorambucil and COP regimen in intermediate stage of chronic lymphocytic leukemia. *Blood* 1986; 68(Suppl 1): 218a.

(201) French Cooperative Group on CLL. Effectiveness of CHOP polychemotherapy in advanced untreated chronic lymphocytic leukemia: results from randomized clinical trial. *Blood* 1986; 68(Suppl): 219a.

(202) French Cooperative Group on CLL. Long-term results of the CHOP regimen in stage C chronic lymphocytic leukaemia. *Br J Hematol* 1989; 73: 334–40.

(203) Hansen MM. CHOP versus prednisolone + chlorambucil in chronic lymphocytic leukemia (CLL) preliminary results of a randomized multicenter study. *Nouv Rev Fr Hematol* 1988; 30: 433–6.

(204) Kempin S, Schiff R, Koziner B et al. *Blood* 1985; 66(Suppl. 1): 202a.

(205) Velasquez WS, McLaughlin P, Swan F et al. Dexamethasone, high dose ara-C and cisplatin (DHAP) combination for progressive chronic lymphocytic leukemia. *Blood* 1986; 68(Suppl 1): 234a.

Clinical and molecular aspects of Philadelphia chromosome positive acute lymphoblastic leukemia

C A WESTBROOK and W STOCK

Introduction

Advances in molecular biology have helped understanding of the molecular basis of the Philadelphia chromosome (Ph[1]) in myeloid and lymphoid leukemias. These studies have led to an improved understanding of the biology of these diseases and to better diagnostic methods; both have contributed to a deeper understanding of the clinical features of these diseases. In this chapter, the contributions of molecular biology to the understanding of Philadelphia chromosome positive acute lymphoblastic leukemia will be discussed.

The molecular basis of Ph[1] ALL

The Philadelphia chromosome was the first cytogenetic abnormality to be specifically associated with a cancer.[1] The molecular basis of this translocation was first elucidated by Heisterkamp and Groffen,[2] and now most clinical oncologists are familiar with its basic principles.[3,4]

The Ph[1] is formed by a reciprocal translocation between chromosomes 9 and 22, within the ABL proto-oncogene and the BCR gene, respectively. The translocation thus results in the BCR–ABL fusion gene, from which is transcribed the BCR–ABL fusion messenger RNA, and resultant chimeric protein. This chimeric protein of 210 kD (p210), is present in virtually every case of chronic myelogenous leukemia (CML), and is felt to be the cause of the disease. The detection of the BCR-ABL fusion gene, either cytogenetically as the Ph[1] chromosome, or by molecular methods, is now recognized to be an important diagnostic criteria for CML. In this review, we will use the terms BCR–ABL and Ph[1] interchangeably.

The Ph[1] is also seen in acute leukemias, both acute myeloid (AML) and

All correspondence to: Dr W Stock, 5841 S Maryland, MC2115, Chicago, Il, 60637, USA.

Cambridge Medical Reviews: Haematological Oncology Volume 2

acute lymphoblastic leukemia (ALL). In the acute leukemias, the BCR–ABL fusion can give rise to either the p210 typical of CML, or a smaller BCR–ABL fusion protein of 190 kilodaltons. The smaller protein species differs from the larger in that it contains less of the BCR gene because the breakpoint occurs further toward the 5' end of the gene.[5-9] This difference in gene structure cannot be detected cytogenetically, but is important to molecular diagnosis, as will be discussed below. Both proteins, like their normal ABL gene counterpart, and the closely related retroviral v-abl, are tyrosine kinases. The relative tyrosine kinase activity of the ABL fusion gene products correlates well with transforming ability; for example, the p190 is a more active tyrosine kinase than the p210, and is 100-fold more active in inducing transformed foci of rat fibroblast cells than the p210.[10]

Diagnosis of the BCR–ABL fusion gene in ALL

One of the major contributions of molecular biology to the clinical management of Ph[1] ALL is in the area of diagnosis. Better diagnostic tools have resulted in more accurate detection of this abnormality and in the specific detection of the p190 or p210 molecular subtypes.[11] Correlations between these parameters and clinical behavior can be made, resulting in improved monitoring of treatment and evaluation of residual disease.

Molecular diagnosis of the BCR–ABL fusion gene is now straightforward in CML, but it is still difficult in ALL.[12] Cytogenetic analysis is the standard diagnostic technique for detection of the Ph[1] in CML. In ALL, however, this technique often yields inadequate results because metaphases are difficult to obtain in lymphoid cells. This relatively low yield with cytogenetics contributes to a significant under-estimation of the prevalence of Ph[1] in adult ALL.[12]

The first molecular test for CML was based on the observation that breakpoints within the BCR gene tended to cluster, and could be detected as gene rearrangements on Southern analysis of DNA extracted from CML cells.[13] This test, now called the 'BCR rearrangement test' was found to be more sensitive than cytogenetics when the two methods were directly compared, as it could demonstrate the presence of a BCR–ABL fusion in up to 10% of cases which did not have a cytogenetically visible Ph[1].[14] While highly sensitive for detection of the p210 rearrangement, the BCR test is completely insensitive for the detection of the p190 molecular subtype. The p190 rearrangement is more difficult to detect because the locations of the breakpoints within the BCR gene occur over too wide an area for the probe to detect. While there are some areas of breakpoint clustering and new probes are being produced which can detect up to 80% of p190 cases,[15] Southern analysis is still limited in ALL. An alternative approach is to perform Southern analysis using pulsed field gel electrophoresis; this method produces restriction fragments much larger than those on the standard Southern blot, and enables one to survey the entire BCR gene for rearrangements.[16] In our experience, this method detects virtually all cases including both p190 and p210 subtypes, and is considerably more sensitive than cytogenetics.

The polymerase chain reaction (PCR), has become an important test in clinical CML[17] because of its rapidity and extreme sensitivity. Early experience with this method in ALL showed a high rate of false negatives,[18] but better selection of primer sequences has improved the sensitivity to close to 100%.[19] The PCR test may now be able to detect the BCR–ABL fusion product in one cell in 100,000, and will thus have an important role in the investigation of residual disease.

The most recent new diagnostic test for the BCR–ABL fusion is based on cytogenetics, using fluorescent probes for in situ hybridization. With probes labelled with two colors, red for ABL and green for BCR, the BCR–ABL fusion gene is easily detected as a red–green doublet in patient cells, either directly on metaphase spreads, or on interphase cells.[20,21] Recently, the addition of new probes has made it possible to distinguish the p190 from the p210.[22] The sensitivity of two color in situ hybridization has been reported to be about one in 100 cells. Because these probes detect the BCR–ABL fusion rather than the Ph[1], we are able to detect additional cases that would be missed using classical cytogenetics. The major advantage of this test is that it will allow the direct detection of the BCR–ABL fusion in individual non-dividing cells, including terminally differentiated cells in the peripheral circulation.

Biological activity of the BCR–ABL fusion genes

The biological activity of the p190 and the p210 have been studied in vitro and in vivo. BCR–ABL can transform direct cultures of murine bone marrow, although the resultant clones tend to be lymphoid, even under conditions favoring myeloid growth.[23,24] In these experiments, the transformed hematopoietic cells represent clonal or oligoclonal outgrowths from the mass population of infected cells, suggesting that additional events are required.

There is a particular interest in developing cellular and animal systems to model chronic phase CML. The models produced, however, more frequently resemble blast-transformed CML or acute leukemia than they do chronic phase CML, and will be useful for the study of Ph[1] ALL.

Early attempts to study the BCR–ABL fusion gene made use of transgenic animals. Hariharan et al. used a BCR–ABL construct which was under the control of the immunoglobulin gene enhancer, specifically restricting its expression to lymphoid cells. The resultant transgenic mice showed B-cell and T-cell neoplasms.[25] Use of the BCR–ABL p190 construct under conditions that were not lineage-restricted resulted in progeny that were either moribund or died of acute myeloid or lymphoid leukemia 10–58 days after birth.[26] These experiments demonstrate the ability of the BCR–ABL gene to cause acute transformation in lymphoid cells, but did not result in chronic phase CML.

More recently, model systems have used a 'reverse bone marrow transplant', in which murine bone marrow is infected with a retrovirus containing the BCR–ABL gene, then used to reconstitute lethally irradiated syngeneic mice. Using the p210 gene in this system, Daley et al. observed the development of three types of hematologic disease: a CML-like myeloproliferative syndrome, an acute lymphoblastic leukemia, and a malignant tumor that appeared to be of macrophage origin.[27] In a similar experiment Kelliher et al. produced some mice with myeloproliferative syndromes, as well as tumors of other lineages.[28] Elefanty et al. reported development of tumors of macrophage, erythroid, mast cell, and lymphoid lineages; but his animals did not develop a chronic myeloproliferative disorder.[29] In the Kelliher experiments, the spectrum of malignancy seen with the p190 was identical to that seen with the p210, although the time to transformation was shorter in the p190 group.

Experiments like these are helping us to better understand the molecular basis of neoplasia associated with the BCR–ABL genes. It is becoming apparent that transformation is a multistep process, with multiple genetic events being required. There is no evidence that p190 directs transformation of lymphoid cells and p210 of myeloid cells; on the contrary, the same spectrum of malignancies is seen with both, although the latency to acute transformation may be shorter with p190. When acute transformation is achieved, the transformed cells appear to be the same regardless of whether the p190 or p210 is the underlying event. This would predict that p190 and p210 Ph[1] ALL would have the same clinical behavior; at present, there is not enough clinical data available yet to assess whether the clinical features differ between the two.

Relationship of ALL to CML
The clinical relationship of Ph[1] ALL to lymphoid blast crisis of CML is not clear. It is simplistic to assume that all cases which contain the p210 were derived from CML, while those which contain the p190 arose de novo in lymphoid cells. Experience holds that some cases of Ph[1] ALL revert to chronic phase CML after treatment, and almost certainly arose within the context of CML. It has been possible to demonstrate the Ph[1] in the myeloid cells of some cases.[30] In other cases, the p210 protein was found to be restricted to lymphoid cells, with the stem cells being unaffected.[31] The results of the in vivo experiments presented above show that the p190 can transform both myeloid and lymphoid cells in model systems; thus the lineage of origin of p190 in human disease might be variable as well, although no one has yet demonstrated the presence of the p190 in myeloid cells of ALL. What is at issue is whether the BCR–ABL fusion arose in a

160

hematopoietic stem cell capable of repopulating the marrow; such a finding may be important for treatment decisions for an individual patient, especially if autologous transplant or marrow purging techniques are considered. Current molecular techniques would be capable of answering this question if properly applied to individual cases, but it is difficult to generalize at the present time.

Clinical features of Ph¹ ALL

Pediatric ALL

The Ph chromosome is uncommon in childhood ALL. Estimates of incidence range from 2.3 to 5.7%.[32-34] Its presence, unfortunately, signifies an extremely poor prognosis in a disease that is often curable with today's therapy. The most comprehensive description of the clinical features of childhood Ph¹ ALL is given by Crist et al., based on a large consecutive series of over 3000 cases enrolled on Pediatric Oncology Group (POG) protocols.[34] In this series, successful cytogenetics were available for 2516 cases (70% of children enrolled), of which 58 (2.3%) showed the Ph¹. The cases were all identified cytogenetically; no molecular studies were performed. Compared to cases which did not contain the Ph¹, these patients had higher leukocyte counts (median, 33 × 10 9/L vs 12, P = .002), older age (9.6 yrs vs 4.8 yrs, median, P <.001), a higher proportion of L2 morphology (by FAB criteria) and a lower frequency of mediastinal mass. Immunologic marker studies showed that most cases were of B-lineage, which probably explains the low incidence of mediastinal mass (which is usually associated with T-cell leukemias); 75% were early pre-B, and 16% were pre-B; only 9% were T-cell.

Early studies suggested that the Ph¹ carries an especially poor prognosis in childhood ALL.[35] This impression is confirmed by recent studies.[34,36] In the Dana Farber Cancer Institute/Boston Children's Hospital program, complete remission was successful in 99% of Ph¹ negative cases, but in only 80% of Ph¹ positive cases (P = .003). Four year event-free survival and overall survivals were 81% and 88%, respectively, in 419 Ph¹− children, but only 0% and 20% in the 15 children with Ph¹. This poor outcome was notable because of the use of intensive therapeutic approaches that resulted in excellent event-free survival for other high-risk patients.[37] Similarly, the POG study[34] reported a CR rate of 78% vs. 96%, for Ph¹ positive and Ph¹ negative cases, respectively, and event free survival was much worse in the Ph¹ positive cases regardless of the treatment regimen (P =<.001, combined data not given). Most relapses occurred within 2 years of remission. Of 7 cases who entered remission and subsequently received allogeneic transplantation, only 3 have extended survival, 3 having died of recurrent disease.

The Ph[1] in adult ALL

The impact of the Ph[1] on adult ALL is only now being appreciated. Though earlier studies suggested an incidence of about 20% in adults, the use of improved molecular methods shows that fully one-third of all adults with ALL may have this genetic abnormality.[12] In a recent study of 56 consecutive cases of adults with ALL entered on treatment protocols for CALGB,[38] 17 were identified with the BCR–ABL fusion using molecular diagnosis (Southern blot and pulsed field electrophoresis); cytogenetics detected only 12 cases with the Ph[1] in the same group. Of 15 cases that were immunophenotyped, 11 showed a B-lineage phenotype, with a small number being mixed, myeloid, or undifferentiated; there were no T-cell cases. FAB subtypes of the BCR–ABL positive and negative groups were similar. There were no significant differences seen in the age, sex, or presenting blood counts of the BCR–ABL positive and BCR–ABL negative cases. There was a complete absence of mediastinal mass, and a relative lack of lymphadenopathy in the BCR–ABL positive group compared to the BCR–ABL negative group, though not statistically significant. As in childhood ALL, this probably represents a lack of T-cell cases in the group.

In these cases of adult ALL, the overall complete remission rate was 73%, as aggressive multiagent chemotherapy was used.[39] Interestingly, the rate of achieving complete remission is virtually the same for both the BCR–ABL positive and negative cases, 71% and 74%, respectively. It appears, however, that relapse occurs much earlier in the BCR–ABL positive group, with a median remission duration of only 10.2 months, compared to a median duration of remission that has yet not been achieved in the BCR–ABL negative group ($P = 0.16$, log rank). The BCR–ABL positive group also has a shorter median survival (11.2 vs 19.4 months), though statistical significance has not yet been achieved ($P = 0.27$, log rank). It is difficult to associate a poor prognosis with the Ph[1] in adult ALL, in part because the comparison group, those without the Ph[1], includes many other patients in poor prognostic cytogenetic subsets. If, however, the comparison group is limited, it is found that the BCR–ABL has an important prognostic impact in certain subgroups such as in B-lineage cases (median remission duration of 10.2 months was shorter for these B-lineage, BCR–ABL positive patients than it was for the BCR–ABL negative patients whose median has not yet been reached, $P=0.38$) or in CALLA positive cases (8.1 months for BCR–ABL positive vs median not reached for BCR–ABL negative $P=0.013$, log rank) and survival (11.1 months for BCR–ABL positive vs. median not reached for BCR–ABL negative, $P=0.055$, log rank).

Although the Ph[1] chromosome is not the only indicator of poor prognosis in adult ALL, its high incidence, combined with the poor outcome associated with its presence, suggests that it is one of the main factors responsible for the poor clinical behavior of adult ALL.

Are pediatric and adult Ph¹ ALL the same disease?

The above comparisons point out many similarities between childhood and adult Ph¹ positive ALL. These similarities are often obscured because the background of Ph¹ negative cases differs greatly between the two age groups, and the incidence differs as well. The clinical features of the two groups appear to be very similar. The immunophenotype of the cells is predomi-nantly B-lineage in both groups, which is reflected in the absence of mediastinal mass and adenopathy. Outcome is also consistently similar: remission rates with intensive therapy are in the 75% range in both children and adults, but remission duration is short and early relapse is the rule. The molecular features of childhood and adult ALL are also the same. Though it was initially felt that the p210, or CML-like translocation, is more common in adults and the p190 more common in children,[40] careful prospective studies have shown that the primary molecular subtype in both groups is p190: 23% p210 and 77% p190 were found in adult ALL[38] which compares well with 15% p210 and 85% p190 reported in pediatric ALL by Suryanarayan[19] using PCR methods. These molecular and clinical findings underscore the relationship of adult to pediatric Ph¹ positive ALL, and suggest that the two diseases are more similar to each other than they are to other types of ALL in the same age-groups.

Implications for treatment

The treatment of children with standard-risk ALL has made considerable progress over the last few years. (No attempt here will be made exhaustively to review the literature of ALL treatment, which is covered in great detail in general oncology textbooks, and in reference 41). The combination of vincristine and prednisone induces remission in over 90% of cases, while addition of L-asparaginase or an anthracycline such as daunorubicin or doxorubicin extends duration and improves disease-free survival, such that some subgroups of children, particularly those with good cytogenetic findings, can be considered cured of their disease. Ph¹ ALL has traditionally fared poorly with these regimens.[32,33]

Recently, two groups reported the use of very intensive therapy for children with poor prognosis ALL, including multi-drug schemes and prolonged treatment.[34,37] These studies resulted in improved survival for many cytogenetic subgroups which were previously considered high risk, such as the t(1;19). However, Ph¹ positive ALL uniformly fared badly, with higher failure of induction and early relapse. Virtually the only patients with prolonged survival were those who went on to allogeneic transplantation.

As a group, adults fare worse than children with ALL. This is partly due to poor treatment tolerance with advancing age, but also because they include a disproportionate number of poor prognosis cytogenetic subgroups. Intensification of treatment has led to improved survival in some subgroups.[42,43]

These more intensive protocols use multiple active drugs in various combinations, doses, and schedules for induction, followed by maintenance therapy for as long as 2 to 3 years, and are comparable to protocols used for high risk children. As discussed above, such protocols had little impact on Ph[1] positive ALL in adults.

Conclusions

Current intensive, multiagent chemotherapy is inadequate for achieving long-term remission of Ph[1] ALL in any age-group. Maintenance of remission is especially difficult in these groups. Both Fletcher et al. and Crist et al. recommended that children with ALL be identified early, treated with agressive induction, and go on to allogeneic transplantation.[34,36] In adults, the same recommendation might be made. Forman et al.[44] have reported on the outcome of 10 adults who received allogeneic bone marrow transplantation for Ph[1] ALL. Four patients died of transplant-related complications, but 6 patients achieved a complete remission with a reported median survival of 19 months. No relapses were reported. The results of this early study are encouraging and future studies to determine the efficacy of allogeneic bone marrow transplantation in Ph[1] adults in first remission are recommended.

Allogeneic transplantation, however, is often not an option. In these instances, treatment alternatives range from palliation to highly experimental approaches. It is intriguing to consider a role for highly experimental treatment in Ph[1] ALL. With continued advances in molecular biology of the BCR–ABL genes come experimental methods to specifically reverse its effects, and relapsed Ph[1] ALL, which is highly resistant to drug treatment or transplantation, might be considered an ideal setting in which to implement new approaches.

Ideally, all new treatment studies should be combined with close monitoring by molecular methods; such monitoring will help to elucidate the effects of treatment and the extent of residual disease, confirm remission, and predict relapse. Continued use of molecular diagnosis in the clinical setting will help to better elucidate the biology and clinical features of Ph[1] positive ALL, and improve our care of patients with this disease.

References

(1) Nowell PC, Hungerford DA. A minute chromosome in human chronic granulocytic leukemia. *J Natl Cancer Inst* 1960; 25: 85–109.
(2) Heisterkamp N, Stephenson JR, Groffen J et al. Localization of the c-abl oncogene adjacent to a translocation breakpoint in chronic myelocytic leukemia. *Nature* 1983; 306: 765–7.
(3) Kurzrock R, Gutterman JU, Talpaz M. The molecular genetics of Philadelphia chromosome-positive leukemias. *New Eng J Med* 1988; 319: 990–8.
(4) Westbrook CA. The ABL oncogene in human leukemias. *Blood Rev* 1988; 2: 1–8.

(5) Hermans A, Heisterkamp N, Von Lindernn M et al. Unique fusion of bcr and c-abl genes in Philadelphia-chromosome acute lymphoblastic leukemia. *Cell* 1987; 51: 33–40.

(6) Rubin CM, Carrino JJ, Dickler MN, Leibowitz D, Smith SD, Westbrook CA. Heterogeneity of genomic fusion of BCR–ABL in Philadelphia chromosome-positive acute lymphoblastic leukemia. *Proc Natl Acad Sci USA* 1988; 85: 2795–9.

(7) Fainstein E, Marcelle C, Rosner A et al. A new fused transcript in Philadelphia chromosome positive acute lymphoblastic leukemia. *Nature* 1987; 330: 386–8.

(8) Clark SS, McLaughlin J, Crist WM, Champlin R, Witte OLN. Unique forms of the abl tyrosine kinase distinguish Ph^1-positive CML from Ph^1-positive ALL. *Science* 1987; 235: 85–7.

(9) Kurzrock R, Shtalrid M, Romero P et al. A novel c-abl protein product in Philadelphia-positive acute lymphoblastic leukemia. *Nature* 1987; 325: 631–5.

(10) Lugo TG, Pendergast M-M, Muller J, Witte ON. Tyrosine kinase activity and transformation potency of bcr–abl oncogene products. *Science* 1990; 247: 1079–81.

(11) Hooberman AL, Westbrook CA. Molecular Diagnosis of the Philadelphia Chromosome in Acute Lymphoblastic Leukemia. *Leukemia and Lymphoma* 1989; 1: 3–10.

(12) Hooberman AH, Westbrook CA, Davey F et al. Molecular detection of the Philadelphia chromosome in adult lymphoblastic leukemia. *Blood* 1989; 74: 769.

(13) Groffen J, Stephenson JR, Heisterkamp N et al. Philadelphia chromosomal breakpoints are clustered within a limited region, bcr, on chromosome 22. *Cell* 1984; 36: 93–9.

(14) Blennerhasset GT, Furth M, Anderson A et al. Clinical evaluation of a DNA probe assay for the Philadelphia (Ph^1) translocation in chronic myelogenous leukemia. *Leukemia* 1988; 2: 648–57.

(15) Goldman JM, Grosveld G, Baltimore D, Gale RP. Chronic myelogenous leukemia – the unfolding saga. *Leukemia* 1990; 4: 163–7.

(16) Hooberman AL, Rubin CM, Barton KP, Westbrook CA. Detection of the Philadelphia chromosome in acute lymphoblastic leukemia by pulsed-field gel electrophoresis. *Blood* 1989; 74: 1101–7.

(17) Kawasaki ES, Clark SS, Coyne MY, Smith SD, Champlin R, Witte ON, McCor-mich FP. Diagnosis of chronic myeloid and acute lymphocytic leukemias by detection of leukemia-specific mRNA sequences amplified in vitro. *Proc Natl Acad Sci USA* 1988; 85: 5898–702.

(18) Hooberman AL, Carino JJ, Leibowitz D et al. Unexpected heterogeneity of BCR–ABL fusion mRNA detected by polymerase chain reaction in Philadelphia chromosome-positive acute lymphoblastic leukemia. *Proc Natl Acad Sci USA* 1989; 86: 4259–63.

(19) Suryanarayan K, Hunger SP, Kohler S et al. Consistent involvement of the BCR gene by 9;22 breakpoints in pediatric acute leukemias. *Blood* 1991; 77: 324–30.

(20) Tkachuk DC, Westbrook CA, Andreef M et al. Detection of bcr–abl fusion in chronic myelogenous leukemia by in situ hybridization. *Science* 1990; 250: 539–62.

C A Westbrook and W Stock

(21) Arnoldus EPJ, Weigant J, Noordermeer IA et al. Detection of the Philadelphia chromosome in interphase nuclei. *Cytogenet Cell Genet* 1990; 54: 108–11.
(22) Yaremko ML, Westbrook CA, Hooberman AH. Rapid diagnosis of the Philadelphia chromosome in acute lymphoblastic leukemia by direct DNA fluorescence in situ hybridization. *Am Assn for Cancer Res* 1991; 32: 164.
(23) McLaughlin J, Chianese E, Witte ON. In vitro transformation of immature hematopoietic cells by the p210 BCR/ABL oncogene product of the Philadelphia chromosome. *Proc Natl Acad Sci USA* 1987; 84: 6558–62.
(24) Young YC, Witte ON. Selective transformation of primitive lymphoid cells by the BCR–ABL oncogene expressed in long-term lymphoid or myeloid cultures. *Mol Cell Biol* 1988; 8: 4079–87.
(25) Hariharan IK, Harris AW, Crawford M et al. A bcr-v-abl oncogene induces lymphomas in transgenic mice. *Mol Cell Biol* 1989; 9: 2798–805.
(26) Heisterkamp N, Jenster G, ten Hoeve J, Zovich D, Pattengale PK, Groffen J. Acute leukemia in bcr/abl transgenic mice. *Nature* 1990; 344: 251–3.
(27) Daley GQ, Van Etten RA, Baltimore D. Induction of chronic myelogenous leukemia in mice by the p210$^{bcr/abl}$ gene of the Philadelphia chromosome. *Science* 1990; 247: 824–30.
(28) Kelliher MA, McLauthlin J, Witte ON, Rosenberg N. Induction of chronic myelogenous leukemia-like syndrome in mice with v-abl and BCR/ABL. *Proc Natl Acad Sci USA* 1990; 87: 6649–53.
(29) Elefanty AG, Hariharan IK, Cory S. bcr–abl, the hallmark of chronic myeloid leukaemia in man, produces multiple haemotpoietic neoplasms in mice. *EMBO J* 1990; 9: 1069–78.
(30) Turhan AG, Eaves CJ, Kalousek DK, Eaves AC, Humphries RK: Molecular analysis of clonality and bcr rearrangements in philadelphia chromosome-positive acute lymphoblastic leukemia. *Blood* 1988; 71: 1495.
(31) Secker-Walker LM, Cooke HMG, Browett PJ, Shippey CA, Norton JD, Corestan-Smith E, Hoffbrant AV. Variable Philadelphia breakpoints and potential lineage restriction of bcr rearrangement in acute lymphoblastic leukemia. *Blood* 1988; 72: 784.
(32) Third International Workshop on Chromosomes in Leukemia: Chromosomal abnormalities and their clinical significance in acute lymphoblastic leukemia. *Cancer Res* 1983; 43: 8686.
(33) Ribiero RC, Abromowitch M, Raimondi SC, Murphy SB, Behm F, Williams DL. Clinical and biologic hallmarks of the Philadelphia chromosome in childhood acute lymphoblastic leukemia. *Blood* 1990; 70: 948.
(34) Crist W, Carroll A, Shuster J et al. Philadelphia chromosome positive childhood acute lymphoblastic leukemia: clinical and cytogenetic characteristics and treatment outcome. A Pediatric Oncology Group Study. *Blood* 1990; 76: 486–94.
(35) Bloomfield CD, Goldman AI et al. Chromosomal abnormalities identify high-risk and low-risk patients with acute lymphoblastic leukemia. *Blood* 1986; 67: 415–20.
(36) Fletcher JA, Lynch EA, Kimball VM, Donnelly M, Tantravahi R, Sallan SE. Translocation (9;22) is associated with extremely poor prognosis in intensively treated children wtih acute lymphoblastic leukemia. *Blood* 1991; 77: 435–9.
(37) Fletcher JA, Kimball VM, Lynch E, Donnelly M, Pavelka K, Gelber RD,

Tantravahi R, Sallan SE. Prognostic implications of cytogenetic studies in an intensively treated group of children with acute lymphoblastic leukemia. *Blood* 1989; 74: 2130–5.

(38) Westbrook CA, and Hooberman AH, manuscript in preparation.

(39) Larson RA. Acute leukemia in adults. In: Rakel RE, ed. *Conn's current therapy*, 1991. Philadelphia, WB Saunders, 1991: 352–7.

(40) Bartram CR. Rearrangement of the c-abl and bcr genes in Ph-negative CML and Ph-positive acute leukemias. *Leukemia* 1988; 2: 63–4.

(41) Champlin R, Gale RP. Acute lymphoblastic leukemia: recent advances in biology and therapy. *Blood* 1989; 73: 2051–66.

(42) Radford JE, Jr, Burns CP, Jones MP et al. Adult acute lymphoblastic leukemia: results of the Iowa HOP-L Protocol. *J Clin Oncol* 1989; 7: 58–66.

(43) Kantarjian HM, Walters RS, Keating MJ et al. Results of the vincristine, doxorubicin, and dexamethasone regimen in adults with standard and high-risk acute lymphoblastic leukemia. *J Clin Oncol* 1990; 8: 994–1004.

(44) Forman SJ, O'Donnell MR, Nademanee AP et al. Bone marrow transplantation for patients with philadelphia chromosome-positive acute lymphoblastic leukemia. *Blood* 1987; 70: 587–8.

Bone marrow transplantation in the management of advanced Hodgkin's disease

G L PHILLIPS, D E REECE and J M CONNORS

Introduction

During the past decade, myeloablative therapy and bone marrow transplantation (BMT) – either allogeneic (Allo) or autologous (Au), but especially the latter – has been employed increasingly for the treatment of certain Hodgkin's disease (HD) patients.[1] To understand the role of BMT in the therapy of HD, it is important to appreciate the impact of current conventional therapy, specifically 7–8 drug regimens such as MOPP/ABVD (mechlorethamine, vincristine [Oncovin], procarbazine, prednisone/doxorubicin [Adriamycin], bleomycin, vinblastine, dacarbazine) and MOPP/ABV 'Hybrid' in the therapy of patients with disseminated HD. Recently, we have reviewed the results of 165 such patients, aged 16–65, who were treated in Vancouver with MOPP/ABV Hybrid between 1980 and 1989. An initial CR was achieved by 158 (93%); the actuarial failure-free survival (FFS) was 72% at 8 years. There were only 3 toxic deaths (1.8%), and only the presence of 'B' symptoms at diagnosis was identified as a negative prognostic feature for FFS, although even patients with B symptoms had an FFS of 62%.[2] Conversely, patients who fail such regimens are occasionally curable with alternative therapies (containing putatively noncross-resistant agents).[3] In contrast with these results are those of numerous series[1,4] suggesting a durable CR rate of >30% in similar patients following BMT in this situation. Nevertheless, it is at least possible that patient selection influences these results to a degree, and a formal randomized trial may be necessary to demonstrate the relative effectiveness of each modality.

In any case, the above results indicate the likely superiority of BMT regimens, and the task for the clinical investigator in this area is now to ensure the availability of BMT for all suitable HD patients, to define optimal patient selection and timing criteria, to develop better methods of ridding the patient

All correspondence to: Dr GL Phillips, Leukemia/Bone Marrow Transplantation Program of British Columbia, Vancouver General Hospital, 910 West 10th Avenue, Vancouver, BC, V5Z 4E3, Canada.

Cambridge Medical Reviews: Haematological Oncology Volume 2
© Cambridge University Press 1992

of HD and to do so with minimal toxicity. The latter consideration involves both increasing the therapeutic index of current cytotoxic regimens and choosing an optimal source of hematopoietic stem cell (HSC) support.

Issues

The critical issues regarding BMT for HD include patient selection, timing considerations, cytoreduction (especially in vivo and, for AuBMT, potentially ex vivo as well) and source of HSC. For the reasons discussed below, the majority of BMTs in HD have been performed using AuBMT, and this chapter is 'weighted' with that fact in mind. Stimulation of marrow recovery by hematopoietic growth factors (usually following, but potentially in lieu of, BMT) is an additional topic of increasing relevance, and clearly influences certain of the above issues. Finally, the economic consequences of BMT will be considered in general terms.

Patient selection and timing considerations

The question of optimal timing for BMT is important, and is often discussed in relationship to considerations of conditioning regimens. In this regard, it is useful to remember that although the AuBMT procedure depends entirely, and the AlloBMT partially, on the conditioning regimen for resultant anti-tumor effects, the degree of dose escalation achieved with many of these drugs used in current conditioning regimens is usually less than anticipated.[5] It is naive to expect these regimens to reliably rescue patients from HD refractory to conventional chemotherapy – it is much more likely that AuBMT regimens will be most successful in a group of patients having at least a degree of curability with conventional dose therapy.

It is easiest to consider the issue of timing in terms of disease status. While an evaluation of disease status is only an estimate of the extent, bulk, and especially the degree of chemoresistance and cumulative toxicity due to prior therapy, it is usually the simplest assay of these parameters. In theory, BMT may be used: 1) as initial therapy; 2) after primary therapy has failed to produce CR; 3) during an initial CR; 4) after relapse, in the place of conventional salvage therapy; and 5) after relapse, following the use of conventional salvage therapy. As noted previously, the influence of primary therapy is potentially very important; for this discussion, we will assume that current optimal primary chemotherapy consists of 7–8 drug regimens, as indicated in several recent trials.[6–8] If less effective primary therapy (such as MOPP or ABVD alone) is used, the role of BMT may be altered, as salvage chemotherapy in standard dose has (at least in some series) been variably effective[9] and the optimal timing of BMT is more controversial.

BMT regimens could be used as initial therapy in HD patients. This approach would have the practical advantage of shortening the treatment duration and the theoretical advantages of minimizing the development of drug resistance and cumulative hematologic and nonhematologic toxicity.

However, it seems unlikely that the use of only a single course of current myeloablative regimens would be much more successful than conventional therapy using the current regimens. The use of more than one BMT procedure is possible (as discussed below) but difficult. Even if BMT regimens were more effective (e.g. by reducing the failure rate by half), a randomized trial of more than 400 patients would be needed to substantiate this point. Using BMT as primary therapy also neglects the potential of conventional therapy to produce a minimal residual disease state and to exploit the putative noncross-resistance of these modalities. It would also be more toxic and more expensive. All in all, it is most unlikely that BMT will replace regimens such as MOPP/ABV Hybrid as primary therapy in HD patients.

Of course, not all patients who are treated with MOPP/ABV Hybrid achieve an initial CR. However, the difficulty is frequently in determining the degree of residual tumor, as radiologically evident residual masses may merely be composed of fibronecrotic material and available diagnostic testing may not be helpful.[10] In any case, patients who are left with radiologically evident viable HD usually progress within a short time, and no significant difference in long-term outcome has been found between those transplanted with less than a CR vs those treated for early relapse (< 1 year after completion of primary chemotherapy).[11]

The use of myeloablative therapy and BMT as consolidation therapy, a frequent strategy for other diseases, is appealing, particularly in patients with poor prognostic signs at diagnosis. While such use of BMT is very likely to produce a decreased rate of relapse, the attendant toxicity may minimize potential gains. For instance, a reduction in the relapse rate by 50% using MOPP/ABV Hybrid followed by BMT (compared with Hybrid alone) could potentially increase the number of cured patients by 10% (50% of the relapses after Hybrid alone would be prevented); however, if the toxic death rate produced is increased to even 5%, curability increases to only 75% from 70%. Considered only in those patients more likely to relapse (as determined in our experience by the presence of B symptoms at diagnosis), if the 20–25% relapse rate could be reduced by 50%, even with a 5% mortality due to toxicity, 70% of patients could be cured, as opposed to the 60% cured by the primary chemotherapy alone. Again, a convincing demonstration of this gain would be difficult, likely requiring a randomized clinical trial, and even such a trial could be complicated in its interpretation by the fact that relapses in a conventional therapy arm could be successfully salvaged with BMT regimens.

Experience using AuBMT during an initial CR has been reported by Carella et al.[12]; 15 patients with an anticipated high risk of relapse despite attaining an initial CR following MOPP/ABVD received a CBV regimen (i.e. cyclophosphamide, BCNU [carmustine] and VP16–213 [etoposide]) and AuBMT 9–13 months after CR was achieved. At the time of their report, 13 patients were alive in CR at a median of 36 months (range 10–64 months) after AuBMT; 1 patient relapsed and another died of interstitial pneumonitis. In their historical experience using MOPP/ABVD alone, only 8 of 24 such patients (33%) would be expected to be in continuous CR at this time. Although interesting, these results are not altogether surprising; a critical point is the verification of the outcome with conventional therapy in poor prognosis patients, a feature that can be addressed most definitively in a randomized trial.

In more advanced disease states, the optimal time to employ BMT with curative intent is likely at the first sign of recurrence or progression after exposure to 7–8 drug induction therapy. This strategy will expose only a very few patients who could be cured with conventional salvage regimens to the inherent risks of BMT, while later use would increase the probability of the presence of resistant tumor cells and increase cumulative hematologic and nonhematologic toxicity. Also, if one awaits the more advanced disease status with which the use of additional salvage therapy is usually associated, then it is inevitable that patients will be lost before BMT can be undertaken.

However, data from various AuBMT studies[13–17] support this postulate only indirectly. These results should not be taken to indicate the lack of validity of this recommendation, however, as virtually all of these studies indicated some advantage for patients with less advanced disease status. The lack of statistical significance may be related to the limited statistical power associated with small sample size and/or heterogeneity in the untreated initial relapse group. Such heterogeneity regarding both the quantity and degree of chemoresistance of the residual tumor burden – and possibly the biological aggressiveness of the HD at the time of relapse or proven persistence – is not easily quantified, and must be evaluated by indirect (i.e. clinical) methods. To this end, we have evaluated the factors which predict for efficacy of salvage therapy for British Columbia HD patients in first relapse after primary chemotherapy. Not unexpectedly, the predictors of success of the salvage therapy are indicators of a lower tumor burden and, perhaps, reduced biological aggressiveness of the tumor and include: 1) less than Stage IV disease at the time of primary diagnosis, 2) longer than one year's duration of CR after the end of primary chemotherapy[11], and 3) the absence of B symptoms at relapse. Although myeloablative chemoradiotherapy and BMT was the only treatment effective in the presence of one or more of these negative prognostic factors, its effectiveness in this group was substantially less than in patients who lacked such characteristics. Therefore, the close association between tumor burden and efficacy of BMT argues strongly for use of such treatment in the overall management of HD as soon as it becomes clear that the primary chemotherapy will not cure the disease. Methods to produce more effective cytoreduction can be focused on such patients.

Despite the absence of randomized clinical trials indicating the superiority of AuBMT regimens compared with conventional salvage chemotherapy, the favorable effects of AuBMT regimens in HD patients not cured by optimal conventional regimens, plus the ability to perform AuBMT in most patients ≤ 60 years of age (~80% of HD patients) indicates that such therapy may none the less be considered a standard approach. (As discussed below, data from the authors' center suggest that patient selection is not a major factor regarding the differences in results between these two modalities.) If so, the simplest goal may be identification of those patients curable with additional conventional therapy, in whom BMT is therefore not indicated. It is believed that only one group clearly falls into this category: those few patients potentially curable with radiotherapy following the failure of 7–8 drug primary chemotherapy. This group can be identified by the absence of B symptoms at the time of relapse, the degree to which the relapsed disease is confined to nodal sites and relapse occurring more than a year after completion of primary chemotherapy.[11] Therefore, other than obvious comorbid illness, there appear to be few obvious contraindications to the use of AuBMT regimens for HD. This is borne out by local experience; of 25 British Columbia patients (during the years 1985 to 1988) aged ≤60 years who were eligible for AuBMT by virtue of not being cured with Hybrid, only 3 were not transplanted. In 2 of these cases, the decision not to perform AuBMT was due to patient refusal (of any therapy), while in the other an initial misdiagnosis of large cell lymphoma and inappropriate chemotherapy prompted the use of Hybrid chemotherapy as salvage treatment. Interestingly, none of these patients had documented bone marrow involvement at the time of protocol entry. Therefore, virtually all of these patients could have undergone AuBMT. If such therapy is not administered at the first sign of incurability with conventional chemotherapy, it is likely that fewer patients will be eligible for AuBMT.

In vivo cytoreduction

There is little doubt regarding the importance of optimal cytoreduction by cytotoxic agents – especially in the AuBMT setting – in producing the bulk of observed antitumor effects. There is strong evidence supporting the use of escalated dose cytotoxic therapy, specifically, for ionizing radiotherapy as well as single and multiagent conventional dose chemotherapy.[18–21]

There are a number of considerations regarding the construction of conditioning regimens for HD. Firstly, the agents employed should be active in conventional dose, and even more effective in escalated dose.[22] Secondly, drugs should be selected such that severe overlapping nonhematologic toxicity is avoided. Thirdly, agents should be selected to minimize the presence of extreme tumor resistance. This usually involves choosing drugs to which the patient is unlikely to have been exposed (a consideration also related to resistance) or which have specific pharmacologic or perhaps synergistic considerations. (It should be noted in passing that very few studies have used AuBMT to support a conditioning regimen composed entirely of multiple myelosuppressive agents in conventional dose; however, the use of agents in conventional dose added to augmented-dose agents is relatively common.)[4]

Finally, the BMT patient must be considered as representing a paradoxical relationship between the disease status (especially but not exclusively considering prior treatment history) and BMT-related toxicity, in that those patients with more advanced disease are precisely those who require more potent cytoreduction – but are less likely to be able to tolerate the resultant side effects.[23] Accordingly, if an untested regimen is assessed in very heavily pretreated patients, excessive nonhematologic toxicity may produce a high treatment-related death rate and give an overestimate of the regimen's toxicity – and an underestimate of its usefulness – compared with a less heavily treated population.

Given these considerations, the alkylating agents (as a class) are the agents probably best suited to BMT, and the specific alkylating agents that are the most attractive for inclusion into conditioning regimens for HD include the chloroethylnitrosoureas, melphalan, carboplatin and thio-TEPA; cyclophosphamide may also be useful (despite the widespread use of mechlorethamine in primary regimens), both for cytoreduction and especially when immunosuppression is needed for allogeneic BMT. Also, other agents (e.g. cisplatin, cytarabine, etoposide, etc.) may be considered in certain cases.

Although the use of BMT involves the use of myeloablative therapy, it should be remembered that conventional-dose cytotoxic therapy (both chemo- and radiotherapy) is frequently used near the time of BMT and may influence post-BMT outcome. Therefore, the following discussion has been divided into sections on myeloablative therapy (i.e. conditioning regimens) and nonmyeloablative therapy that may be a useful adjunct to myeloablative therapy. (The term myeloablative is used with the full realization that true myeloablation is not universally observed with current regimens,[24] but the term will be used herein to refer to therapy in which stem cell support is utilized, and will be used in preference to the term intensive – which is admittedly no more descriptive, but has been used to describe therapy in which stem cell support is not utilized.)

Myeloablative conditioning regimens
Although the combination of cyclophosphamide and total body irradiation (TBI) is frequently used as conditioning for many hematologic malignancies,[25] this regimen has been used infrequently in HD patients undergoing BMT,[4] probably due to the increased incidence of pulmonary toxicity noted in patients previously exposed to thoracic radiotherapy who receive conditioning with TBI.[26] However, regimens including TBI may be both safe and effective in patients who have not had prior mediastinal radiotherapy,[16,27,28] except perhaps in the situation of end-stage HD.[29] The majority of patients have received conditioning regimens consisting of myeloablative combination chemotherapy alone, most of which are derivations of BACT (carmustine [BCNU], arabinosyl cytosine [ara-C], cyclophos-

174

phamide and thioguanine) developed at the NCI nearly 20 years ago.[30] As indicated in Table 1 in a simplified fashion, the most popular combination of drugs, cyclophosphamide, carmustine (BCNU) and etoposide (VP16–213) – CBV – has been used in varying doses and schedules: Wheeler et al.[31] have performed a Phase I study of this combination and suggested that the BCNU dose is critical regarding pulmonary toxicity. The popularity of this regimen probably is due to activity of these drugs as single agents, the infrequency of use of these agents in primary chemotherapy regimens, and the relatively low degree of overlapping nonhematologic toxicity of the combination.

In the absence of comparative trials, it is most difficult to accurately assess the relative superiority of the various CBV regimens. That said, it may be observed that the various CBV regimens can be roughly divided into two groups, those using higher versus those using lower (i.e. more conventional) doses of all agents (especially VP16–213 and to a lesser degree, BCNU). Although only the roughest comparison can be made, it does appear that the antilymphoma effects are greater with the higher-dose regimens, but that, as expected, toxicity is also increased.[33] In any case, the high-dose regimen should be used primarily in those patients likely to survive and benefit from its use – namely, less heavily pretreated patients.

The other BACT variant to be widely used is carmustine (BCNU), etoposide (VP16–213), cytarabine (ara-C) and melphalan – BEAM. This regimen has many of the features of CBV and combines high dose intravenous melphalan[34] and high dose carmustine,[35] single agents shown to produce durable CR in the AuBMT setting.

Whether or not the CBV and BEAM regimens could be improved by further manipulation of these agents or by the addition or substitution of other cytotoxic agents is unknown, but modifications should be evaluated (despite the difficulty in so doing) as all of these regimens fail to cure a substantial fraction of patients. Also, other standard conditioning regimens should be considered for clinical testing; for example, Jones et al.[16] have reported that the combination of busulfan and cyclophosphamide (cumulative doses of 16 mg/kg and 200 mg/kg, respectively) originally developed to treat acute myelogenous leukemia[36] is active in BMT regimens for HD as well. This is somewhat surprising, as busulfan is not considered an active agent in standard therapy for HD[37] and it is unlikely that cyclophosphamide alone could produce satisfactory results.

A somewhat different strategy is that of the sequential use of two conditioning regimens and AuBMTs. This approach potentially allows the use of a greater number of cytotoxic agents in augmented dose and has been employed by Ahmed et al.,[32] who used a CBV-like regimen followed by a second regimen consisting of agents less frequently used in conditioning regimens, namely vinblastine, cytarabine (or thio-TEPA), mitoxantrone and carboplatin. These results require further evaluation.

Table 1. Reported conditioning regimens in autologous bone marrow transplantation studies for Hodgkin's disease

Author (reference)	ARA-C (mg/m²)	BCNU (mg/m²)/(mg/kg)	CDDP (mg/m²)	CY (mg/m²)/(mg/kg)	MEL (mg/m²)	VP16-213 (mg/m²)/(mg/kg)
Carella[13] (1988)	–	600/-	–	-/150	–	600/-
Jagannath[14] (1989)	–	300/-	–	6000/-	–	600–900/-
Gribben[15] (1989)	800–1600	300/-	–	–	140	400–800/-
Russell[34] (1989)	–	–	–	–	140–220	–
Wheeler[a][31] (1990)	–	450/-	–	7200/-	–	2000/-
Harden[b][76] (1990)	–	600/-	–	7200/-	–	2400/-
Horning[28] (1991)	–	-/15	–	-/100	–	-/60
Ahmed[c][32] (1991)	–	400–600/-	–	5000/-	–	1800/-
Lazarus[77] (1991)	–	600–1050/-	200	–	–	2400–3000/-
Reece[d][17] (1991)	–	600	–	7200/-	–	2400/-
Reece[e][78] (1991)	–	500/-	150	7200/-	–	2400/-

[a] Maximum tolerated dose in Phase I study.

[b] VP16-213 given as continuous infusion over ~34 hours.

[c] First of two AuBMT regimens; second included thioTEPA 900 mg/m², vinblastine 400–600 mg/kg, ± Ara-C 3- 6 g/m² or thioTEPA 750 mg/m², mitoxantrone 40 mg/m², and carboplatin 1 g/m².

[d] VP16-213 given as twice daily infusion × 3 days.

[e] VP16-213 as per Harden et al.[76] (above).

CDDP = cisplatin

An alternative approach to the improvement of conditioning regimens merely by the addition or substitution of other drugs is that of immune targeting with isotopes or toxins. This approach is hampered somewhat by a lack of definition of the stem cell for HD and therefore its antigenic characteristics. Nevertheless, it potentially allows a large increase in the therapeutic index. Previously, yttrium-90 labelled antiferritin has been used in advanced HD,[38] and recently Bierman et al.[39] treated 11 patients with far-advanced HD with this agent before a CBV regimen and AuBMT. Calculated radiotherapy doses of 400–1500 cGy were achieved. Although the contribution of the radioimmunotherapy to antitumor activity was difficult to ascertain, additional toxicity appeared minimal, and further studies of this type would be of interest.

In any case, the question of whether conditioning regimens can be made more effective by any means is critical; it has been assumed, perhaps optimistically, that the immediate problem is not the intrinsic incurability of certain HD patients with current modalities but rather the increasingly severe extramedullary toxicity that usually accompanies dose escalation. (As an aside, it is possible that hematologic toxicity might also be magnified due to increased damage to the hematopoietic microenvironment associated with such regimens.) In any case, there is no clear solution to this problem, but several approaches are suitable for exploration. First, a surprising result from a study using hematopoietic growth factors (i.e. granulocyte–macrophage colony-stimulating factor – GM-CSF) in an allogeneic BMT trial suggests that earlier count recovery is associated with less hepatotoxicity.[40] While the etiology of this effect is obscure, it may merely relate to decreased use of supportive care measures (specifically, certain antimicrobials) after BMT. Also, the cytokine inhibitor pentoxifylline (PTX) may ameliorate the toxic effects of cyclosporine[40,41]; its ability to block toxic and/or antitumor effects by these same mechanisms is not clear but should be evaluated. In any case, the use of these or other protectives may allow additional dose exploration.

Non-myeloablative therapy

Conventional therapy may be given before the conditioning regimen, either as a probe for residual chemosensitivity before BMT (i.e. as a device for patient selection) or for cytoreduction to produce a state of minimal residual disease – ideally, of course, both functions would be accomplished. Such therapy could be given post-BMT, but any myelosuppressive activity might be amplified in such cases. In any case, probing for chemosensitivity, with the general supposition that patients resistant to such therapy would not be advanced to BMT, is used much less commonly for HD than for the non-Hodgkin's lymphomas (NHL)[1] as it is clear that (in contrast to the NHL[42]) some HD patients in chemotherapy-refractory relapse can be cured with BMT,[27,43] and that such therapy may prejudice post-BMT results by producing more toxicity.

In Vancouver, we have used conventional MVPP (mechlorethamine, vinblastine, prednisone, procarbazine) chemotherapy for several cycles immediately before BMT in selected patients (i.e. those previously achieving CR and remaining free of relapse for greater than 3 months)—not to probe for chemosensitivity, as all such patients so treated proceeded directly to BMT, but to attempt to produce a state of minimal residual disease. Although not all of these patients were meticulously restaged after MVPP, fewer than 5% clearly progressed during MVPP treatment. This strategy also allowed some flexibility regarding timing of admission to transplant facilities. Whether or not it improved outcome cannot be directly evaluated.

As with salvage chemotherapy in conventional dose (as discussed above), the precise role of local radiotherapy as an additional cytoreductive element is unclear. (In theory, local radiotherapy could be used either before or after BMT; the problem with post-BMT therapy would be the possibility of additional myelosuppression.) In any case, the use of local radiotherapy is common, especially in patients with bulky disease, for the following reasons: 1) patients tend to relapse in sites of bulky disease; 2) local radiotherapy (in sufficient doses) can eradicate even bulky HD;[18] 3) durable CR can be obtained in some patients given local radiotherapy to areas of residual disease while in a PR post-AuBMT; and 4) the toxicity of 1500–3000 cGy local radiotherapy, even to the mediastinum, is acceptable in patients who do not receive TBI-containing regimens – although regimens such as CBV may also increase lung toxicity, albeit likely to a lesser degree than TBI.[17] It follows that mediastinal irradiation should be used selectively in patients eligible for AuBMT, especially when used beyond initial therapy. The radiation dose should not be excessive and meticulous care should be directed to minimizing irradiation of uninvolved tissue, especially pulmonary, when the treatment fields are planned.

Another topic considered in this general area is that of biologic response modifiers; these are usually considered as post-BMT modalities. In this regard, a number of alternatives have been (or are in the process of being) explored. First, α-interferon is active in HD,[44] and it may be of some use in the post-AuBMT situation[45] – similar to the apparent beneficial effect of this agent (in the purified, not the recombinant form) after AlloBMT in acute lymphoblastic leukemia patients.[46] Also, it is possible that interleukin-2 (IL-2) or LAK cells[47] may be used post-BMT.

In any case, a direct evaluation of a graft-vs-HD effect seems worthwhile. If graft-vs-HD requires the presence of graft-vs-host disease (GVHD), the simplest approach is the more widespread use of allogeneic BMT. However, as noted below, it is difficult to visualize how allogeneic BMT could be applied to an increased number of patients without increasing mortality and thus sacrificing the graft-vs-HD effect. An alternative approach has been suggested by Jones et al. to produce a state of autologous GVHD,[48] and Phase II clinical trials are underway in NHL.

Source of stem cells

By far the majority of HD patients have received autologous marrow; roughly equal numbers of patients have received autologous peripheral blood (PB) HSC and allogeneic BMT. Few have received high dose conditioning regimens without added HSC support,[49,50] although in theory such endogenous reconstitution could be utilized with therapy that was not truly myeloablative if appropriate hematopoietic growth factor support were available.

Autologous BMT

A primary concern of any AuBMT regimen in HD is the ability of the marrow, especially after having been exposed to multiple chemotherapy agents, to ensure a sustained hematologic recovery. Failure to achieve such recovery is generally assumed to reflect quantitative and/or qualitative damage to the repopulating cells of the marrow, although this has been difficult to test in a definitive way due to a lack of qualitative assays for such cells. In any case, the routine use of unpurified cryopreserved marrow will produce reasonable recovery; in our experience using AuBMT for HD, data from 75 patients who had all been previously exposed to MOPP/ABV(D) showed insufficient graft function (defined as absolute neutrophil count [ANC]$<0.5 \times 10^9$/L by day +30) in~3%. Platelet recovery was slower, but 77% of these patients were free of the need for platelet transfusions by day +30, and 93% by day +45 (Phillips GL: unpublished observations). However, one may assume that more heavily pretreated patients have delayed hematologic toxicity.[51]

There are several other potential limitations to the use of AuBMT, including the possibility of contamination with occult HD cells, loss of a potential allogeneic antitumor (i.e. graft-vs-HD) effect[16,52] as discussed below, incomplete immunologic recovery, and in certain cases, inadequate harvestable marrow due to prior pelvic radiotherapy or involvement.

The most obvious of these considerations pertains to marrow contamination. Although not proven to be of clear benefit in any circumstance, one would intuit that ex vivo cytoreduction would be of primary importance when contamination of the marrow space is frequent. Whether or not this is true in HD depends to some degree on disease status[53,54]; autopsy series have reported marrow involvement in a relatively high percentage of patients[55] but, and as noted above, none of the 25 Vancouver patients seen between 1985 and 1988 in an initial relapse was found to have documented marrow involvement.

Moreover, some HD patients with a prior history of marrow involvement have undergone harvest and cryopreservation of remission bone marrow and have subsequently been autotransplanted at the time of progression using unpurified marrow, without recurrence, suggesting that a history of contaminated marrow does not preclude successful AuBMT.[27] Therefore, the biologic significance of the reinfusion of variable numbers of 'HD' stem cells is not known with certainty.

There have been only a small number of HD patients reported who have received an AuBMT purified ex vivo (i.e. purged) to remove contaminating HD cells. Jones et al.[16] reported the use of 4-hydroperoxycyclophosphamide (4-HC) purging in 28 HD patients; although the 4-HC purged AuBMT patients had delayed engraftment as compared with the allogeneic BMT patients (median absolute neutrophil count [ANC] recovery on days +32.5 and +14, respectively), there was no increased mortality or even prolonged duration of hospitalization in the AuBMT group. Also, it must be recognized that even if these patients did less well than those without marrow involvement, it would not prove that reinoculated tumor cells in the marrow were responsible, only that HD patients with marrow involvement may have a poorer prognosis.[56]

In addition, the ability of primary chemotherapy to induce leukemogenesis must be considered; Chao et al.[57] reported on the presence of clonal abnormalities in the pre-harvest marrow that may have predicted the development of myelodysplasia or leukemia, and cytogenetic analysis should be added to other methods to ensure the health of the marrow before harvest.

Autologous peripheral blood (PB) HSC

It is now clear that PBHSC can be used to successfully reconstitute hematopoiesis in some situations in which AuBMT cannot be employed due to therapy-related marrow damage or involvement with HD. Körbling et al.[58] used PBHSC mobilized by either chemotherapy or granulocyte–macrophage colony-stimulating factor (GM–CSF) for autotransplantation after CBV in 12 HD patients in whom marrow harvest was not feasible due to pelvic irradiation. As with other PBHSC studies that include mobilization, hematologic recovery time was relatively short: ANC recovered to $>0.5 \times 10^9/l$ at a median of 20.5 days post-transplant; even more interestingly, 2 patients did not require platelet transfusions. More recently, Kessinger et al.[59] reported their experience using steady-state PBHSC harvests followed by CBV and subsequent transplantation in 56 HD patients in whom a major bone marrow abnormality (including involvement with HD) precluded a marrow harvest. Although such comparisons are somewhat problematic, the 3-year event-free survival of 37% was similar to that observed in their previous experience using identical conditioning and AuBMT. Not surprisingly, patients with a history of marrow involvement at the time of PBHSC harvest had poorer results, although, as noted above, it is unclear whether this represents a distinct biology or occult contamination of the blood and the negative impact of its subsequent reinfusion.

A true HSC transplant need not be performed if the conditioning chemotherapy does not eliminate all endogenous HSC. It could be envisaged that a sufficient number of more differentiated progenitor cells might provide transient hematopoietic support until residual HSC could repopulate the marrow. Until HSC can be differentially isolated and genetically marked, this will remain unproven, although considerable data in support of such a possibility have already been obtained from experiments with mice.[60-63] Alternatively, PBHSC may be solely responsible for hematologic recovery, as murine studies have shown that HSC can also be demonstrated in the PB of mice treated with granulocyte-colony stimulating factor (G-CSF).[64] In any case, it has been established that PBHSC transplants in man can be used successfully in lieu of AuBMT and may even be considered in preference to marrow in some instances, especially if it could be shown that occult contamination of remission marrow with HD was less than that of the PB, or if hematopoietic recovery was markedly shorter after PBHSC transplants.

Allogeneic BMT

As expected from work with other hematologic malignancies, allogeneic BMT can be used successfully in selected cases (i.e. usually those patients aged no more than ~50 years and with suitably [HLA] matched donors). While most patients do not have histocompatible related donors, the expanded use of mismatched related donors[65] and the further development of registries of volunteer donors[66] makes allogeneic BMT a more frequent option.

Only three series (comprising a total of 36 patients) dealing more-or-less specifically with allogeneic BMT for HD have been published.[16,67,68] The results have been relatively poor, but expectedly so, due to the advanced disease status of these patients. While these series provide data that indicate allogeneic BMT can be successfully used in HD, they do not address the question of whether allogeneic BMT should be used in preference to AuBMT. Nevertheless, this approach is at least arguable, especially in a patient with a relatively high risk of relapse post-BMT but who might be expected to survive an episode of GVHD. As noted above, the presence of a graft-vs-HD effect[52] will only have a survival advantage if GVHD deaths are not increased. Unfortunately, the very nature of allogeneic BMT makes it unlikely that a truly randomized study versus AuBMT will be performed; the best one can hope for is that an allocated study (similar to those done for acute myelogenous leukemia[69]) will be performed. Until then, it is likely that the centers that prefer one source of marrow over another will continue those efforts without definitive data.

Hematopoietic growth factors

As of this writing, several studies have evaluated either GM- or G-CSF in enhancing hematologic recovery in the AuBMT setting, including some studies specifically in HD.[70,71] Although one would anticipate that diagnosis alone would generally not greatly influence such recovery, the treatment peculiarities of an individual disease, such as the more frequent use of extensive radiotherapy and certain stem cell poisons used to treat HD could affect both marrow repopulating cells and the microenvironment. Phase I-II trials of these agents given by infusion have been found to usually produce earlier ANC recovery as compared with historical series, but with no hastening of platelet recovery. Complications of these growth factors themselves have generally been minor, and their effects on morbidity and hospitalization (and therefore cost) have been variable although often marginally favorable. Fewer Phase III studies have been reported; although Nemunaitis and co-workers[72] noted favorable effects of yeast GM-CSF at a dose of 250 µg/day × 14–21 days on the kinetics of ANC recovery in a group of patients with lymphoid malignancy, no benefit was shown in the subgroup of HD patients.

It is not surprising that the results of these trials have been relatively marginal, given the still-evolving knowledge as to how best to use the growth factors now available. It now seems clear that currently available hematopoietic growth factors can be clinically useful to augment the progenitor content of peripheral blood harvests. The use of similar treatments either in vivo or possibly ex vivo to enhance the effectiveness of marrow harvests are possibilities currently being investigated. Finally, it now also seems likely from laboratory studies that combinations of growth factors not yet tested clinically will enable significant improvements to be made in stimulating hematopoietic recovery in patients given myeloablation and AuBMT.[73] However, it is important to note that even dramatic changes in hematopoietic recovery are unlikely to influence the treatment results in HD to a great degree. For instance, we have documented a death rate due to infection (≤ 30 days post-BMT) of only ~2% in 88 consecutive Vancouver patients given a CBV regimen and an unpurged AuBMT (although most of these patients did not have advanced or refractory disease) (Phillips GL: unpublished data).

Other relevant uses of growth factors are also being explored but the data are still too early to evaluate. For example, growth factors are being tested for their ability to sensitize malignant stem cells to chemotherapy[74] particularly in patients with AML. While the ultimate outcome of this strategy is unknown, it is an attractive concept and, especially with the introduction of other growth factors, may be applicable to other diseases as well.

In summary, the relatively minor impact of current growth factor protocols on outcome should not blunt enthusiasm for a continued search to develop new strategies for their use, both as single agents and more importantly as combined factor protocols. And, despite the above qualifying statement regarding mortality, the virtual elimination of severe pancytopenia would undeniably be a major advance, with important economic implications in favor of their use, as detailed below.

Economic considerations

Although not diretly related to the issue of increasing the cure rate in patients with HD who require BMT, the changing climate of medical economics is such that this issue bears discussion. Relatively little on this topic has been published,[75] probably due to the disparity between the cure rates using conventional chemotherapy and AuBMT regimens in patients with relapsed HD and the assumption that saving lives is ultimately cost-effective. Nevertheless, in an attempt to apply this therapy more widely, it would clearly be desirable to decrease the unit cost of BMT. This can be done most simply by optimal patient selection, especially by avoiding end-stage patients unlikely to be cured and most likely to die as a result of toxicity. Also, the use of various measures to ameliorate hematologic toxicity (primarily utilizing hematopoietic growth factors) as well as nonhematologic toxicity will be crucial, reducing hospitalization and the use of various supportive resources.

Conclusions

Certain recent developments in HD have implications for routine management of these patients, and also provide direction for future clinical research. First, and probably most importantly, oncologists who manage HD patients primarily should be aware that the vast majority of HD patients < 60 years of age who fail conventional chemotherapy need to be evaluated promptly for BMT, with the understanding that most patients should be transplanted at that time. Secondly, in vivo cytoreduction needs to be improved, although it is not clear how this is to be done, as severe nonhematologic toxicity may preclude further dose escalation. Thirdly, the role of both PBHSC and allogeneic BMT should be evaluated more fully; either technique may replace AuBMT in situations of marrow contamination, and perhaps in other cases as well. It is likely that the use of hematopoietic growth factors will be increasingly useful, both by reducing toxicity and perhaps by allowing certain patients to be transplanted who cannot at present.

References

(1) Armitage JO. Bone marrow transplantation in the treatment of patients with lymphoma. *Blood* 1989; 73: 1749–58.

(2) Hoskins P, Klimo P, Fairey R, O'Reilly SE, Voss N, Connors JM. MOPP/ABV Hybrid chemotherapy for advanced Hodgkin's disease (HD). 7 year experience at a single centre. (Abstract presented at the Fourth International Conference on Malignant Lymphoma; 1990 June 6–9; Lugano, Switzerland.)

(3) Bonadonna G, Viviani S, Valagussa P, Bonfante V, Santoro A. Third-line salvage chemotherapy in Hodgkin's disease [Abstract]. *Semin Oncol* 1985; 12 (suppl 2): 23–5.

(4) Phillips GL, Reece DE. Clinical studies of autologous bone marrow transplantation in Hodgkin's disease. *Clin Haematol* 1986; 15: 151–66.

183

(5) Herzig GP. Autologous marrow transplantation in cancer therapy. *Prog Hematol* 1981; 12: 1–23.

(6) Canellos GP, Propert K, Cooper R et al. MOPP vs. ABVD vs. MOPP alternating with ABVD in advanced Hodgkin's disease: A prospective randomized CALGB trial [Abstract]. *Proc Am Soc Clin Oncol* 1988; 7: 230.

(7) Glick J, Tsiatis A, Chen M, Rassiga A, Mann R, O'Connell M. Improved survival with MOPP-ABVD compared to BCVPP ± radiotherapy (RT) for advanced Hodgkin's disease: 6-year ECOG results [Abstract]. *Blood* 1990; 76 (suppl 1): 350a.

(8) Glick J, Tsiatis A, Schilsky R et al. A randomized Phase III trial of MOPP/ABVD Hybrid vs sequential MOPP-ABVD in advanced Hodgkin's disease: Preliminary results of the intergroup trial. ECOG, CALGB, and SWOG, Philadelphia, PA, Boston, MA, Chicago, IL [Abstract]. *Proc Am Soc Clin Oncol* 1991; 10: 271.

(9) Santoro A, Bonfante V, Bonadonna G. Salvage chemotherapy with ABVD in MOPP-resistant Hodgkin's disease. *Ann Intern Med* 1982; 96: 139–43.

(10) Canellos GP. Residual mass in lymphoma may not be residual disease. *J Clin Oncol* 1988; 6: 931–3.

(11) Lohri A, Barnett M, Fairey RN et al. Outcome of treatment of first relapse of Hodgkin's disease after primary chemotherapy: Identification of risk factors from the British Columbia experience 1970 to 1988. *Blood* 1991; 77: 2292–8.

(12) Carella AM, Carlier B, Congiu A et al. Autologous bone marrow transplantation as adjuvant treatment for high-risk Hodgkin's disease in first complete remission after MOPP/ABVD protocol. *Bone Marrow Transplant* 1991; 8: 31–5.

(13) Carella AM, Congiu AM, Gaozza E et al. High-dose chemotherapy with autologous bone marrow transplantation in 50 advanced resistant Hodgkin's disease patients: An Italian Study Group report. *J Clin Oncol* 1988; 6: 1411–6.

(14) Jagannath S, Armitage JO, Dicke KA et al. Prognostic factors for response and survival after high-dose cyclophosphamide, carmustine, and etoposide with autologous bone marrow transplantation for relapsed Hodgkin's disease. *J Clin Oncol* 1989; 7: 179–85.

(15) Gribben JG, Linch DC, Singer CRJ, McMillan AK, Jarrett M, Goldstone AH. Successful treatment of refractory Hodgkin's disease by high-dose combination chemotherapy and autologous bone marrow transplantation. *Blood* 1989; 73: 340–4.

(16) Jones RJ, Piantadosi S, Mann RB et al. High-dose cytotoxic therapy and bone marrow transplantation for relapsed Hodgkin's disease. *J Clin Oncol* 1990; 8: 527–37.

(17) Reece DE, Barnett MJ, Connors JM et al. Intensive chemotherapy with cyclophosphamide, BCNU and etoposide followed by autologous bone marrow transplantation for relapsed Hodgkin's disease. *J Clin Oncol* 1991; 9: 1871–9.

(18) Kaplan HS. Evidence for a tumoricidal dose level in the radiotherapy of Hodgkin's disease. *Cancer Res* 1966; 26: 1221–4.

(19) Brindley CO, Salvin LG, Potee KG et al. Further comparative trial of triethylene thiophosphoramide and mechlorethamine in patients with melanoma and Hodgkin's disease. *J Chronic Dis* 1964; 17: 19–30.

(20) Frei III E, Spurr CL, Brindley CO et al. Clinical studies of dichloromethotrexate (NSC 29630). *Clin Pharmacol Ther* 1965; 6: 160–71.

(21) Carde P, MacKintosh FR, Rosenberg SA. A dose and time response analysis of the treatment of Hodgkin's disease with MOPP chemotherapy. *J Clin Oncol* 1983; 1: 146–53.

(22) Frei III E, Canellos GP. Dose: a critical factor in cancer chemotherapy. *Am J Med* 1980; 69: 585–94.

(23) Bearman SI, Appelbaum FR, Back A et al. Regimen-related toxicity and early posttransplant survival in patients undergoing marrow transplantation for lymphoma. *J Clin Oncol* 1989; 7: 1288–94.

(24) Gale RP, Butturini A. The role of hematopoietic growth factors in nuclear and radiation accidents. *Exp Hematol* 1990; 18: 958–64.

(25) Thomas ED. The use and potential of bone marrow allograft and whole-body irradiation in the treatment of leukemia. *Cancer* 1982; 50: 1449–54.

(26) Pecego R, Hill R, Appelbaum FR et al. Interstitial pneumonitis following autologous bone marrow transplantation. *Transplantation* 1986; 42: 515–17.

(27) Phillips GL, Wolff SN, Herzig RH et al. Treatment of progressive Hodgkin's disease with intensive chemoradiotherapy and autologous bone marrow transplantation. *Blood* 1989; 73: 2086–92.

(28) Horning SJ, Chao NJ, Negrin RS et al. The Stanford experience with high-dose etoposide cytoreductive regimens and autologous bone marrow transplantation in Hodgkin's disease and non-Hodgkin's lymphoma: Preliminary data. *Ann Oncol* 1991; 2 (suppl 1): 47–50.

(29) Philip T, Dumont J, Teillet F et al. High dose chemotherapy and autologous bone marrow transplantation in refractory Hodgkin's disease. *Br J Cancer* 1986; 53: 737–42.

(30) Graw Jr RG, Lohrmann H-P, Bull MI et al. Bone-marrow transplantation following combination chemotherapy immunosuppression (B.A.C.T.) in patients with acute leukemia. *Transplant Proc* 1974; 6: 349–54.

(31) Wheeler C, Antin JH, Churchill WH et al. Cyclophosphamide, carmustine, and etoposide with autologous bone marrow transplantation in refractory Hodgkin's disease and non-Hodgkin's lymphoma: A dose-finding study. *J Clin Oncol* 1990; 8: 648–56.

(32) Ahmed T, Feldman E, Ciavarella D et al. Sequential autologous bone marrow transplantation (BMT) for high risk Hodgkin's disease (HD) [Abstract]. *Proc Am Soc Clin Oncol* 1991; 10: 223.

(33) Phillips GL, Reece DE. High-dose chemotherapy with cyclophosphamide, BCNU and VP16-213 (CBV) and bone marrow transplantation for advanced Hodgkin's disease. In: Zander AR, Barlogie B, eds. *Proceedings of the International Symposium on Autologous Bone Marrow Transplantation in Lymphoma, Hodgkin's Disease and Multiple Myeloma*. Springer-Verlag (in press).

(34) Russell JA, Selby PJ, Ruether BA, et al. Treatment of advanced Hodgkin's disease with high dose melphalan and autologous bone marrow transplantation. *Bone Marrow Transplant* 1989; 4: 425–9.

(35) Carella AM, Santini G, Santoro A et al. Massive chemotherapy with non-frozen autologous bone marrow transplantation in 13 cases of refractory Hodgkin's disease. *Eur J Cancer Clin Oncol* 1985; 21: 607–13.

(36) Santos GW, Tutschka PJ, Brookmeyer R et al. Marrow transplantation for acute nonlymphocytic leukemia after treatment with busulfan and cyclophosphamide. *N Engl J Med* 1983; 309: 1347–53.

(37) Kaplan HS. Chemotherapy. In: *Hodgkin's Disease*. 2nd ed. Cambridge, Mass.: Harvard University Press, 1980: 442–77.

(38) Vriesendorp HM, Blum JE, Herpst JM et al. Refractory Hodgkin's disease: Treatment with polyclonal yttrium labeled antiferritin [Abstract]. *Proc Am Soc Clin Oncol* 1990; 9: 256.

(39) Bierman PJ, Vriesendorp HM, Vose JM et al. High-dose chemotherapy and polyclonal yttrium-90 labeled antiferritin (Y-90) followed by autologous bone marrow transplantation (ABMT) for Hodgkin disease (HD) [Abstract]. *Blood* 1990; 76(suppl 1): 528a.

(40) Bianco JA, Appelbaum FR, Nemunaitis J et al. Phase I-II trial of pentoxifylline for the prevention of transplant-related toxicities following bone marrow transplantation. *Blood* 1991; 78: 1205–11.

(41) Bianco J, Singer J, Ballard B, Almgren J, Appelbaum F, Storb R. Pentoxifylline prevents cyclosporine and amphotericin B induced acute renal failure in patients undergoing allogeneic bone marrow transplantation. (Abstract presented at the 13th International Congress of the Transplantation Society, August 19–24, 1990, San Francisco.)

(42) Philip T, Armitage JO, Spitzer G et al. High-dose therapy and autologous bone marrow transplantation after failure of conventional chemotherapy in adults with intermediate-grade or high-grade non-Hodgkin's lymphoma. *N Engl J Med* 1987; 316: 1493–8.

(43) Bierman PJ, Vose JM, Armitage JO. Chemotherapy sensitivity predicts a better outcome with high-dose therapy and autotransplantation in Hodgkin disease (HD) [Abstract]. *Proc Am Soc Clin Oncol* 1990; 9: 259.

(44) Redman J, Hagemeister F, McLaughlin P et al. α-interferon treatment of Hodgkin's disease (HD) [Abstract]. *Proc Am Soc Clin Oncol* 1990; 9: 256.

(45) Klingemann H-G, Grigg AP, Wilkie-Boyd K et al. Treatment with recombinant interferon (α-2B) early after bone marrow transplantation in patients at high risk for relapse. *Blood* 1991; 78: 3306–11.

(46) Meyers JD, Flournoy N, Sanders JE et al. Prophylactic use of human leukocyte interferon after allogeneic marrow transplantation. *Ann Intern Med* 1987; 107: 809–16.

(47) Higuchi CM, Thompson JA, Petersen FB, Buckner CD, Fefer A. Toxicity and immunomodulatory effects of interleukin-2 after autologous bone marrow transplantation for hematologic malignancies. *Blood* 1991; 77: 2561–8.

(48) Jones RJ, Vogelsang GB, Hess AD et al. Induction of graft-versus-host disease after autologous bone marrow transplantation. *Lancet* 1989; i: 754–7.

(49) Fouillard L, Gorin NC, Laporte JP, Douay L, Isnard F, Najman A. Recombinant human granulocyte-macrophage colony-stimulating factor plus the BEAM regimen instead of autologous bone marrow transplantation [Letter]. *Lancet* 1989; i: 1460.

(50) Neidhart J, Mangalik A, Kohler W et al. Granulocyte colony-stimulating factor stimulates recovery of granulocytes in patients receiving dose-intensive chemotherapy without bone marrow transplantation. *J Clin Oncol* 1989; 7: 1685–92.

(51) Brandwein JM, Callum J, Sutcliffe SB, Scott JG, Keating A. Analysis of factors affecting hematopoietic recovery after autologous bone marrow transplantation for lymphoma. *Bone Marrow Transplant* 1990; 6: 291–4.

(52) Jones RJ, Ambinder RF, Piantadosi S, Santos GW. Evidence of a graft-versus-lymphoma effect associated with allogeneic bone marrow transplantation. *Blood* 1991; 77: 649–53.

(53) Rosenberg SA. Hodgkin's disease of the bone marrow. *Cancer Res* 1971; 31: 1733–6.

(54) Bartl R, Frisch B, Burkhardt R et al. Assessment of bone marrow histology in Hodgkin's disease: Correlation with clinical factors. *Br J Haematol* 1982; 51: 1852–62.

(55) Colby TV, Hoppe RT, Warike RA. Hodgkin's disease at autopsy: 1972–1977. *Cancer* 1981; 47: 1852–62.

(56) Longo DL, Young RC, Wesley M et al. Twenty years of MOPP therapy for Hodgkin's disease. *J Clin Oncol* 1986; 4: 1295–306.

(57) Chao NJ, Nademanee AP, Long GD et al. Importance of bone marrow cyto-genetic evaluation before autologous bone marrow transplantation for Hodgkin's disease. *J Clin Oncol* 1991; 9: 1575–9.

(58) Korbling M, Holle R, Haas R et al. Autologous blood stem-cell transplantation in patients with advanced Hodgkin's disease and prior radiation to the pelvic site. *J Clin Oncol* 1990; 8: 978–85.

(59) Kessinger A, Bierman PJ, Vose JM, Armitage JO. High-dose cyclophos-phamide, carmustine, and etoposide followed by autologous peripheral stem cell transplantation for patients with relapsed Hodgkin's disease. *Blood* 1991; 77: 2322–5.

(60) Ploemacher RE, Brons NHC. Isolation of hemopoietic stem cell subsets from murine bone marrow: II. Evidence for an early precursor of day-12 CFU-S and cells associated with radioprotective ability. *Exp Hematol* 1988; 16: 27–32.

(61) Szilvassy SJ, Humphries RK, Lansdorp PM, Eaves AC, Eaves CJ. Quantitative assay for totipotent reconstituting hematopoetic stem cells by a competitive repopulation strategy. *Proc Natl Acad Sci USA* 1990; 87: 8736–40.

(62) Jones RJ, Celano P, Sharkis SJ, Sensenbrenner LL. Two phases of engraftment established by serial bone marrow transplantation in mice. *Blood* 1989; 73: 397–401.

(63) Magli MC, Iscove NN, Odartchenko N. Transient nature of early haematopoietic spleen colonies. *Nature* 1982; 295: 527–9.

(64) Molineux G, Pojda Z, Hampson IN, Lord BI, Dexter TM. Transplantation potential of peripheral blood stem cells induced by granulocyte colony-stimulat-ing factor. *Blood* 1990; 76: 2153–8.

(65) Beatty PG, Clift RA, Mickelson EM et al. Marrow transplantation from related donors other than HLA-identical siblings. *N Engl J Med* 1985; 313: 765–71.

(66) Nitzberg MC, Newburger PE, Raymond J. Marrow donors and international cooperation. *Lancet* 1988; i: 117–18.

(67) Phillips GL, Reece DE, Barnett MJ et al. Allogeneic marrow transplantation for refractory Hodgkin's disease. *J Clin Oncol* 1989; 7: 1039–45.

(68) Appelbaum FR, Sullivan KM, Thomas ED et al. Allogeneic marrow transplan-tation in the treatment of MOPP-resistant Hodgkin's disease. *J Clin Oncol* 1985; 3: 1490–4.

(69) Appelbaum FR, Fisher LD, Thomas ED. Chemotherapy v. marrow transplantation for adults with acute nonlymphocytic leukemia: A five-year follow-up. *Blood* 1988; 72: 179–84.

(70) Devereaux S, Linch DC, Gribben JG, McMillan A, Patterson K, Goldstone AH. GM-CSF accelerates neutrophil recovery after autologous bone marrow transplantation for Hodgkin's disease. *Bone Marrow Transplant* 1989; 4: 49–54.

(71) Taylor KM, Jagannath S, Spitzer G et al. Recombinant human granulocyte colony-stimulating factor hastens granulocyte recovery after high-dose chemotherapy and autologous bone marrow transplantation in Hodgkin's disease. *J Clin Oncol* 1989; 7: 1791–9.

(72) Nemunaitis J, Rabinowe SN, Singer JW et al. Recombinant granulocyte-macrophage colony-stimulating factor after autologous bone marrow transplantation for lymphoid cancer. *N Engl J Med* 1991; 324: 1773–8.

(73) Moore MAS. Clinical implications of positive and negative hematopoietic stem cell regulators. *Blood* 1991; 78: 1–19.

(74) Bettelheim P, Valent P, Andreeff M et al. Recombinant human granulocyte-macrophage colony-stimulating factor in combination with standard induction chemotherapy in de novo acute myeloid leukemia. *Blood* 1991; 77: 700–11.

(75) McMillan A, Goldstone A. What is the value of autologous bone marrow transplantation in the treatment of relapsed or resistant Hodgkin's disease? *Leuk Res* 1991; 15: 237–43.

(76) Harden E, Bolwell B, Fay J et al. Treatment of progressive Hodgkin's disease (HD) with cyclophosphamide (C), BCNU (B) and continuous infusion etoposide (V): CBVi and autologous marrow transplantation (AMT) [Abstract]. *Proc Am Soc Clin Oncol* 1990; 9: 271.

(77) Lazarus HM, Crilley P, Ciobanu N et al. High-dose BCNU, etoposide, cisplatin and autologous bone marrow transplant (ABMT) for relapsed lymphoma [Abstract]. *Proc Am Soc Clin Oncol* 1991; 10: 275.

(78) Reece DE, Barnett MJ, Connors J et al. Intensive therapy with cyclophosphamide, BCNU, VP-16-213 ± cisplatin (CBV±P) and autologous bone marrow transplantation (AuBMT) for advanced Hodgkin's disease (HD): Outcome and prognostic factors in 90 patients (pts) [Abstract]. *Blood* 1991; 78(suppl 1): 273a.

Clinical features and management of localized extranodal lymphomas

S B SUTCLIFFE and M K GOSPODAROWICZ

Introduction

Malignant lymphomas account for about 5% of human cancers with an age-standardized incidence of approximately 17 per 100 000 of the population. Non-Hodgkin's lymphomas are about four times more common than Hodgkin's disease and have an age-peak in the over-50 years age group. Both diseases share similar symptomatology in terms of characteristic symptoms (fever, night sweats, and weight loss) and with respect to nodal enlargement as the most common form of presentation. Both share a common staging classification which is based upon anatomical distribution of disease. A major difference occurs, however, in the frequency with which non-Hodgkin's lymphomas present with apparently localized disease in extranodal sites – primary extranodal lymphoma – a circumstance of extreme rarity in Hodgkin's disease.

Primary extranodal non-Hodgkin's lymphoma

The evolution of histological classifications of non-Hodgkin's lymphoma has followed from largely morphological observation stressing architecture and cytology to functional and biological measurements recognizing lineage and differentiation of lymphoma cells. Much of the controversy of lymphoma classification is illustrated in the histology of primary extranodal non-Hodgkin's lymphoma:

- extranodal sites rarely align themselves with lymph node structure, thus the majority of primary extranodal lymphomas manifest 'diffuse' effacement of tissue architecture.
- lymphoid aggregates within extranodal tissue may lack characteristic features of lymphoma in terms of invasion and mitotic activity. Such aggregates have been considered pseudotumors and have charac-

All correspondence to: Dr SB Sutcliffe, Department of Radiation Oncology, Princess Margaret Hospital, 500 Sherbourne Street, Toronto, Ontario M4X 1K9, Canada.

Cambridge Medical Reviews: Haematological Oncology Volume 2
© Cambridge University Press 1992

teristically been recorded in orbital, pulmonary and gastrointestinal sites. Current functional characterization of the cells within such aggregates to define clonality should resolve the issue of 'benign' versus 'malignant' lymphoid infiltrates.

- certain extranodal sites clearly have a spectrum of lymphoma histology from low to high grade within the International Working Formulation e.g. orbit, head and neck, gastrointestinal tract, lung and skin. Other sites have a highly skewed representation of intermediate and high grade tumors e.g. extradural, brain, testis and bone lymphomas. The basis for this variable distribution of histology by geographic or anatomic site is unknown.
- certain extranodal sites have characteristic spectra of B- or T-cell disease. Cutaneous lymphoma clearly comprises a range of lymphomas of T-cell origin which demonstrate a preferential localization for the skin for long periods of the natural history of the disease. Similarly, the gastrointestinal tract favours a subset of lymphomamucosa associated lymphoid tissue lymphoma (MALT lymphoma) demonstrating preferential traffic patterns influencing localization and recurrence within the gastrointestinal tract. Similar analogies apply to thyroid and lung lymphoma.
- whereas the existing histological classifications apply satisfactorily to nodal and B-cell lymphoma, the histological classification of T-cell disease within nodes and in extranodal sites is less satisfactory. The diversity of T-cell disease is demonstrated in primary cutaneous lymphoma with a disease spectrum ranging from chronic, indolent lichenoid eruptions through to lymphoblastic disease with a fulminant natural history. Even within a single disease entity – lymphomatoid granulomatosis – a very wide pattern of clinical behaviour is contained within a seemingly uniform histology.

Thus, in terms of prognostic importance, histology is not only distinguished in its own right, but also in the context of histology in relation to primary extranodal site as a component of therapeutic management.

Despite the obvious clinical diversity of primary extranodal lymphoma, there are many common attributes to define prognosis and management strategy. Stage, in the context of localization, defines those who are potential candidates for radiation as opposed to those who require systemic therapy for more advanced disease. However within localized stage, additional factors – presence or absence of symptoms ('A' or 'B'), tumor bulk, and extent of local invasion – influence the success of local therapies (radiation and/or surgery) with respect to both local tumor control and distant relapse rate. Histology influences management of those with localized or advanced lymphoma. In

190

certain sites where low grade tumors occur, localized or more conservative treatment options may be applicable. In other sites where virtually all tumors are of diffuse, aggressive type, initial systemic therapy is a mandatory component of potentially curative treatment. Finally, advancing age is an independent determinant characterizing poorer survival and disease-free rates.

Whilst the approach to management of localized nodal lymphoma is generally well recognized, there is less familiarity with the management of localized extranodal lymphoma. This, in part, reflects the infrequency of extranodal presentations in certain anatomic sites and the requirement for a significant referral practice to acquire familiarity with management. This chapter will deal specifically with localized extranodal non-Hodgkin's lymphoma, the patterns of disease, and will address three principal questions:

1. To what extent is the natural history and outcome of nodal and extranodal disease similar, given similar management?
2. Are all extranodal sites similar in natural history and outcome, given similar management?
3. Can the same principles of management be applied to extranodal lymphoma, as are applied to nodal lymphoma?

In addressing these questions, data will be reviewed from the world literature and also from the experience at the Princess Margaret Hospital.

General features of extranodal non-Hodgkin's lymphoma

During the period 1967–1988, the referral of patients for radical treatment of non-Hodgkin's lymphoma at Princess Margaret Hospital was approximately 62% Stage I–II and 38% Stage III–IV (Fig. 1). The composition of the stage I–II cohort is shown in Table 1 and Fig. 2.

The representation of stage I–II extranodal lymphomas by site is shown in Table 2 and Fig. 3. In descending order of frequency, the most common extranodal presentations were gastrointestinal tract, Waldeyer's ring, brain, head and neck, thyroid, soft tissue and testis. Symptomatic presentations (B symptoms) were uncommon. Certain presentations were frequently associated with clinical or surgically defined regional adenopathy, e.g. Waldeyer's ring, thyroid, gastrointestinal tract. Others were infrequently associated with regional adenopathy, e.g. eye and orbit, head and neck, testis, brain and other rare sites. This difference may, in part, reflect the higher probability of recording nodal disease in sites presenting primarily through surgical management.

The cause-specific survival rates (i.e. death from lymphoma as the end point of analysis) from the time of diagnosis for extranodal and nodal presen-

191

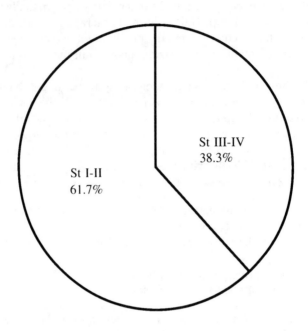

St III-IV
38.3%

St I-II
61.7%

*Does not include 79 pts with 1° brain lymphoma

Fig. 1. Non-Hodgkin's lymphoma: PMH 1967–1988. Distribution by clinical stage.

Table 1. *Stage I and II non-Hodgkin's lymphoma: PMH 1967–1988*

Number of patients	1391*	Nodal	49.1%
Male : female	1.17 : 1.0	Extranodal	50.9%
Low grade	27.5%	B symptoms	6.8%
Intermediate and high grade	69.5%		

* Excluding patients with primary brain lymphoma.

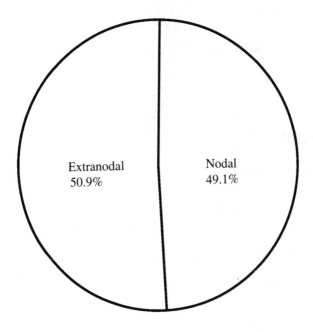

Extranodal
50.9%

Nodal
49.1%

*Does not include 79 pts with 1° brain lymphoma

Fig. 2. Stage I and II non-Hodgkin's lymphoma: PMH 1967–1988. Distribution by nodal or extranodal site of presentation.

Table 2. *Stage I and II head and neck lymphoma presenting extranodal sites: PMH 1967–1988*

Waldeyer's ring		Non-Waldeyer's ring	
Tonsil	35.0	Oral cavity	16.0
Nasopharynx	17.5	Salivary glands	9.6
Base of tongue	5.2	Paranasal sinuses	8.0
Larynx and hypopharynx	1.3	Nasal cavity	2.2

S B Sutcliffe and M K Gospodarowicz

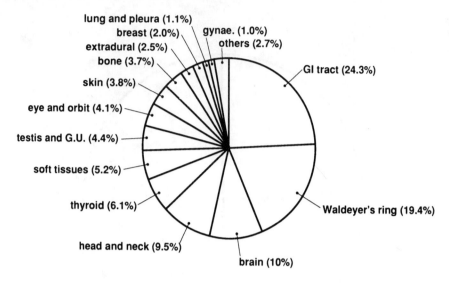

Fig. 3. Stage I and II non-Hodgkin's lymphoma: PMH 1967–1988. Distribution by extranodal site of presentation.

tations demonstrate no significant difference (Fig. 4). These survival analyses do not take into account imbalances in the groups with respect to important prognostic factors including therapy. Table 3 shows the composition of the two groups with the respect to major prognostic variables. Patients with primary brain lymphoma are included in this analysis. There is a slightly higher proportion of patients ≥ 60 years of age in the extranodal group. Other variables are fairly balanced other than for histology, with diffuse large cell (histiocytic) and higher grade histologies accounting for 39% of localized nodal presentations compared with 67% of localized extranodal presentations. Treatment allocations were similar during this time period with two-thirds or more of patients being treated primarily with radiation alone. More patients in the extranodal group received combined modality therapy (25% vs 17%), and surgery alone was the only form of treatment for 4.2% of extranodal presentations compared with 1.6% for the nodal group. Despite these imbalances, no significant difference in death from lymphoma was apparent within the overall analysis of nodal versus extranodal presentation of lymphoma.

If, indeed, there is no overall difference in outcome, between nodal and extranodal disease, are all sites of extranodal lymphoma comparable in terms

194

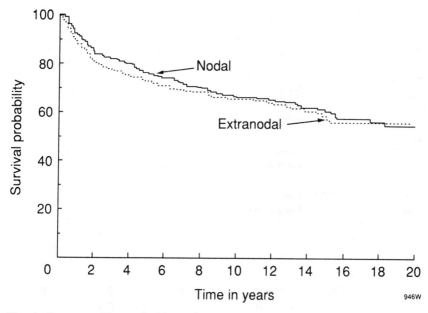

Fig. 4. Cause specific survival rates from the date of diagnosis for extranodal and nodal presentations of Stage I and II non-Hodgkin's lymphoma.

Table 3. *Prognostic factor distribution nodal and extranodal lymphoma – stage I and II: PMH 1967–1988*

	Nodal	Extranodal
Age >60 years	57	49
Stage IA & IIA	95	92
Histology =>DLC	39	67
Bulk >5 cm	30	27
Treatment XRT alone	72	63

of outcome? The cause specific survival rates for various sites of localized extranodal lymphoma is shown in Table 4. Outcomes vary from a 5-year actuarial cause-specific survival of >75% for skin, eye and orbit, thyroid and gastrointestinal lymphoma to <50% for testis, bone and brain lymphoma. Although these results are cause-specific actuarial survivals, given the distribution of prognostic factors including treatment allocation, it is unlikely

S B Sutcliffe and M K Gospodarowicz

Table 4. *Localized[1] extranodal lymphoma cause-specific 5-year survival: PMH 1967–1988*

Skin	92%	Waldeyer's[2]	72%
Thyroid	76%	Non-Waldeyer's[2]	67%
Gastrointestinal	77%	Breast	63%
Soft tissue	77%	Genitourinary[3]	52%
Orbit	76%	Bone	47%
Gynaecological	75%	Lung and pleura	44%
Extradural	73%	Brain	24%

[1] Clinical stage I & II.
[2] Head and neck lymphoma.
[3] Mostly including testis lymphoma.

that the variable outcomes reflect changing treatment policy or imbalance of prognostic variables.

Given this heterogeneity of outcomes, the various primary extranodal presentations will now be examined, particularly with respect to factors in the natural history that should influence management strategy.

Primary gastrointestinal lymphoma
The gastrointestinal tract is the most frequent site of presentation of localized extranodal lymphoma in adults. In the Western world, the most common locations are stomach (approximately 50–60%), small intestine (approximately 30%), large intestine (approximately 10%). Localized oesophageal lymphoma is extremely rare. Within the small intestine, ileal (ileocecal) presentations are most common (approximately 60%), followed by jejunal (approximately 30%) and duodenal sites (approximately 10%). These proportions differ by ethnic group and geography with small intestinal lymphomas being more common than gastric lymphoma in the Middle East. In such Mediterranean lymphomas, not only is there a background of malabsorption related to immunoproliferative small intestinal disease, but also a similar proportion of presentations in jejunum and ileum and an equal proportion (approximately 30%) of presentations at multiple sites within the small bowel. Colorectal lymphomas occur most commonly in the cecum, although this may be somewhat artificial due to the higher frequency of ileocecal presentation. The rectum is the site of presentation in approximately 20% of large bowel presentations with equal (5–10%) incidence in the ascending, transverse and descending colon. Presentation frequencies of large bowel lymphomas in association with ulcerative colitis show a higher proportion of recto-sigmoid and transverse colon lesions.[1]

Presenting symptoms are most frequently due to the local lesion (pain, obstruction, haemorrhage). Symptoms of lymphoma (fever and night sweats) are uncommon, however, weight loss associated with anorexia, pain or obstructive symptomatology are frequent and are more likely related to the primary presentation rather than a symptom of lymphoma per se.

Radiological procedures commonly identify the site and nature of disease. Within the stomach, lymphoma is most common at the pyloric antrum, followed by the body, then the cardia. Lesions may appear polypoid, ulcerative or diffusely thickening the stomach wall giving rise to rigidity and alteration of mucosal texture. Whilst computed tomography is not well suited to imaging of the intraluminal component of lymphoma, visualization of wall thickening is possible as well as commentary on regional node size. Imaging of small bowel lymphoma more commonly illustrates luminal narrowing or obstruction with the more gross impact of mass size and mesenteric node status being defined by computerized tomography. In both large and small bowel, lesions may be annular, ulcerative, proliferative or polypoid.

Diagnosis is made by examination of an adequate tissue sample most commonly obtained by endoscopy. Given access to fresh, frozen and fixed material with availability of immunophenotyping or genotypic studies, a preoperative diagnosis should be achievable on most patients with gastrointestinal lymphoma. Optimal histological classification remains controversial. The vast majority of tumors have a diffuse architectural pattern and are of predominantly large cell type, i.e. intermediate grade tumors within the Working formulation. Both low grade (follicular or small cleaved cell tumors) and high grade lymphomas (Burkitt, undifferentiated non-Burkitt) occur less frequently. The overwhelming majority of tumors are of B-cell origin although there is a distinct, small subset of T-cell tumors of pleomorphic type ranging from low to high grade.[1-4] True histiocytic lymphoma is not recorded in circumstances where accurate lineage definition is available. A further caveat to the histological classification is provided by the concept of mucosa-associated lymphoid tissue.[5] Based upon clinical features suggesting preferential patterns of response and failure (clinical inference of homing), the presence of evolutionarily conserved endothelial antigens involved in preferential lymphocytic traffic between gastrointestinal and nodal sites,[6] and the distinction of T. lymphocytic recognition systems that differ between gut and nodal sites,[7,8] it has been suggested that within the histogenesis of gastrointestinal lymphoma, MALT lesions be recognized within existing histological classification schemes. The validity and utility of such modifications remain to be seen.[1,9]

Prognostic factors for survival include stage, nodal status and extent of nodal disease for localized presentations, ESR, and histological subtype. The role of tumor bulk, a highly significant prognostic factor in lymphoma, has to be evaluated in GI lymphoma in light of the fact that the majority of lesions are surgically excised prior to any additional therapy. There is little indication that the size of the primary lesion is of prognostic significance, as long as complete surgical resection has been achieved. Other factors are also controversial: site within GI tract, depth of tumor penetration through bowel wall, and presentation with perforation.[10,11] In part, the role of factors characterized by the primary tumor is influenced by the fact that virtually all patients receive therapy in addition to initial surgery.

Historically, surgery has been the initial procedure of choice for management of primary bowel lymphoma. This has been predicated on an overall surgical cure rate of the order of 25–40%;[12] an operative mortality of 5–20%; a procedure which can define accurate staging information; an effective debulking mechanism; and a means of restoring bowel integrity with avoidance of spontaneous or treatment-induced perforation. Whilst the indications for surgery remain unchanged, it is rarely the sole form of therapy. Postoperative radiation therapy has been commonly applied to fields involving the tumor bed or the whole abdomen with an expectation of cause-specific survival rates in excess of 70% at 10 years of follow-up. In the most favourable circumstances of totally resected disease or microscopic residual disease (Stage IA, IIA stomach and IA small bowel) surgery and radiation therapy resulted in cause-specific survival of 80% and a relapse rate of less than 15%. The prognosis was less favorable for Stage IIA small bowel lymphoma with a relapse rate of 45%.[11] More recently, surgery and chemotherapy have been employed given the relapse rate of approximately 30–35% for unselected patients with Stage I–II gastrointestinal lymphoma and the predominantly extraabdominal pattern of relapse, in those with complete resection of the primary tumor. With this approach, cause-specific survival rates in excess of 75% at 5 years have been achieved.[13,14]

Whilst it is now clear that combination chemotherapy is required for patients with advanced local (residual local disease, Stage II with multiple involved nodes) and disseminated disease, the effectiveness of this treatment has engendered a reconsideration of the role of primary surgery. In principle, chemotherapy is effective for both debulking localized disease and for control of occult or overt disseminated disease. It might be argued that enhanced local control could be achieved with radiation to the tumor bed as part of a combined modality approach with the only principal additional morbidity from radiation. This approach has been pursued by the MD Anderson group with apparent success.[15] Such a management plan is based upon effective endoscopic diagnosis and removes detailed pathologic information. It does not deal with the issue of perforation, however, this risk may have been overestimated. In addition, it removes the place of radiation therapy from an adjuvant to surgery to an adjuvant to a combined modality role. The optimal approach remains to be established. For patients with surgically resected primary bowel lymphoma (Stage I and IIA), a cause-specific survival rate and relapse-free rate of approximately 80% should be achieved for selected patients receiving postoperative chemotherapy. Preliminary data suggest a similar prognosis for patients receiving combined chemo-radiation in the absence of primary surgery.

Upper aerodigestive tract

Non-Hodgkin's lymphoma occurring in the head and neck region is the second most frequent site of localized extranodal presentation. In practice, it is preferable to restrict the term head and neck lymphoma to those presentations occurring in the upper aerodigestive tract and to consider thyroid, brain, orbit and ocular, skin and cervical nodal lymphoma as separate sites.

The localization of tumor presentation by site reveals tonsil to be the most common, followed by nasopharynx, oral cavity, salivary glands (probably incorporating nodal lymphoma presenting within salivary tissue), paranasal sinuses and base of tongue (Table 2). Thus, excluding multiple sites of presentation, lymphomas involving Waldeyer's ring constitute the majority (almost 60%) of upper aerodigestive tract localized lymphomas as in other series.[16,17] In the Princess Margaret series, localized disease with involvement confined to the first echelon draining lymph nodes accounted for 82% of cases and intermediate grade histologies were present in 75% of patients. Localized presentation with B symptoms are unusual. The precise definition of disease bulk poses some difficulty with upper aerodigestive tract presentations. Advances in imaging, particularly computerized tomography (CT) and magnetic resonance imaging (MRI) have greatly assisted the definition of disease extent.[18] Even so, documentation of margins and establishing the correlation of all abnormalities to malignancy, e.g. paranasal sinus opacification, constitute problems with description of tumor bulk.

Traditionally, radical radiation employing involved or extended field techniques to tumor doses of 35 Gy or more has been the treatment method of choice. Retrospective analysis of such an approach reveals:[16,19–25]

- head and neck; – actuarial survival 25–60%
  upper aero-digestive – relapse-free
  tract rate/survival 38–50%
- Waldeyer's ring – actuarial survival 25–70%
  – relapse-free
  rate/survival 25–65%

The wide range in survival and relapse-free rate largely reflects the effect of stage of disease with most series observing that nodal involvement effectively halves the results obtained for Stage I disease. In addition, the use of TNM staging has indicated a substantial effect of primary tumor size and extent. Prognostic factor analysis commonly identifies stage as the most significant factor. In the PMH series, lymphomas at sites other than Waldeyer's ring had a significantly higher relapse rate compared with Waldeyer's ring, although this is not a uniform experience. The prognosis for paranasal sinus tumors also appears to be within the expected range for other aero-digestive sites with more extensive local tumors (T_3 and T_4) clearly having an inferior survival compared with T_{1-2} lesions.[25,26] Following irradiation, the isolated local failure rate is low (13% at 10 years in the PMH series), and the vast majority of failures are distant.

More recently, chemotherapy usually in combination with radiation, has been employed as primary management. In retrospective analysis this approach has generally resulted in superior overall survival and relapse-free rates: 60–80% and 56–100% respectively (PMH series 1967–86).[19,22,27] The benefits of combined modality are most evident in patients with Stage II disease. In addition, the advantage of initial control of disease by combined modality therapy almost certainly outweighs a strategy of chemotherapy for salvage of radiation failure given a relatively unfavourable survival rate from relapse after radiation.

An important aspect of the natural history of primary upper aerodigestive tract lymphoma is its relationship to gastrointestinal (GI) tract involvement, either concurrently at presentation or at subsequent relapse. The association at presentation was noted in 11 of 292 cases reported by Banfi et al. (1972). Although it is common practice to perform investigation of the GI tract in patients with apparently localized upper aerodigestive tract presentations, the yield is usually low.[21] The GI tract as a site of first relapse is clearly acknowledged and, indeed, is commonly the most frequent extranodal site of disease progression beyond the primary site.[16,20,22–24,28] There is no apparent predilection for any other extranodal site of relapse – particularly, central nervous system progression is not an identified pattern of failure.

Primary thyroid lymphoma

Primary thyroid lymphoma commonly presents as a rapidly enlarging neck mass producing local obstructive and infiltrative symptomatology. The median age at presentation is in the mid-60 years and women are more commonly affected than men (M:F :: 4:1). Approximately 90% of tumors are of diffuse architecture and of intermediate or high grade classification. Tumors are often bulky and complete or total thyroidectomy is rarely accomplished (approximately 10–20% of patients). Clinical Stage I and II disease accounts for approximately 80% of thyroid lymphomas. Involvement of the adjacent neck nodes is common. The predictive association of pre-existing chronic lymphocytic thyroiditis and subsequent lymphoma of the thyroid gland is well documented.[29]

Overall 5-year survival rates for patients with localized thyroid lymphoma range from 40–72%.[30–33] The cause-specific survival rate at 10 years (survival rate based on mortality directly due to lymphoma) is 64%, indicating the significant age-related mortality in a patient population with a median age of 65 years. Relapse-free rates vary from 38–64%. The majority of patients in these reports were treated with radical radiation therapy alone. Local control of neck disease was achieved in >70% of patients. Overall survival and relapse-free rates of 93% and 78% are quoted for the MD Anderson series.[33] More recently, chemotherapy has been incorporated into the management plan. In the MD Anderson series, overall survival and relapse-free rates were 77% respectively for combined modality and 53% and 30% for chemotherapy alone.[33] The role of primary chemotherapy alone for unselected patients with thyroid lymphoma remains to be defined[34] given that most experience to-date probably reflects outcome for patients with adverse prognostic factors.

Prognostic factor analysis commonly reveals that age and histology are not significant – a reflection of the advanced age of patients with thyroid lymphoma and the dominance of diffuse large cell histology. Most reports clearly define the role of stage and tumor bulk either as size, unresected neck disease, extrathyroid invasion or tumor fixation. In addition, retrosternal nodes or mediastinal mass are defined as adverse, bearing in mind the predominant role of radiation therapy in most of the reported results.[31–33]

Patterns of failure analysis record recurrence in the abdomen with gastrointestinal, liver and splenic disease. Tonsillar recurrence is recorded and also lung and bone sites. The patterns of recurrence linking Waldeyer's ring and gastrointestinal sites accord with the view that primary thyroid lymphoma is a tumor of mucosa-associated lymphoid tissue.[35] As such, a preferential lymphocyte traffic may exist for sites of common embryologic origin. Disease progression in the central nervous system is noted very rarely.

In current practice, the role of surgery is largely diagnostic and modern histopathologic techniques applied to fine-needle aspiration specimens or tissue biopsies should render thyroidectomy unnecessary. Radiation is highly effective for local tumor control and is a curative treatment for patients with limited, small bulk neck disease. In all other circumstances, combined modality therapy would appear to be optimal therapy with an anticipated cure rate of 80% for localized disease. The role of adjuvant radiotherapy in a combined modality regimen remains to be defined by prospective study, however, the high local control rate with modest dose radiation (35–40 Gy) is largely without significant acute or chronic morbidity.

Primary central nervous system (CNS) lymphoma

Central nervous system involvement by non-Hodgkin's lymphoma is not uncommon, however, secondary involvement subsequent to, or concurrent with, presentation at other nonneurological sites is the usual circumstance. The probability of CNS involvement may be predicted based upon certain presentation parameters – diffuse, high grade histology, extensive bone marrow involvement particularly with circulating lymphoma cells, certain extra-nodal presentations e.g. testis, intraocular or epidural lymphoma and widespread, particularly progressive, advanced disease.[36-38]

Lymphoma involving the central nervous system in the absence of overt systemic disease comprises two major types of presentation:

- primary CNS lymphoma
- primary leptomeningeal lymphoma

Primary CNS lymphoma

Primary parenchymal lymphoma of the brain is rare, usually comprising about 1–2% of all lymphomas and approximately 1% of primary brain tumors. It commonly presents in the 50–70 year age group and gives rise to symptomatology based upon raised intracranial pressure, cranial nerve palsies, neurologic deficit and, commonly, a significant impairment of mental function. Primary CNS lymphoma occurs almost exclusively in the brain with spinal cord presentation being extremely rare.[39] The incidence of primary parenchymal brain lymphoma has increased in the last decade as a result of HIV/AIDS, thereby establishing clearly the association previously observed in the organ transplantation setting, that primary CNS lymphoma is associated with immunodeficiency and immunoincompetence. CNS lymphoma in association with HIV infection differs from the non-HIV associated disease inasmuch as the age of presentation is younger, patients commonly have lymphoma symptomatology (approximately 40% with B symptoms), performance status is commonly poorer, and prognosis is significantly worse.[40] Computerized tomography usually reveals a hyperdense or isodense, enhancing mass lesion in the white matter with or without surrounding oedema. Calcification is not seen. In HIV-associated CNS lymphoma, lesions are more commonly hypodense with ring enhancement, thereby resulting in diagnostic overlap with benign conditions such as cerebral abscess, toxoplasmosis, etc. MRI-appearances commonly reveal isointense or hypointense lesions on T-1 weighted imaging. Appearances on T-2 weighted images may tend to isointensity associated with the tumor or hyperintensity reflecting the associated oedema. Both imaging techniques have considerably improved tumor visualization and knowledge of multifocality and direct routes of intracerebral spread.[40-42] In the absence of mass lesion, CT findings may be minimal and nonspecific. MRI may add additional information in cases with negative and positive CT examinations.

Histologically, the substantial majority of lesions are of diffuse large cell or immunoblastic type and of B-cell lineage. T-cell tumors have been recorded in non-HIV-related primary CNS lymphoma. Admixture of small lymphocytes, mitotic figures and necrosis are common, necrosis being particularly evident in HIV-related CNS lymphoma. CSF studies are commonly abnormal with respect to elevated protein level and increased cell count, however, cytology diagnostic of lymphoma is unusual (approximately 10–20% of cases). The application of molecular techniques may increase the diagnosis of leptomeningeal disease associated with primary parenchymal disease.[40,42]

Historically, the majority of patients reported have received irradiation to the whole brain following a tissue biopsy or cytological confirmation of diagnosis. In practice, a surgical procedure more definitive than biopsy is rarely indicated, given the usually poor performance status, frequent extensive invasion and multifocality of the tumor and short survival independent of extent of surgical resection.[43] An improved, albeit poor, prognosis may be achieved with radiation therapy. Whilst most agree that whole brain radiation is appropriate, there is controversy surrounding the optimal dose and whether the spinal cord should be treated in continuity. There is general consensus that cranial radiation dose should not be less than 40 Gy. Despite this dose, which will give local control rates for localized non-Hodgkin's lymphoma at other sites, the principal site of failure is local (90% first failure or progression in the brain or neuraxis), and there is no persuasive evidence of higher local control rates with higher dose. The argument for craniospinal radiation is cogent based upon involvement of the pia-arachnoid in up to 25% of cases and a recognized first failure in the non-irradiated neuraxis in a significant proportion of patients. In practice, however, craniospinal irradiation is less rarely employed given an increasing emphasis on the use of adjunctive systemic and intrathecal chemotherapy in combination with whole brain irradiation. With the use of radical irradiation alone for unselected patients with non-HIV-associated CNS lymphoma, the 5-year survival rate is 5–15% with a median survival in the 12–24 month range. The median survival for HIV-associated CNS lymphoma is 2–4 months.[38,40,42–45]

Several factors have indicated that a combined modality approach to management of primary CNS lymphoma might be beneficial – a local failure or recurrence rate of approximately 90%, a systemic progression rate of approximately 10% and a tumor that is highly chemosensitive in non-CNS sites. Whilst there are anecdotal, retrospective reports of improved local control and survival (50th percentile survival: 20–30 months; 25th percentile survival: 25–50 months), the extent to which this constitutes a real change in the natural history of disease or a sample or selection bias is conjectural.[46,47] There is certainly an equal literature to indicate that patterns of local failure and overall survival rates have not been materially influenced. In practice, therefore, standard therapy might be considered to be radical whole brain irradiation to doses of 40–50 Gy with intrathecal chemoprophylaxis/therapy. Optimization of systemic chemotherapy and the impact of combined modality therapy on survival remains to be defined.

Primary leptomeningeal lymphoma

Rarely, malignant lymphoma may present as a localized leptomeningeal disease in the absence of parenchymal brain involvement and without an antecedent history of lymphoma, AIDS or organ transplantation.[48-50] The neurological features may include raised intracranial pressure, encephalopathy, and cranial or spinal nerve root dysfunction. Imaging may reveal hydrocephalus, intradural nodule formation, thickened nerve roots or may show either no abnormalities or non-specific changes. Diagnosis is commonly by positive CSF cytology (either cytologic or immunophenotypic) or less frequently by spinal nerve root biopsy. Treatment has comprised intrathecal chemotherapy with craniospional or regional neuraxis irradiation. The prognosis is poor with a median survival of 8 months and few survivors beyond 24 months. The majority of deaths represent disease progression within the neuraxis and systemic relapse is rare within the short survival time thereby rendering the role of systemic therapy of limited value.

Primary exradural lymphoma

Spinal cord or cauda equina compression is a well-recognized, albeit relatively uncommon, presentation of non-Hodgkin's lymphoma. In the PMH experience, extranodal presentations accounted for 2.5% of localized extranodal disease and approximately 1% of all Stage I and II non-Hodgkin's lymphoma. The lesion is commonly imaged by myelography. Significant additional information relating to extent of extradural disease, associated bone or soft tissue extension, optimal route for decompression and/or reconstructive surgery and otherwise inapparent nodal or systemic involvement may be obtained by CT or MRI. The diagnosis is usually by tissue biopsy at the time of decompressive surgery. CSF studies are usually negative. Diffuse large cell lymphoma is the most common histology.

Overall survival for radically treated patients at PMH was 55% at 10 years with a relapse-free rate of 54%. The survival rate at 10 years was 31% for those treated with radiation alone versus 86% for those receiving combined modality therapy. The distant relapse-free rate for the XRT alone group was 33%, compared to 100% for the combined modality group.

Whilst there is no doubt that combined modality therapy is the optimal initial management, the role of intrathecal therapy is less clear. In the PMH series, only a few patients developed recurrence in either CSF or other extradural sites. Other retrospective analyses have identified the predictive role of extradural involvement with respect to subsequent CNS lymphoma.[38] The favourable results with combined modality therapy and the high rates of local control within radically irradiated fields contrast sharply with primary parenchymal and leptomeningeal lymphoma and clearly align the natural history of primary extradural lymphoma with other non-CNS extranodal lymphomas.

Primary orbital lymphoma

Primary lymphomas of the orbit and eye account for about 4.0% of all primary extranodal Stage I and II non-Hodgkin's lymphoma and 2.0% of all Stage I and II lymphoma in the PMH experience. Lymphoma of the extraocular orbital space is considerably more common than lymphoma of the eye (intraocular lymphoma) and the two types of presentation should be distinguished by virtue of their clearly different natural history.

Primary orbital lymphomas consist of those involving the anterior compartment of the orbital cavity: the eyelids, lacrimal gland and conjunctiva, and those in the posterior or retrobulbar compartment. Lesions in the eyelid and lacrimal gland present as mass lesions, while conjunctival involvement presents as fleshy, salmon pink tumors visible externally or following eversion of the eyelid. Retrobulbar lymphoma presents as exophthalmos. Chemosis, oedema of the eyelids and pain may accompany rapidly growing lesions and diplopia or dysconjugate extraocular movement reflect extensive proptosis or muscle dysfunction. Vision is not usually impaired unless papilloedema or optic nerve dysfunction is apparent. Imaging techniques including ultrasound, CT and MRI may all yield information regarding site, extent and invasion of orbital lymphoma. Bilateral localized orbital disease is also well recognized.

Traditional histopathological classification has proved complex due to the absence of naturally occurring nodal tissue at this site, the frequent small size of biopsies often providing only cytological information without architectural distinction and the heterogeneity of cytological appearance from pseudotumor to monomorphic lymphoma. The confusion engendered by reactive lymphoid hyperplasia and inflammatory pseudotumor may now, in large part, be overcome by immunophenotypic and genotypic diagnosis.[51–53] Whilst a proportion of such benign lesions will be reclassified as lymphoma either at presentation or progression, the heterogeneity of cytological appearance indicates that a higher proportion of orbital lymphomas are of indolent type, compared with the usual histological spectrum of extranodal lymphoma. This may be reflected in the 75% 10-year survival for primary orbital lymphoma seen in the PMH experience.[54]

Radiation therapy has been the common form of treatment for primary orbital lymphoma with survival rates of 60–75%[54,55] and high local control rates with moderate dose radiation (25–35 Gy). Progression rates of up to 50% reflect failure outside the radiation field, either in the contralateral orbit or as systemic disease. Retrobulbar involvement carries a higher risk of disease failure than anterior compartment disease.[54] There is little literature regarding combined modality therapy, although this would clearly be a consideration for histologically aggressive lymphoma.

Primary ocular lymphoma

Primary ocular lymphoma is well documented but extremely rare. Bilateral involvement is common and symptomatology comprises decreased visual acuity, uveitis, vitritus or glaucoma. Concurrent central nervous system disease at presentation or with disease progression is common, whilst systemic disease is unusual.[56] Examination reveals a picture resembling diffuse uveitis with yellow or white chorioretinal infiltrates, vitreous cellular opacities and rarely, hypopyon and/or hyphema. Diagnosis is by anterior chamber or vitreous fine-needle aspiration cytology with recourse to appropriate immunocytochemical or molecular techniques thereby removing the need for open biopsy or enucleation. In addition to systemic evaluation, detailed imaging of the neuraxis and CSF cytological examination should be performed.

Although the literature defines a high mortality rate for patients with intraocular lymphoma, certain principles of therapy are apparent. The natural history defines a high probability of bilateral ocular disease, a very high risk of CNS involvement and a significant risk of systemic disease at presentation or with disease progression.[56-59] Treatment should, therefore, be directed to securing control of local disease by irradiation to both orbits in conventional dose for lymphoma (approximately 30–35 Gy) with prophylactic whole brain irradiation, intrathecal chemotherapy or high dose systemic therapy with agents achieving high CSF or intraocular concentration, e.g. cytosine arabinoside or methotrexate.[60] Clearly, considerations related to symptomatic care of the eye (cataract formation, lacrimation and retinal neovascular proliferation) and CNS toxicity of combined therapy are appropriate. In addition, systemic chemotherapy would appear warranted based upon the significant risk of occult systemic disease, at presentation, or upon disease progression in those surviving with local tumor control.

Primary lymphoma of the genito-urinary tract

Localized genito-urinary lymphomas are rare, constituting approximately 5% of all localized extranodal lymphomas and 2.5% of all localized lymphomas in the PMH series. Testicular lymphomas comprise the vast majority of localized genito-urinary presentations, all other sites being particularly rare. Involvement of genito-urinary sites in advanced lymphoma is more common.

Primary testicular lymphoma

The literature regarding the natural history of testicular lymphoma is relatively homogeneous. Although it is a rare, primary testicular malignancy (<5%), it is the most common primary testicular tumor in men over 60 years of age. The usual presentation is a painless testicular swelling. Whilst the differential diagnosis of such swellings can be classified by ultrasonography and fine needle aspiration cytology, the definitive diagnosis is almost always obtained by high inguinal orchiectomy. The tumor predominantly involves the body of the testis with a largely intact tunica vaginalis. The spermatic cord and epididymis are commonly involved and vascular invasion is frequent. Haemorrhage and necrosis is commonly seen macroscopically. Virtually all tumors are of diffuse type and over 90% are type intermediate or high grade. The tumor infiltrate penetrates the tissue spaces diffusely separating, but not obliterating, the basic architecture and retaining the tubular structure to varying extent.

Detailed staging evaluation is mandatory given a high propensity for the disease to involve the contralateral testis, paraaortic nodes, liver and spleen. The natural history also defines a significant risk for involvement of mediastinal nodes, Waldeyer's ring, bone marrow, lung, skin and CNS.

Whilst it is apparent that a small cure rate follows orchiectomy alone for Stage IEA disease, the ability to predict such cases and the high progression rate associated with orchiectomy with radiation for patients with apparently localized disease militates strongly against attempting curative surgery. In several cases reported up to the early 1980s, the traditional therapy for Stage I and II disease comprised orchiectomy plus paraaortic and pelvic irradiation. A cause-specific survival of 30% at 10 years in the PMH series is typical of that experience. Overall survival rates of 16–50% at 5 years with relapse rates in excess of 50% are commonly reported.[61–67] Salvage following first progression has been poor with progression-free rates approximating overall survival rates. Factors prognostic for improved survival include age and stage of disease. The patterns of disease control and failure are also well defined with a synchronous and metachronous involvement of the contralateral testis in 5–35% of patients, and disease progression in extranodal sites including Waldeyer's ring, bone marrow, liver, spleen, lung and bone. CNS progression has been noted in up to 30% of patients.[64]

The role of systemic chemotherapy in patients with localized testicular lymphoma as part of a combined modality program incorporating orchiectomy, paraaortic and pelvic radiation for patients with Stage II disease, and irradiation to the remaining testis for all patients has been demonstrated by Connors et al.,[68] with an overall survival and relapse-free survival of 93% at 4 years. Given an historic overall survival rate of 16–50% and a median survival of 12–24 months, the impact of systemic chemotherapy upon prevention of systemic failure is clear. In addition, no evidence of CNS progression was apparent despite no inclusion of prophylactic CNS therapy in Connors series.

In practice, therefore, a combined modality approach utilizing orchiectomy and systemic chemotherapy can be advocated for all patients with localized testicular lymphoma. The role of paraaortic and pelvic irradiation is now more conjectural – it was not employed in Stage IEA disease in the Connors report,[68] however, given the limited morbidity of moderate dose radiation and the high rate of local control, its role can readily be sanctioned. Central

S B Sutcliffe and M K Gospodarowicz

nervous system prophylaxis is almost certainly not warranted in Stage I and II disease, given a combined modality approach. The high incidence of CNS progression for patients with systemic disease would argue, however, for the incorporation of CNS prophylaxis into the management of Stage III and IV disease. There is no unanimity on the role of irradiation to the contralateral testis. Several factors would, however, indicate its usefulness in management: the high incidence of metachronous involvement, the sanctuary nature of the testis with respect to chemotherapy, and the low morbidity and high local control probability with radiation to moderate dose (approximately 25–30 Gy).

Primary lymphoma of the kidney

Primary lymphoma of the kidney is extremely rare, if, indeed, it is ever a localized tumor arising within the kidney.[69] Involvement by haematogenous spread in patients with advanced disease[70,71] or contiguous involvement from perirenal tissue/nodes is a much more recognized association.[72] The radiologic aspects of genitourinary tract lymphoma have been well reviewed by Chamsangavej.[73] In the circumstance of apparent primary renal lymphoma, management would almost certainly comprise chemotherapy. Irradiation would require individualized consideration given the limited radiation tolerance of the kidney. There is no information on patterns of failure following therapy for primary renal lymphoma.

Primary lymphoma of the bladder, prostate and urethra

Primary lymphoma of the bladder is very rare, accounting for less than 1% of all bladder tumors. Symptomatology comprises haematuria, frequency and dysuria. On cytoscopic examination the tumor is usually lobulated and spares the overlying epithelium. Hydronephrosis is common.[74] Tumors are usually of diffuse type although intermediate and low grade tumors are recorded.[75-78] Primary prostate lymphomas are rarely recorded, although secondary involvement, particularly in low grade lymphoma may be more common than clinically apparent.[77,79,80] Primary lymphoma of the urethra has been reported by Simpson et al.[78] There is little experience upon which to base treatment recommendations, however, there would appear to be no rationale for surgery beyond biopsy and considering the paucity of localized presentations, the management should be similar to treatment policy for advanced disease.

Primary lymphoma of the female genital tract

Primary lymphoma of the female genital tract is uncommon[81] and presents both clinical and histopathologic dilemmas with respect to the interpretation of 'lymphoma-like' lesions simulating malignant lymphoma.[82] The most common site reported is the uterine cervix. There is a clearly distinguishable group of patients with an evident cervical mass, often barrel-shaped expansion of the cervix without surface ulceration, deep infiltration and a diffuse infiltrate of large cells with mitotic activity. A second category comprises patients with superficial, commonly erosive, inflammatory lesions, and patients in whom lymphocytic aggregates are defined within an apparently normal cervix examined following hysterectomy for reasons unrelated to malignancy. This dichotomy impacts upon the interpretation of the natural history of uterine lymphoma in reported series.

There would appear to be no rationale for hysterectomy where the diagnosis of primary uterine lymphoma is clinically and histologically secure. For lesions of intermediate or high grade type, combined modality therapy would appear appropriate. Radiation therapy alone may be considered for primary low grade lymphoma of the cervix.[83] There is no information regarding failure patterns following therapy. The radiation therapy approaches employed have comprised fields covering the pelvis plus paraaortic and pelvic irradiation to 35 Gy. Local control rates are high. Hormonal replacement therapy is indicated in those of appropriate age if oophorepexy is not performed.

Primary lymphoma of the ovary

Involvement of the ovary by lymphoma is not uncommon in patients with advanced disease. Significant ovarian involvement occurs most commonly in high grade lymphoma of Burkitt or undifferentiated non-Burkitt type.[84–86] Primary presentations are very uncommon[85,87] and are usually of intermediate or high grade type. The approach to management would appear to have many parallels with testicular lymphoma with survival rates in the pre-chemotherapy era being extremely poor.

Primary lymphoma of bone

Non-Hodgkin's lymphoma involving bone is relatively common in patients with advanced disease, but constitutes less than 5% of localized extranodal presentations[69] and comprised 3.7% of the PMH series.[90] The most common sites of presentation are the femur and long bones followed by the ilium and scapula. Pain is the usual symptom and radiological findings comprise a lytic and, less commonly, a sclerotic or mixed lesion with or without a pathological fracture. Lymphoma symptomatology is unusual and loco-regional nodal disease occurs infrequently.

Whilst surgical cure is recognized, the majority of patients reported have received additional radiation therapy or, more recently, combined modality treatment. Overall survival rates of 45–65% at 5 years of follow-up are reported with cause-specific, overall and relapse-free survival rates being roughly comparable indicating little non-tumor related mortality and little effective salvage of relapse. Local failure rates following radiation have been in the 14–40% range (20% in-field and 20% loco-regional in the PMH experience). Some reports advocate dose–response data supporting irradiation doses of ≥ 50 Gy[88] whilst most series do not define an advantage for doses in excess of 40 Gy.[89,90] Prognostic factors adverse for loco-regional failure in the PMH series included large tumor bulk and the use of radiation fields restricted to gross disease with a limited margin. In this context, the role of CT and MRI relative to conventional planar imaging in defining disease extent both within and outside the bone cortex is particular relevant.

Despite high local control rates, the long-term relapse-free rate following radiation alone is around 40–50% (27% in the PMH series). In common with several reports, the use of combined modality therapy provides significant survival and relapse-free advantage both in the context of enhanced local control and reduced systemic failure with overall survival and relapse-free rates in excess of 85% at 5 years.[89–92] Patterns of failure and the natural history of the disease do not indicate a risk of CNS progression that warrants CNS prophylaxis. Long-term follow-up also reveals modest morbidity related to the site of presentation and radiation field disposition but no indication of second tumor, either of bone or soft tissue, as a result of therapy.

Primary cutaneous lymphoma

Whereas many extranodal presentations of non-Hodgkin's lymphoma present a fairly homogenous picture with respect to clinical features and management, primary cutaneous lymphoma comprises a remarkably heterogeneous group of lymphoid malignancies at the level of clinical presentation, histology, immunophenotyping and natural history. To quote an overall or median survival for patients with cutaneous lymphoma is essentially meaningless unless more distinction is provided with respect to the composition of the group.

The frequency with which lymphoma presents in the skin is quoted at 5%,[93] and was 3.8% in the PMH series. This frequency reflects referral to a tertiary cancer centre and, as such, may underestimate the true frequency given that many more indolent lesions hitherto not recognized to be clonal malignant lymphomas prior to immunophenotypic or molecular analysis are probably managed in non-cancer centre settings.

Additional complexity is provided by the representation of three cell lineages in cutaneous lymphoma: true histiocytic, B- and T-cell malignancies, and by presentation as unifocal and multi-centric disease within one organ system within the term primary cutaneous lymphoma. The survival figure of 90% in the PMH series (Fig. 2) reflects unicentric or localized primary cutaneous lymphoma and, almost certainly, a predominance of B-cell tumors with a lesser representation of true histiocytic or cutaneous T-cell lymphomas. As such its interpretation is subject to considerable selection bias.

True histiocytic tumors are rare and localization to the skin despite presentation as cutaneous disease is unusual. More commonly, this disease presents as a fairly fulminating malignant histiocytosis with florid symptomatology, extensive dissemination and a poor prognosis despite intensive systemic therapy.

The introduction of techniques to define lineage and clonality has clearly distinguished primary B-cell from primary T-cell cutaneous lymphoma. The clinical spectrum of B-cell lymphoma appears more restricted with a common presentation of single or multiple cutaneous nodules, usually without epithelial breakdown or ulceration. The histological spectrum ranges from small to large follicular centre cell type, the former being more commonly associated with systemic disease. These lesions are readily controlled locally by radiation to doses from 25–35 Gy. A distant relapse rate of up to 50% may be anticipated either as further cutaneous disease or systemic lymphoma.[94] Primary erythrodermic B-cell lymphoma of low grade type is also a rare but well-documented disorder.

Cutaneous T-cell lymphomas cover a wide spectrum of disorders from chronic diseases with a long natural history: mycosis fungoides, Sezary syndrome, lichenoid papulosis, pagetoid reticulosis, chronic lymphocytic vasculitis, to more aggressive peripheral T-cell lymphomas presenting in the skin: angiocentric and angiodestructive lesions such as lymphomatoid granulomatosis and also tumor lesions previously described as diffuse mixed, poorly differentiated lymphocytic or pleomorphic lymphoma, to frankly aggressive high grade T-cell lesions of immunoblastic or lymphoblastic type.[95] A subset of large cell anaplastic cutaneous lymphoma – the Ki-I positive large cell lymphoma – is also a distinguishable entity with a potentially more favourable prognosis than pleomorphic or immunoblastic subtypes.[96,97] Clear precedents exist for the treatment of mycosis fungoides and Sezary syndrome with superficial electron beam irradiation,[98] topical nitrogen mustard, photo chemotherapy,[99] and alpha interferon either alone or in combination with existing superficial therapies or etretinate.[101,101] Such treatments can induce prolonged remission of superficial disease consonant with a natural history expressed over several years. The treatment of disseminated, visceral mycosis fungoides with systemic chemotherapy has largely been of palliative benefit with a median survival of 2–3 years from the documentation of tumor stage disease.[102]

Primary peripheral T-cell cutaneous lymphoma of large cell type is rarely localized and is most commonly approached with intensive systemic therapy. The risk of CNS involvement is well recognized and CNS prophylaxis is a significant consideration. There is some evidence to suggest that peripheral T-cell lymphoma has a worse prognosis than B-cell lymphoma given equivalent therapy.[103]

There is no uniform opinion on the optimal management of angiocentric peripheral T-cell lymphoma (predominantly lymphomatoid granulomatosis) which appears to have a variable and unpredictable natural history with or without treatment. Localized lesions may be controlled by radiation therapy, however, the more common presentation is with more extensive disease involving the airway and lung, kidney and central nervous system and, whilst responsive to combination chemotherapy, it is unclear what proportion and which patients derive long-term benefit from this approach.

In summary, the management of primary cutaneous lymphoma depends greatly upon accurate histological classification, detailed staging and extent within the skin. Radiation therapy readily controls localized skin lesions but survival is determined by the management of systemic dissemination given that the majority of patients will either present with, or progress to, systemic disease. Whilst a proportion of patients with large cell lymphoma may be effectively treated with intensive chemotherapy, the definition of prognostic subsets within peripheral T-cell lymphoma of pleomorphic and angiocentric type and the derivation of optimal therapy remains to be determined.

Primary extranodal lymphoma – other sites

Primary lymphoma in soft tissues
Approximately 5% of primary localized lymphoma in the PMH series arose in soft tissues, location otherwise unspecified. The majority of these are in subcutaneous tissue, retroperitoneum or muscle without clear indication of association with skin or lymph nodes. Various histologic subtypes are included and determination of bulk is often imprecise. The overall survival of approximately 50% at 10 years is characteristic of unselected localized extra-nodal lymphoma. The management of these lesions is largely determined by histologic subtype, with large cell lesions being optimally approached with combined modality therapy given high rates of local control with radiation and control of occult systemic disease with chemotherapy. Localized low grade lesions are effectively controlled locally with radiation.

Primary lymphoma of the breast
Primary lymphoma of the breast comprises approximately 2% of all localized extranodal presentations,[17,69] and approximately 0.17% of breast tumors.[104] The presentation is with a breast mass, frequently large, with or without ipsilateral adenopathy. The mammographic appearances simulate carcinoma although calcification is not seen. Lesions are commonly excised in the absence of a definitive diagnosis of lymphoma although a preoperative diagnosis by fine needle aspiration cytology with appropriate cytological and cytochemical should be attainable. Excision commonly achieves a debulking procedure at the primary site. Large cell lymphoma is the most common histological type although low grade lesions are seen.

Traditionally, radical radiation therapy has been employed following surgery. Fields have incorporated the breast plus the regional lymph nodes to doses of 35–40 Gy. Local control is achieved in approximately 80% of patients and overall survival rates of 40–65% at 10 years are recorded.[104-107] Despite high local control rates, distant failure occurs in approximately 50% of patients. Prognostic factors for disease progression at local and distant sites include large tumor bulk and nodal involvement. No preferential distant sites of failure are apparent, e.g. contralateral breast, CNS, to indicate particular approaches to prophylaxis other than systemic chemotherapy.

In practical terms, for patients with large cell lesions, a combined modality approach would appear to offer optimal management given a progression rate of 50–60% over 10 years of follow-up using radiation alone.

Primary lymphoma of the liver

Traditionally, lymphoma of the liver has been considered in the context of Stage IV (disseminated) disease. Isolated involvement of the liver does, however, occur.[108,109] The principal characteristics include pain, hepatomegaly, palpable mass, jaundice and lymphoma symptoms. Presentation simulating chronic active hepatitis, granulomatous cholangitis, inflammatory pseudotumor or Budd–Chiari syndrome is also documented.[110] Gross appearances may comprise single or multiple tumor masses or diffuse infiltration of the liver in the absence of any evidence of systemic lymphoma. Microscopic features include replacement of liver architecture by lymphoma, destructive sinusoidal and portal tract infiltrates with necrosis and haemorrhage. Diffuse large cell morphology is characteristic. Both T- and B-cell tumors are reported.[110]

The cumulative anecdotal literature defines a 5-year survival in the 40–50% range. The most favourable outcomes appear to be associated with partial hepatectomy for solitary lesions. Given a secure diagnosis, frequent extensive intrahepatic disease, and a mortality rate in excess of 50%, the addition of chemotherapy in addition to any surgical procedure would be justified given appropriate consideration to the choice of agents/regimen in patients with potential or overt liver dysfunction.

Primary lymphoma of the lung

Involvement of the lung by disseminated lymphoma is common. Isolated pulmonary lymphoma is rare comprising 1% of all extranodal localized disease in the PMH series. Three categories of pulmonary lymphoma should be recognized: T-cell lymphoma occurring usually as a component of a more widespread angiocentric and angiodestructive process such as lymphomatoid granulomatosis; large cell lymphoma presenting primarily in the lung; and the more common lymphocytic or lymphoplasmacytoid lymphoma previously considered a reactive infiltrate or a pseudotumor. The presenting features comprise pain, fever and cough, dyspnoea, recurrent pulmonary infections, haemoptysis, or an asymptomatic finding on routine chest radi-

S B Sutcliffe and M K Gospodarowicz

ography. Radiological features include pulmonary consolidation, solid pulmonary opacities, associated hilar adenopathy or pleural effusion. The diagnosis is commonly made by aspiration cytology or open biopsy or excision. Immunocytochemical or molecular techniques are essential to define clonal evidence of malignancy particularly with respect to distinguishing low grade lymphoma from lymphocytic interstitial pneumonia.

A chronic natural history is characteristic of the low grade lymphocytic or lymphoplasmacytoid primary lung lesions even when dissemination to nodes or peripheral blood has been demonstrated. Lesions frequently remain confined to the lung over long periods and local recurrence following resection or irradiation is characteristic. Anecdotal association with subsequent development of gastrointestinal lymphoma is recorded and has led to the development of a BALT hypothesis (bronchus-associated lymphoid tissue) as part of the wider MALT (mucosa-associated lymphoid tissue) theory.[5] This hypothesis would suggest preferential homing of bronchus derived lymphoid cells to the lung or mucosal sites thereby conferring preferential localization of tumors in these sites. Circulating cells would have limited proliferative potential in non-BALT/MALT sites thereby focusing clinical management at the level of the local lesion rather than at systemic dissemination.[111] This hypothesis is compatible with the long natural history of primary low grade lymphoma of lung and would suggest that local treatment approaches may be optimal, e.g. lung resection, partial lung irradiation. The radiosensitivity of these lesions is well-recognized and significant local palliation accompanies its use. Chemotherapy appropriate to management of low grade lymphoma is appropriate for multifocal or extensive intrapulmonary low grade disease.

Conclusions
It has been traditional practice to treat patients with Stage I and II non-Hodgkin's lymphoma with radiation therapy following a diagnostic biopsy or more definitive surgical procedure for some extranodal presentations. The Princess Margaret Hospital experience with such an approach has defined that radiation therapy is effective in achieving a high level of progression-free survival providing that selection according to defined prognostic parameters takes place: age $\leq$ 60 years, Stage IA disease or first echelon nodal extent in Stage IIA, and tumor bulk of 0–2.5 cm residuum prior to radiation.[112] Through such selection, cause-specific survival and relapse-free rates of 90% and > 75% at 10 years can be achieved with radiation alone for patients with either low or intermediate and high grade histology. In practice, such selection identifies a small proportion of patients with localized Stage I and II lymphoma who do very well with radiation. Patients failing to meet these criteria have cause-specific survival and relapse-free rates of 50% or less with radiation, and given effective chemotherapy for those with intermediate and

high grade lymphoma, such patients are more optimally treated with combined modality therapy.

In the previously reported analysis, no distinction was made between nodal and extranodal presentation. We have, however, drawn attention to the variation in prognosis between different extranodal presentations within clinical Stage I–II non-Hodgkin's lymphoma.[113] The question, therefore, arises as to whether the natural history of nodal and extranodal disease is similar. In terms of comparability of presentations, Table 4 has defined that the prognostic factor distribution between nodal and extranodal groups is generally equivalent other than for a much higher representation of diffuse large cell histology or higher grade lesions in the extranodal category. Given some imbalance in the allocation of treatment, the cause-specific survival curves for aggregated Stage I and II nodal and extranodal lymphoma are superimposable (Fig. 4). When distinguished by stage, the cause-specific survival of Stage I extranodal lymphoma is inferior to that of nodal lymphoma whilst the Stage II extranodal survival is superior to that of nodal disease. Thus, in very broad terms, the overall prognosis for extranodal disease is comparable to nodal disease for the treatments employed during this time period (1967–78) a somewhat surprising finding given the much higher representation of intermediate, predominantly diffuse large cell histology in extranodal presentations.

This should not indicate, however, that site of extranodal disease is unimportant in choice of treatment allocation and prognosis. The very wide range of outcomes by site is shown in Table 3 and ranges from a 90% to a 20% cause-specific survival at 5 years. Clearly, in addition to age, stage, histology and bulk of disease, site of extranodal presentation is an important prognostic factor. In this setting, radiation alone might be considered appropriate therapy for those selected by age, stage and bulk of disease with gastrointestinal, thyroid, orbital (though not intra-ocular) and selected skin presentations. Given that diffuse large cell histology comprises over 75% of histologic subtypes in extranodal lymphoma, a very strong case can be made for treating all patients with localized lymphoma at all other extranodal sites with a combined modality approach.

Even so, this approach would ignore certain other relevant aspects of the natural history of specific extranodal sites. Primary central nervous system lymphoma of parenchymal or leptomeningeal type requires separate consideration given a high local failure rate with radical irradiation and the failure of systemic and/or intrathecal chemotherapy to make a major impact upon a very poor survival rate. Intra-ocular lymphoma, although rare, requires central nervous system prophylaxis over-and-above considerations relating to local tumor control. CNS chemo prophylaxis is also a relevant consideration for primary extradural presentations and also those with advanced testicular presentations. In addition, prophylactic irradiation to the remaining testis for patients with primary testicular lymphoma is a justifiable practice.

A study of the natural history of treated extranodal lymphoma has also indicated that there may be preferential localization of disease for certain sites – G.I. tract stage, low grade pulmonary lymphoma, thyroid, orbital and skin lymphoma, perhaps reflecting biologic properties, e.g. homing, the understanding of which may subsequently be important in defining the risk of distant metastatic potential of apparently localized lymphoma.

References

(1) Levison DA, Hall PA, Blackshaw AJ. The gut-associated lymphoid tissue and its tumours. *Curr Topics Path* 1990; 81: 133–75.

(2) Grody WW, Magidson JG, Weiss LM, Hu E, Warnke RA, Lewin KJ. Gastro-intestinal lymphoma. Immunohistochemical studies on the cell of origin. *Am J Surg Path* 1985; 9: 328–37.

(3) Isaacson PG, Spencer J. Malignant lymphoma of mucosa-associated lymphoid tissue. *Histopathology* 1987; 11: 445–62.

(4) Laszewski MJ, Kamat D, Kemp JD et al. Immunophenotypic and genotypic characterization of primary non-Hodgkin's lymphoma of the gastrointestinal tract. *Mod Path* 1990; 3: 423–8.

(5) Isaacson P, Wright DH. Malignant lymphoma of mucosa-associated lymphoid tissue. *Cancer* 1983; 52: 1410–16.

(6) Wu NW, Jalkanen S, Streeter PR, Butcher EC. Evolutionary conservation of tissue-specific lymphocyte-endothelial cell recognition mechanisms involved in lymphocyte homing. *J Cell Biol* 1988; 107: 1845–51.

(7) Spencer J, Cerf-Bensussan N, Jarry A, Brousse N, Guy-Grand D, Krajewski AS. Enteropathy associated T-cell lymphoma (malignant histiocytosis of the intestine) is recognized by a monoclonal antibody (HML-1) that defines a membrane molecule on mucosal lymphocytes. *Am J Path* 1988; 132: 1–5.

(8) Stein H, Dieneman D, Sperling M, Zeitz M, Rieken EO. Identification of a T-cell-derived lymphoma derived from intestinal mucosa associated T-cells. *Lancet* 1988; ii: 1053–4.

(9) Van Krieken JH, Otter R, Hermans et al. Malignant lymphoma of the gastro-intestinal tract and mesentery. A clinico-pathological study group of the comprehensive cancer centre west. *Am J Path* 1989; 135: 281–9.

(10) Azab MB, Henry-Amar M, Rougier P et al. Prognostic factors in primary gastrointestinal non-Hodgkin's lymphoma. A multivariate analysis, report of 106 cases, and review of the literature. *Cancer* 1989; 64: 1208–17.

(11) Gospodarowicz MK, Sutcliffe SB, Clark RM et al. Outcome analysis of localized gastrointestinal lymphoma treated with surgery and post-operative irradiation. *Int J Rad Oncol Biol Phys* 1990; 19: 1351–5.

(12) Jaser N, Sivula A, Franssila K. Primary gastric non-Hodgkin's lymphoma in Finland, 1972–1977. Clinical presentation and results of treatment. *Scand J Gastroenterol* 1990; 25: 1052–9.

(13) Shepherd FA, Evans WK, Kutas G et al. Chemotherapy following surgery for

stages IE and IIE non-Hodgkin's lymphoma of the gastro-intestinal tract. *J Clin Oncol* 1988; 6: 253–60.

(14) Bellesi G, Alterini R, Messori A et al. Combined surgery and chemotherapy for the treatment of primary gastrointestinal intermediate- or high-grade non-Hodgkin's lymphomas. *Br J Cancer* 1989; 60: 244–8.

(15) Fuller LM, Hagemeister FB, Sullivan MP, Velasquez WS. In: *Hodgkin's disease and non-Hodgkin's lymphoma in adults and children*. New York: Raven Press, 1988: 331–2.

(16) Brugere J, Schlienger M, Gerard-Marchant R, Tubiana M, Pouillart P, Cachin Y. Non-Hodgkin's malignant lymphoma of upper digestive and respiratory tract: natural history and results of radiotherapy. *Br J Cancer* 1975; 31. Suppl. 2: 435–40.

(17) Otter R, Gerrits WB, Sandt MM, Hermans J, Willemze R. Primary extranodal and nodal non-Hodgkin's lymphoma. A survey of a population-based registry. *Eur J Cancer Clin Oncol* 1989; 25: 1203–10.

(18) De Pena CA, Van Tassel P, Lee Y-Y. Lymphoma of the head and neck. *Radiol Clinics of N Am* 1990; 28: 723–43.

(19) Ossenkoppele GJ, Mol JJ, Snow GB et al. Radiotherapy versus radiotherapy plus chemotherapy in Stages I and II Non-Hodgkin's lymphoma of the upper digestive and respiratory tract. *Cancer* 1987; 60: 1505–9.

(20) Hoppe RT, Burke JS, Glatstein E, Kaplan HS. Non-Hodgkin's lymphoma, involvement of Waldeyer's ring. *Cancer* 1978; 42: 1096–104.

(21) Conley SF, Staszak C, Clamon GH, Maves MD. Non-Hodgkin's lymphoma of the head and neck: the University of Iowa experience. *Laryngoscope* 1987; 97: 291–300.

(22) Liang R, Ng RP, Todd D, Choy D, Khoo RK, Ho FC. Management of Stage I–II diffuse aggressive non-Hodgkin's lymphoma of the Waldeyer's ring: combined modality therapy versus radiotherapy alone. *Hematol Oncol* 1987; 5: 223–30.

(23) Wulfrank D, Speelman T, Pauwels C, Roels H, De Schryver A. Extranodal non-Hodgkin's lymphoma of the head and neck. *Radiother Oncol* 1987; 8: 199–207.

(24) Banfi A, Bonadonna G, Ricci SB et al. Malignant lymphoma of Waldeyer's ring: natural history and survival after radiotherapy. *Br Med J* 1972; 3: 140–3.

(25) Fuller LM, Hagemeister FB, Sullivan MP, Velasquez WS. *Hodgkin's disease and non-Hodgkin's lymphomas in adults and children*. New York: Raven Press, 1988; 326–31.

(26) Wang CC. Primary malignant lymphoma of the oral cavity and paranasal sinuses. *Radiology* 1971; 100: 151–3.

(27) Teshima T, Chatani M, Inoue T et al. Radiation therapy for primary non-Hodgkin's lymphoma of the head and neck in Stage I–II. *Strahlenther Onkol.* 1986; 162: 478–83.

(28) Ree HJ, Rege VB, Knisley RE et al. Malignant lymphoma of Weldeyer's ring following gastrointestinal lymphoma. *Cancer* 1980; 46: 1528–35.

(29) Holm LE, Blomgren H, Lowhagen T. Cancer risks in patients with chronic lymphocytic thyroiditis. *New Eng J Med* 1985; 312: 601–4.

(30) Makepeace AR, Fermont DC, Bennett MH. Non-Hodgkin's lymphoma of the thyroid. *Clin Radiol* 1987; 38: 277–81.

(31) Blair TJ, Evans RG, Buskirk SJ, Banks PM, Earle JD. Radiotherapeutic management of primary lymphoid lymphoma. *Int J Rad Oncol Biol Phys* 1985; 11: 365–70.

(32) Tupchong L, Hughes F, Harmer CL. Primary lymphoma of the thyroid: clinical features, prognostic factors, and results of treatment. *Int J Rad Oncol Biol Phys* 1986; 12: 1813–21.

(33) Vigliotti A, Kong JS, Fuller LM, Velasquez WS. Thyroid lymphomas Stages IE and IIE: Comparative results for radiotherapy only, combined chemotherapy only and multi-modality treatment. *Int J Rad Oncol Biol Phys* 1986; 12: 1807–12.

(34) Leedman PJ, Sheridan WP, Downey WF, Fox RM, Martin FI. Combination chemotherapy as single modality therapy for Stage IE and IIe thyroid lymphoma. *Med J Aust* 1990; 152: 40–3.

(35) Anscombe AM, Wright DH. Primary malignant lymphoma of the thyroid – a tumour of mucosa-associated lymphoid tissue: review of seventy-six cases. *Histopathology* 1985; 9: 81–97.

(36) Litam JP, Cabanillas F, Smith TL, Bodey GP, Freireich EJ. Central nervous system relapse in malignant lymphomas: risk factors and implications for prophylaxis. *Blood* 1979; 54: 1249–57.

(37) Levitt LJ, Dawson DM, Rosenthal DS, Moloney WC. CNS involvement in the non-Hodgkin's lymphomas. *Cancer* 1980; 45: 545–52.

(38) Mackintosh FR, Colby TV, Podolsky WJ et al. Central nervous system involvement in non-Hodgkin's lymphoma: an analysis of 105 cases. *Cancer* 1982; 49: 586–95.

(39) Hobson DE, Anderson BA, Carr I, West M. Primary Hodgkin's lymphoma of the central nervous system: Manitoba experience and review of literature. *Can J Neurol Sci* 186; 13: 55–61.

(40) Remick SC, Diamond C, Migliozzi JA et al. Primary central nervous system lymphoma in patients with and without the acquired immunodeficiency syndrome. A retrospective analysis and review of the literature. *Medicine* 1990; 69: 345–60.

(41) Zimmerman RA. Central nervous system lymphoma. *Radiol Clinics N Am* 1990; 28: 697–721.

(42) O'Neill BP, Illig JJ. Primary central nervous system lymphoma. *Mayo Clin Proc* 1989; 64: 1005–20.

(43) Murray K, Kun L, Cox J. Primary malignant lymphoma of the central nervous system: results of treatment of 11 cases and review of the literature. *J Neurosurg* 1986; 65: 600–7.

(44) Bonnin JM, Garcia JH. Primary malignant non-Hodgkin's lymphoma of the central nervous system. *Path Ann* 1987; 22: 353–75.

(45) Berry MP, Simpson WJ. Radiation therapy in the management of primary malignant lymphoma of the brain. *Int J Rad Oncol Biol Phys* 1981; 7: 55–9.

(46) Chamberlain MC, Levin VA. Adjuvant chemotherapy for primary Hodgkin's lymphoma of the central nervous system. *Arch Neurol* 1990; 47: 1113–16.

(47) Shibamoto Y, Tsutsui K, Dodo Y, Yamabe H, Shima N, Abe M. Intracranial

lymphoma treated by high-dose radiation and systemic vincristine–doxorubicin–cyclophosphamide–prednisolone chemotherapy. *Cancer* 1990; 65: 1907–12.

(48) Lachance DH, O'Neill BP, MacDonald DR et al. Primary leptomeningeal lymphoma: report of 9 cases, diagnosis with immunocytochemical analysis and review of the literature. *Neurology* 1991; 41: 95–100.

(49) Nguyen D, Nathwani BN. Primary meningel small lymphocytic lymphoma. *Am J Surg Pathol* 1989; 13: 67–70.

(50) Kepes JJ, Maxwell JA, Hedeman L, Slaven J. Primary diffuse malignant lymphoma of the leptomeninges presenting as 'pseudotumour cerebri'. *Neurochirurgia* 1971; 14: 188–96.

(51) Harris NL, Harmon DC, Pilch BZ, Goodman ML, Bhan AK. Immunohistologic diagnosis of orbital lymphoid infiltrates. *Am J Surg Pathol* 1984; 8: 83–91.

(52) Astarita RW, Minckler D, Taylor CR, Levine A, Lukes RJ. Orbital and adnexal lymphomas – a multiparameter approach. *Am J Clin Pathol* 1980; 73: 615–21.

(53) Knowles DM II, Jakobiec FA, Halper JP. Immunologic characterization of ocular adnexal lymphoid neoplasms. *Am J Ophthal* 1979; 87: 603–19.

(54) Fitzpatrick PJ, Macko S. Lymphoreticular tumours of the orbit. *Int J Rad Oncol Biol Phys* 1984; 10: 333–40.

(55) Jereb B, Lee H, Jakobiec FA, Kutcher J. Radiation therapy of conjunctival and orbital lymphoid tumours. *Int J Rad Oncol Biol Phys* 1984; 10: 1013–19.

(56) Trudeau M, Shepherd FA, Blackstein ME, Gospodarowicz M, Fitzpatrick P, Moffatt KP. Intraocular lymphoma: report of three cases and review of the literature. *Am J Clin Oncol* 1988; 11: 126–30.

(57) Qualman SJ, Mendelsohn G, Mann RB, Green WR. Intraocular lymphoma: natural history based on a clinicopathologic study of eight cases and review of the literature. *Cancer* 1983; 52: 878–86.

(58) Simon JW, Friedman AH. Ocular reticulum cell sarcoma. *Br J Opthal* 1980; 64: 793–9.

(59) Rockwood EJ, Zakov ZN, Bug JW. Combined malignant lymphoma of the eye and CNS (reticulum-cell sarcoma). *J Neurosurg* 1984; 61: 369–74.

(60) Baumann MA, Ritch PS, Harde KR, Williams GA, Topping TM, Anderson T. Treatment of intraocular lymphoma with high-dose ara-C. *Cancer* 1986; 57: 1273–5.

(61) Kiely JM, Massey BD Jr, Harrison EG Jr, Utz DC. Lymphoma of the testis. *Cancer* 1970; 26: 847–52.

(62) Sussman EB, Hajdu SI, Lieberman PH, Whitmore WF. Malignant lymphoma of the testis: a clinicopathologic study of 37 cases. *J Urol* 1977; 118: 1004–7.

(63) Duncan PR, Checa F, Gowing NF, McElwain TJ, Peckham MJ. Extranodal non-Hodgkin's lymphoma presenting in the testicle: a clinical and pathologic study of 24 cases. *Cancer* 1980; 45: 1578–84.

(64) Turner RR, Colby TV, MacKintosh FR. Testicular lymphomas: a clinicopathologic study of 35 cases. *Cancer* 1981; 48: 2095–102.

(65) Buskirk SJ, Evan RG, Banks PM, O'Connell MJ, Earle JD. Non-primary Hodgkin's lymphoma of the testis. *Int J Rad Oncol Biol Phys* 1982; 8: 1699–703.

(66) Tepperman BS, Gospodarowicz MK, Bush RS, Brown TC. Non-Hodgkin's lymphoma of the testis. *Radiology* 1982; 142: 203–8.

(67) Doll DC, Weiss RB. Malignant lymphoma of the testis. *Am J Med* 1986; 81: 515–24.

(68) Connors JM, Klimo P, Voss N, Fairey RN, Jackson S. Testicular lymphoma: improved outcome with early brief chemotherapy. *J Clin Oncol* 1988; 6: 776–81.

(69) Freeman C, Berg JW, Cutler SJ. Occurrence and prognosis of extranodal lymphomas. *Cancer* 1972; 29: 252–60.

(70) Richmond J, Sherman RS, Diamond HD, Craver LF. Renal lesions associated with malignant lymphoma. *Am J Med* 1962; 32: 184–207.

(71) Richards MA, Mootoosamy I, Reznek RH, Webb JA, Lister TA. Renal involvement in patients with non-Hodgkin's lymphoma: clinical and pathological features in 23 cases. *Hematol Oncol* 1990; 8: 105–10.

(72) Kandel LB, McCullough DL, Harrison LH. Primary renal lymphoma presenting with perirenal masses. *Br J Radiol* 1988; 61: 1077–8.

(73) Charnsangavej C. Lymphoma of the genitourinary tract. *Radiol Clinics N Am* 1990; 28: 865–77.

(74) Guthman DA, Malek RS, Chapman WR, Farrow GM. Primary malignant lymphoma of the bladder. *J Urol* 1990; 144: 1367–9.

(75) Aigen AB, Phillips M. Primary malignant lymphoma of the urinary bladder. *Urology* 1986; 28: 235–7.

(76) Heaney JA, Delellis RA, Rudders RA. Non-Hodgkin's lymphoma arising in the lower urinary tract. *Urology* 1985; 25: 479–84.

(77) Binkovitz LA, Hattery RR, LeRoy AJ. Primary lymphoma of the bladder. *Urol Radiol* 1988; 9: 231–3.

(78) Simpson RH, Bridger JE, Anthony PP, James KA, Jury I. Malignant lymphoma of the lower urinary tract. *Br J Urol* 1990; 65: 254–60.

(79) Bostwick DG, Mann RB. Malignant lymphomas involving the prostate. *Cancer* 1985; 56: 2932–8.

(80) Sridhar KN, Woodhouse CR. Prostate infiltration in leukemia and lymphoma. *Eur Urol* 1983; 9: 153–6.

(81) Harris NL, Scully RE. Malignant lymphoma and granulocytic sarcoma of the uterus and vagina. A clinicopathologic analysis of 27 cases. *Cancer* 1984; 53: 2530–45.

(82) Young RH, Harris NL, Scully RE. Lymphoma-like lesions of the lower female genital tract: a report of 16 cases. *Int J Gynecol Pathol* 1985; 4: 289–99.

(83) Miketic LM, Carroll R, Harris NL, Linggood RM. Computed tomography in the evaluation of lymphoma of the uterine cervix. *Comput Tomog* 1988; 12: 154–8.

(84) Brew DS, Jackson JG. Lymphosarcoma in the ovary in young African girls in Nigeria. *Br J Cancer* 1961; 14: 621–6.

(85) Paladugu RR, Bearman RM, Rappaport H. Malignant lymphoma with primary manifestation in the gonad: a clinico-pathologic study of 38 patients. *Cancer* 1980; 45: 561–71.

(86) Woodruff JD, Castillord RD, Novak ER. Lymphoma of the ovary. A study of

35 cases from the ovarian tumour registry of the American Gynecological Society. *Am J Obstet Gynecol* 1963; 85: 912–18.

(87) Chorlton I, Norris HJ, King FM. Malignant reticuloendothelial disease involving the ovary as a primary manifestation. A series of 19 lymphomas and 1 granulocytic sarcoma. *Cancer* 1974; 34: 397–407.

(88) Dosoretz DE, Murphy GF, Raymond AK et al. Radiation therapy for primary lymphoma of bone. *Cancer* 1983; 51: 44–6.

(89) Bacci G, Jaffe N, Emiliani E et al. Therapy for primary non-Hodgkin's lymphoma of bone and a comparison of results with Ewing's sarcoma. *Cancer* 1986; 57: 1468–72.

(90) Rathmell AJ, Gospodarowicz MK, Sutcliffe SB, Clark RM. Localized lymphoma of bone: prognostic factors and treatment recommendations. (manuscript submitted 1991).

(91) Mendenhall NP, Jones JJ, Kramer BS et al. The management of primary lymphoma of bone. *Radiother Oncol* 1987; 9: 137–45.

(92) Loeffler JS, Tarbell NJ, Kozakewich H, Cassady JR, Weinstein HJ. Primary lymphoma of bone in children: analysis of treatment results with adriamycin, prednisone, oncovin (APO) and local radiation therapy. *J Clin Oncol* 1986; 4: 496–501.

(93) Rosenberg SA, Diamond HD, Jaslowitz B, Craver LF. Lymphosarcoma: a review of 1269 cases. *Medicine* 1961; 40: 31–84.

(94) Esche BA, Fitzpatrick PJ. Cutaneous malignant lymphoma. *Int J Radiat Oncol Biol Phys* 1986; 12(12): 2111–15.

(95) Jimbow K, Takami T. Cutaneous T-Cell lymphoma and related disorders. *Int J Dermatol* 1986; 25: 485–97.

(96) Agnarsson BA, Kadin ME. Ki-1 positive large cell lymphoma. A morphologic and immunologic study of 19 cases. *Am J Surg Path* 1988; 12: 264–74.

(97) Beljaards RC, Meijer CJLM, Scheffer E, Van Vloten WA, Willemze R. Cutaneous large cell lymphoma of T-Cell origin: diagnosis, classification and prognostic parameters. In: Van Vloten WA, Willemze R, Lange Fejlsgaard G, Thomsen K, eds. *Cutaneous lymphoma. Curr Probl Dermatol* 1990; 19: 144–9.

(98) Hoppe RT, Wood GS, Abel EA. Mycosis fungoides and the Sezary syndrome: pathology, staging and treatment. *Curr Probl in Cancer* 1990; 14: 293–371.

(99) Rosenbaum MM, Roenigk HH Jr, Caro WA, Esker A. Photochemotherapy in cutaneous T-cell lymphoma and parapsoriasis en plaques. *J Am Acad Dermatol* 1985; 13: 613–22.

(100) Roenigk HH Jr, Kuzel TM, Skoutelis AP et al. Photochemotherapy alone or combined with interferon alpha-2A in the treatment of cutaneous T-cell lymphoma. *J Invest Dermatol* 1990; 95: 198S–205S.

(101) Zachariae H, Thestrup-Pederson K. Interferon alpha and etretinate combination treatment of cutaneous T-cell lymphoma. *J Invest Dermatol* 1990; 95: 206S–8S.

(102) Hallahan DE, Griem ML, Griem SF et al. Combined modality therapy for tumour stage mycosis fungoides: results of a 10-year follow-up. *J Clin Oncol* 1988; 6: 1177–83.

(103) Coiffier B, Brousse N, Peuchmaur M et al. for the GELA. Peripheral T-cell

lymphomas have a worse prognosis than B-cell lymphomas: a prospective study of 361 immunophenotyped patients treated with the LNH-84 regimen. *Ann Oncol* 1990; 1: 45–50.

(104) DeBlasio D, McCormick B, Straus D et al. Definitive irradiation for localized non-Hodgkin's lymphoma of breast. *Int J Rad Oncol Biol Phys* 1989; 17: 843–6.

(105) Brustein S, Filippa DA, Kummel M, Lieberman PH, Rosen PP. Malignant lymphoma of the breast. A study of 53 patients. *Ann Surg* 1987; 205: 144–50.

(106) Liu FF, Clark RM. Primary lymphoma of the breast. *Clin Radiol* 1986; 37: 567–70.

(107) Dixon JM, Lumsden AB, Krajewski A, Elton RA, Anderson TJ. Primary lymphoma of the breast. *Br J Surg* 1987; 74: 214–17.

(108) Osborne BM, Butler JJ, Guarda LA. Primary lymphoma of the liver. Ten cases and review of the literature. *Cancer* 1985; 56: 2902–10.

(109) Dement SH, Mann RB, Staal SP, Kuhajda FP, Boitnott JK. Primary lymphoma of the liver. Report of six cases and review of the literature. *Am J Clin Pathol* 1987; 88: 255–63.

(110) Anthony PP, Sarsfield P, Clarke T. Primary lymphoma of the liver: clinical and pathologic features of ten patients. *J Clin Pathol* 1990; 43: 1007–13.

(111) Herbert A, Wright DH, Isaacson PG, Smith JL. Primary malignant lymphoma of the lung: histopathologic and immunologic evaluation of nine cases. *Hum Pathol* 1984; 15: 415–22.

(112) Sutcliffe SB, Gospodarowicz MK, Bush RS et al. Role of radiation therapy in localized non-Hodgkin's lymphoma. *Radiother Oncol* 1985; 4: 211–23.

(113) Gospodarowicz MK, Sutcliffe SB, Brown TC, Chua T, Bush RS. Patterns of disease in localised extranodal lymphoma. *J Clin Oncol* 1987; 5: 875–80.

Index

Index

Index

226

Index

228

AKBAR AND BIRBAL

AKBAR & BIRBAL
TALES OF HUMOUR

Monisha Mukundan

Illustrated by
TAPAS GUHA

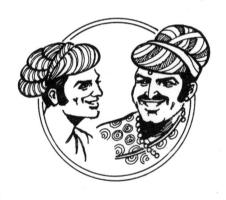

Rupa & Co

An Original Rupa Paperback
First Published 1992
Seventh impression 2000

Published by
Rupa & Co.
7/16, Ansari Road, Daryaganj
New Delhi 110 002

Cover and book design by Tapas Guha

Typeset in 12 pt. Garamond by
Nikita Overseas Pvt Ltd
19A Ansari Road, Daryaganj
New Delhi 110 002

Printed in India by
Gopsons Paper Ltd
A-14 Sector 60
Noida 201 301

ISBN 81-7167-086-5

To
Muk
Govind and Vasundhara

CONTENTS

Introduction

Akbar, the third Mughal emperor, had many talented and clever people at his court. Among them was a man called Raja Birbal, who was a special favourite of the emperor because of his quick wit. Raja Birbal wrote poetry, and Akbar gave him the title of Poet Laureate. He liked to have Birbal near him, because he enjoyed his conversation and his clever way with words.

In the four hundred years since Emperor Akbar ruled India and since Birbal's poems and sayings and ready answers made the great emperor laugh and think, many stories have been told about them. Some may be true, many are not. They are folk tales, or stories that people have passed on from one generation to the next, by telling them again and again. Storytellers have added to the stories and changed them. Nevertheless, they remain popular because they are fun to hear and to

AKBAR & BIRBAL

read and they make us laugh. And, sometimes, they make us think about what is true and good in our lives.

How They Met

Emperor Akbar loved to go hunting. Even as a child, he would run away from his lessons and his tutors in order to go riding and hunting. When he grew up, he was a better rider and a more fearless hunter than any of his courtiers. One day, chasing a tiger, Akbar and a few brave soldiers rode so fast that they left all the others behind. They had gone a long distance from the royal capital at Agra and, as evening came, they realised that they were lost. They went on slowly. They were hot, dusty, and tired. Presently, they reached a place where three roads met. "Ah, at last", the emperor exclaimed. Then, turning to his men, he asked, "Which way shall we go? Which road goes to Agra?"

The roads all looked the same. It was hard to tell which road led to Agra. The men looked at each other. They looked at the road. Then they looked at the dust

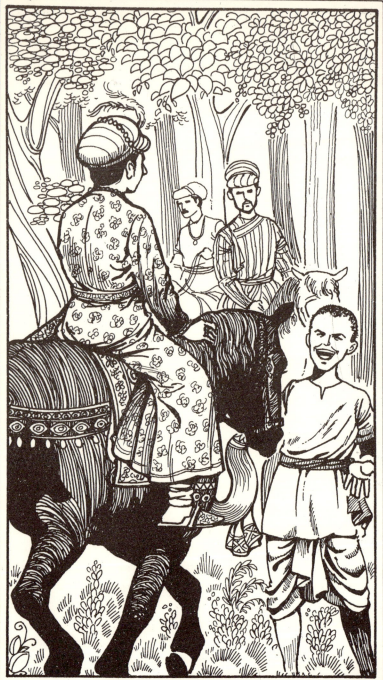

beneath their horses' hooves. Nobody said a word.

Just then, a young man came walking down one of the roads. Glad to have something to do, the Emperor's men called out to him and ordered him to come forward. He did so, looking up at the richly-dressed hunters with bright, curious eyes. "Tell us, boy", said Emperor Akbar, "which road goes to Agra?"

The young man began to smile. "Huzoor, everybody knows that roads cannot move. How can this road go to Agra, or go anywhere else?" he said, and he chuckled delightedly at his own joke.

There was absolute silence. The emperor stared down at the youth. His soldiers held their breath. They knew the emperor's temper. Not one of them dared to say a single word. "People travel", the boy went on, not seeming to notice the ominous silence, "roads, don't, do they?"

"No, they don't", the emperor cried suddenly and began to laugh. Nervously, his soldiers began to laugh too. The youth ignored them and continued to look up at the emperor with twinkling eyes. "What's your name?" Emperor Akbar asked the young man. "Mahesh Das", he replied. "And what is your name, Huzoor?" The emperor pulled off an enormous emerald ring which he wore on his hand. Leaning down, he gave it to the young man.

"You are speaking to Akbar, Emperor of Hindustan", he said. "We need fearless young men such as you at our court, Mahesh Das. Bring this ring with you when you come, and I shall recognise and remember you. And now, show us the road we must take in order to go to Agra."

Mahesh Das bowed low and pointed towards the capital. The emperor turned his horse and galloped away, followed by his soldiers. Mahesh Das watched until a bend in the road hid them from his sight.

Mahesh Das and the Sentry

A few years later, Mahesh Das decided to travel to the emperor's court at Agra to seek his fortune. He had finished his studies and was ready to see the world. When he arrived at Agra, he walked through the bazaar and past the great havelis in which the nobles lived. It was all very confusing to a young man who had spent all his life in the village. But Mahesh Das was no ordinary individual. He held on to the cloth bag in which he carried the emperor's ring and he looked around him with interest. It was evening by the time he reached the massive fort on the bank of the river Yamuna in which the Emperor of Hindustan lived. Even though he was a brave and resolute young man, Mahesh Das felt very small as he neared the enormous studded gate of the fort. The huge wooden gate was open and important-looking people hurried in and out. Two guards stood outside,

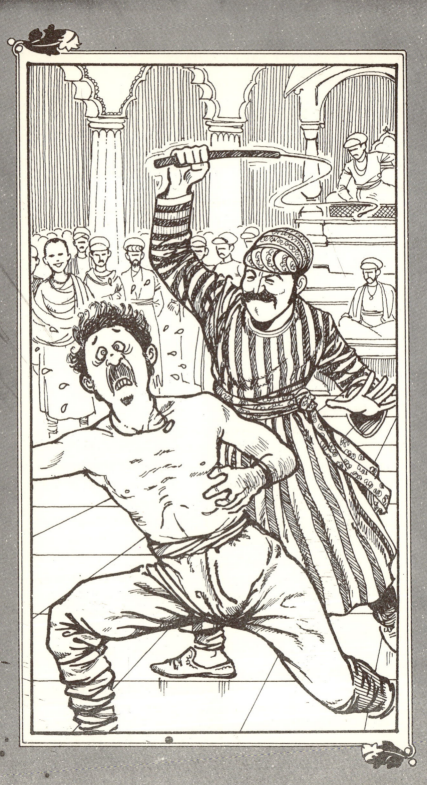

holding spears in their strong, muscular hands. Mahesh Das took a deep breath and then going up to one of the soldiers, he said, "I have come to meet the emperor. He invited me to come to court."

"Ho!" said the soldier, looking at the young man's dusty feet and simple cotton clothes. "So the emperor invited you to his durbar, did he? To the Diwan-i-Khas, no doubt, the Hall of Private Audience, where he meets high-ranking nobles!" A few passersby stopped to watch, smiling at the simple village lad's discomfiture.

"Perhaps", Mahesh Das answered boldly, keeping his voice steady even though he felt very frightened. "And I have his ring to prove it." From his bag, he pulled out the richly worked ring which Emperor Akbar had given him. "Oh", said the guard, in sudden doubt.

"That's no ordinary ring", said a pundit who had stopped to watch. "You'd better let the young man in."

"We-ell", said the guard, sorry to have lost an opportunity to bully and to tease. "I'll let you go in on one condition. When you see the emperor, he is sure to give a gift. I'll let you in if you swear to give me half of whatever the emperor gives you."

People standing nearby began to murmur. They knew the guard and his greedy ways, and wondered how the young man would deal with him. But to their surprise, Mahesh Das agreed at once, without even trying to argue or bargain. The guard said again softly, threateningly, "Don't forget, or I'll make you very, very sorry."

Mahesh Das nodded. "I won't forget", he said, and he walked into the fort.

Emperor Akbar was in the Diwan-i-Am, the Hall of Public Audience. Lamps lit up the carvings on the wall and the rich carpets which were spread on the floor. The great pillared hall was full of courtiers dressed in the finest and most beautifully woven garments. But Mahesh Das had eyes only for the emperor, who sat grandly on a platform at the far end of the hall. Bowing low, he made his way towards the throne. The courtiers murmured to each other in surprise. Who could this be? But Emperor Akbar happened to glance up. He recognised the young man at once and asked him to come forward. "I remember you, Mahesh Das", he said. "And I am pleased that you have come. Ask for anything your heart desires and it shall be yours."

"Jahanpanah is most gracious", Mahesh Das answered. "If Huzoor pleases, my dearest wish is to be given fifty lashes of the whip!"

"Mad, the boy must be mad", people whispered to each other. But the emperor liked the bright, straightforward look in his eyes and he said, "Before we grant this strange wish you must tell us why you want such a gift."

Then Mahesh Das bowed once again and said, "Before the sentry who guards Jahanpanah's fort permitted me to come into the palace, he made me promise that I should give him half the gift that I received. I am ready to bear twenty-five lashes, in order to share this with the guard."

When Akbar heard this, he grew very angry. "Are our people to be kept away by a greedy, wicked guard?" he thundered. "Send for the rascal!"

The guard was sentenced to the entire gift of fifty lashes and never again tried to bully poor people who sought an audience with the emperor. And, Mahesh Das was given a place at the court, with all the comforts that went with it. "We confer on you the

10

title of Raja Birbal from this day on", the emperor declared. "And you shall stay near us and amuse and guide us henceforth!"

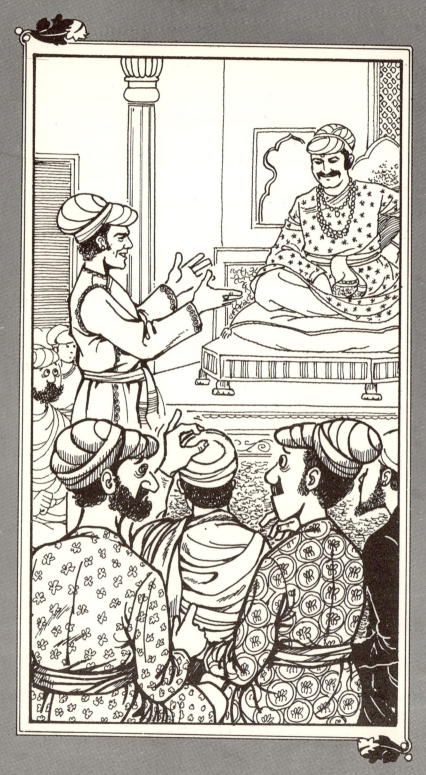

A Matter of Crows

C lose to the emperor's private apartments was the Diwan-i-Khas, the Hall of Private Audience. It was not as large as the Diwan-i-Am, but it was beautifully decorated and luxuriously furnished. Here, special courtiers and the highest nobles in the land met the emperor to discuss matters of state. Sometimes the emperor liked to discuss other things too, such as where the best melons came from or who the wisest sage was. Occasionally, he liked to pose questions which his courtiers thought were unanswerable. To Emperor Akbar's delight, Birbal always had an answer no matter how absurd the question.

One morning, the emperor took his seat on the throne in the Diwan-i-Khas and demanded, "Tell us at once: How many crows are there in all of Agra? It is important that we have this information immediately. And if it is not absolutely correct, there will be serious

13

trouble, I warn you."

The courtiers looked at each other in alarm. What were they to do? Some had a reasonable idea of how many elephants there were in the city. Many knew more or less how many horses there were. One man had even kept track of how many pet parrots there were. But crows? Some courtiers began to pray desperately for a flash of divine inspiration. Others tried to hide behind their friends. A few began to examine the sky anxiously, wondering if they could make a quick count of all the crows they could see and calculate the total on that basis. Only Raja Birbal remained calm and smiling. "Jahanpanah", he said after several minutes. "There are exactly ten thousand, six hundred and sixty-six crows in all of Agra."

"Oh?" said Emperor Akbar with a gleam in his eye. "You shall not bluff your way out of this one, Birbal, my friend. We shall have a proper count to confirm your estimate."

"By all means, Huzoor", Birbal replied, unmoved. "But I cannot vouch for all the crows remaining in Agra until that is done. Some may go away to visit their friends and relatives in Dilli, in which case you may find that there are fewer than the number I gave you. Or, it is possible that their friends and relatives from Dilli and elsewhere may come to pay them a visit, and so increase the number. But I can say with utter certainty that at this exact moment and only at this moment, there are ten thousand, six hundred and sixty-six crows in Agra!"

"Birbal you are incomparable", Akbar exclaimed as he burst out laughing. "And now, let us go on to more important matters."

Inauspicious Omens

Many people at Emperor Akbar's court were superstitious about all kinds of silly things. One popular superstition was that people's faces could be auspicious or inauspicious. If the first person you was in the morning had an auspicious face, it was believed, you would have a happy day. But if you saw someone who had an inauspicious face, things would go wrong all through the day. Emperor Akbar heard of this belief. He wasn't sure whether he believed it or not, but somehow, it stuck in his memory. One morning, he awoke very early and looked out of his window. He saw a poor washerman scrubbing clothes in the river Yamuna. "Hmm", Emperor Akbar mused. "I wonder if it is a good omen or a bad one to see a washerman at the start of the day."

The washerman happened to glance up at the fort just then. He caught a glimpse of the emperor's face

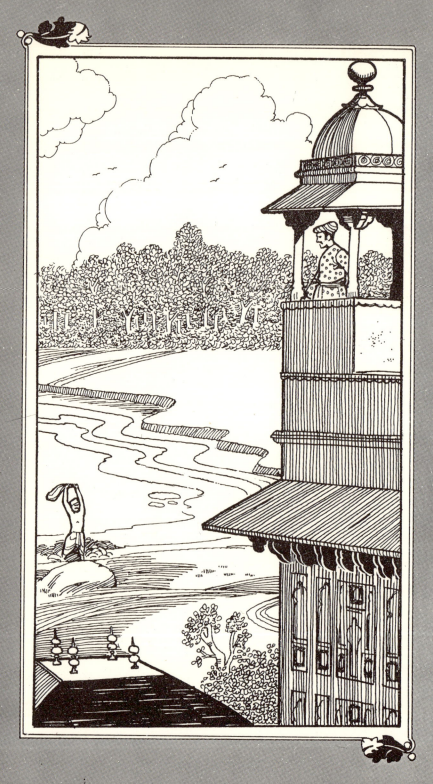

at the window and at once he went down on his knees in joyous respect. The emperor smiled and turned away. Later that morning, as the emperor went up the steps of the Diwan-i-Khas, he tripped and bumped his shin. The royal hakims hurried to apply soothing oils and ointments, but the Emperor's leg was badly bruised and hurt him when he walked. He decided he would not go out riding that day and went for a stroll in the garden instead. He stopped to admire a particularly fine rose and as he bent towards the flower, a bee flew out and stung him on the hand. His attendants rushed around in distress, trying to help him, urging him to go inside, begging him to sit down. "What an ill-omened day, that our Shahanshah should be stung in his own garden", one of them lamented.

Akbar heard him and his face grew thoughtful. "Ill-omened?" He said slowly. "The first person I saw today was the washerman by the river. Perhaps it is he who blighted my day? Perhaps he had an inauspicious face?"

"Oh yes, Jahanpanah" , some silly courtier cried. "It must be so indeed. The inauspicious face of the washerman has brought pain to your royal person."

"May he suffer for his evil presence!" cried another.

"May no unfortunate being ever look upon his ill-starred face", cried a third.

"He doesn't deserve to live!" cried yet another. "One who brings so much misery should certainly die!"

"Put him to death!" rose a babble of voices. "He caused our Shahanshah pain and he should die for it. It was all his fault. Put him to death!"

Birbal arrived as more and more courtiers were raising their voices against the washerman, imploring the emperor to send for him at once in order to sentence him to death. Tansen, the celebrated musician, was standing on the edge of the agitated crowd. He smiled in relief when he saw Birbal arrive. Drawing him aside, he told him all that had happened. Birbal shook his head in amazement. Then he pushed his way to the emperor's side. "Jahanpanah!" he cried in his ringing voice. "I am extremely sad to hear of your injuries." Akbar nodded. "Tell us, Birbal", he said. "Shall we behead this ill-omened washerman?" "Ill-omened, Huzoor?" Birbal asked. "You saw his face and you have a bruised shin and a bee-sting. Jahanpanah, the washerman saw your face early this morning and is now about to lose his head! Which do you think was the more inauspicious of the two?"

Emperor Akbar stared at Birbal for a moment. Then he began to smile. "You are right, Raja Birbal!" he said. "It is really a very foolish belief."

"Jahanpanah", Tansen called. "I have a special song that I would like to present to you to celebrate the victory of sense over nonsense."

"Let us have music, then", Emperor Akbar commanded. "And let us all think as we listen."

The Scribe's Dream

T here was once a poor scribe in the city of Agra. He copied other people's writings and books. He earned barely enough to support his family. But, no matter how difficult it was, he and his wife always managed to feed themselves and their children. The scribe was proud of the fact that he had never borrowed a single copper coin. "We must never fall into the hands of the moneylender", he often told his wife. "For if we do, we will surely be ruined."

The scribe worried so much about his lack of money and his fear of borrowing that his worries even found a place in his dreams. One night he dreamt that he had borrowed one hundred gold coins from the moneylender. He woke up in terror, thinking, "One hundred gold coins! Where, oh where will I ever find such wealth!" Still trembling from his nightmare, he woke his wife and told her all about it. They talked

19

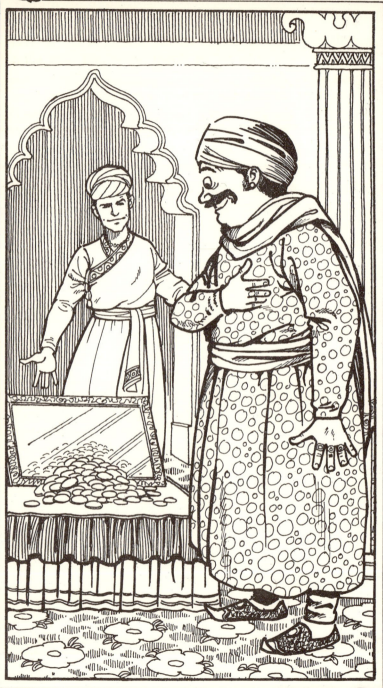

quietly for a while and soon the scribe began to feel better. He was able to lie down again and was soon asleep once more.

The next day, as the scribe's wife drew water from the well at the end of the street on which they lived, she told her friends of her husband's dream. "Imagine!" she exclaimed. "He dreamt that we'd borrowed not one or two, but one hundred gold coins from the moneylender!" Her friends laughed with her. A few of them thought it was a very good story and repeated it to their husbands when they got home. The story spread and a few days later, it reached the moneylender's ears. He laughed when he heard it but his eyes began to glitter greedily. That evening, he put on his turban and, picking up his walking stick, strolled over to the scribe's small house.

"I've come", he announced to the nervous and worried scribe, "to remind you of the money you owe me."

"Money?" squeaked the scribe in a panic. "I owe you?"

"Yes, bhai" , answered the moneylender firmly. "One hundred gold coins. Surely you cannot have forgotten?"

"One-one-one h-h-hundred gold c-c-coins . . ." gasped the scribe in a failing voice, tottering to the nearest chair.

The scribe's wife, who had been listening from an inner room, came hurrying out. "But it was only a dream!" she cried. "You cannot ask us to return money that has only been borrowed in a dream!"

"Money is money", the moneylender said, unmoved. "And money borrowed must be returned. You will have to start tomorrow. I am a kind man, a good-hearted man, and so I shall not demand it all back at once.

One gold coin a month will do. And then there will be the interest above that as well." And with these words, he stood up and left.

The scribe began to moan softly. His wife sat down suddenly, her knees giving way beneath her. They sat in silent despair. Suddenly, from the depths of her misery, the wife had an idea. "Husband", she said, sitting up straight. "We must beg Raja Birbal to help us. Only he can save us from utter ruin." At this, the scribe sat up. Strength and energy seemed to flow into his limbs. "I shall go to his house at once", he said. "If anyone can save us it is he."

Birbal listened to the poor scribe's tale of woe. Then he brought out a bag of gold coins and emptied them on to a table. He counted out a hundred and put the rest away. Then he placed a large mirror in front of the coins.

"Huzoor, huzoor!" the scribe said in a distressed voice. "I did not come here to beg or to ask you to pay the moneylender. Surely there is another way!"

"There *is* another", Birbal answered with a smile. "Compose yourself and go and call the moneylender to my haveli. Tell him his debt is about to be paid."

Full of doubts, the scribe hurried to the moneylender's house with Birbal's message. The moneylender smiled when he heard and got up at once to accompany him.

When they arrived at Birbal's house and were shown in, the moneylender spotted the pile of gold coins on the table. He smiled and smiled, unable to take his eyes off them. The mirror behind the coins made the pile look larger and more glittering.

"So the scribe borrowed a hundred gold coins from you in his dream, did he?"

"That is so", replied the moneylender, never taking his eyes off the coins on the table.

"Well", said Birbal. "You may take all the coins in the mirror," said Birbal. The real coins belong to me, but all those in the reflection are yours in return for the dream loan!"

The moneylender knew he had met his match. Without a word, he turned and left the house. Never again did he try to bully the scribe or anyone else in the city of Agra.

The Best Vegetable of All

One evening, as Emperor Akbar and a group of his courtiers strolled along a terrace which overlooked the river, the emperor remarked, "Brinjals are the finest vegetables, without a doubt." All his courtiers were quick to agree. "Oh", said one. "Brinjal is said to be excellent for one's health." Another commented, "And the taste! Brinjal cooked with lamb or any other meat is delicious."

To everybody's surprise, even Birbal began to praise the brinjal. "What delicacy! What subtle texture! What fine colour!" he cried. "Oh, brinjal is the emperor of vegetables to be sure. It is a veritable gift from heaven!" And he went on and on, even reciting a small poem in praise of the brinjal. This was a bit too much, even for Emperor Akbar, who was accustomed to flattery and to fawning courtiers. He was certain that Birbal was teasing him and mocking all the courtiers who surrounded him. So, a few days later, the emperor declared, "There can be no better vegetable in all the world than spinach!"

At once, all those around him began to praise spinach. "It's so good for the digestion" , said a very fat man who loved to eat. "And full of goodness", said his extremely thin friend. "And it is excellent with meat", added a man whose wife was notorious for her bad cooking.

"Never has there been a tastier vegetable", Birbal's voice rose over all the rest. "What delicacy! What fine colour! Oh, spinach is the emperor of all vegetables. It is a veritable gift of the heavens!"

"Birbal!" Emperor Akbar cried in an outraged voice. "Only last week you were praising the brinjal in exactly the same words. Have you no loyalty to your beliefs, no faithfulness to the truth!"

Birbal's eyes twinkled. "Jahanpanah", he said, bowing very low. "My loyalty and faith are given only to you, my Shahanshah, from whom all bounty flows. What do I care for brinjal and spinach if I may be near you?"

Akbar looked around at all his courtiers, who were too nervous of him to ever question anything he said. He understood that Birbal was mocking their sheep-like behaviour, as he proved his own loyalty in his own witty way. He smiled appreciatively. "Wah, Wah! Birbal", he said. "You never fail to teach us something even when you make us laugh!"

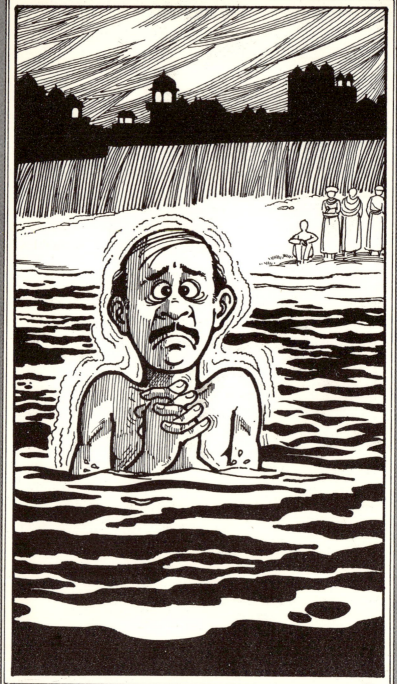

Lamplight

Emperor Akbar was amazingly brave and strong. On one occasion, he fought a tiger · single-handedly. On another, he rode a maddened elephant and brought it under control, even though he almost died in the attempt. The emperor admired those who had as much stamina and courage as he did. One cold January day, he sent messengers through the city of Agra to announce a contest. "He who can spend the entire night standing chest-deep in the icy waters of the Yamuna river", declared the messengers, "shall be awarded one hundred gold coins by the emperor himself!"

There was great excitement all through the city. Athletes and wrestlers and war-toughened soldiers all wanted to try their luck. Some oiled their bodies well so that they would be protected from the cold water. Others ate fistfuls of almonds, which were said to warm the blood. A few drank flasks of wine all through the day in an effort to warm themselves for the ordeal. As night fell, hundreds of men of all ages waded into the river. Among them was a poor stonemason, who needed enough money to pay for his son's education. He was too poor to buy almonds to eat, or oil to rub over himself, but he was determined to win the money for his beloved child.

As night wore on and the river water began to get colder, a large number of men began to leave. By midnight, only a handful were left. Their friends called encouragingly to them from the river bank. One by one, even they began to leave. They could not stand the icy chill that set in during the last few hours before dawn. By the time the first rays of the sun lit the battlements of the fort, only the stonemason was still in the river. He was so cold, he could not move. His friends had to help him out of the water and revive him with a massage and a hot drink and wrap him in a blanket.

That evening, as the emperor prepared for the evening durbar in the Diwan-i-Am, one spiteful courtier said, "Jahanpanah, the prize you are about to award was not won by fair means."

"Oh?" said Emperor Akbar. "And how is that?"

"Huzoor", said the man, his eyes glittering with malice. "It is said that the man drew warmth and comfort from the sight of the lamplight from the palace. If he was warmed by the lamps of the palace, then he did not truly withstand the icy waters of the river. He won the contest by unfair means, Huzoor!"

Emperor Akbar began to think. Could the courtier be right? It *was* strange that the stonemason had succeeded when all the wrestlers and athletes and soldiers had failed. He was so busy thinking and wondering that he did not notice Raja Birbal slipping away.

It was some time later that Akbar decided to ask Birbal for his advice, and found that he was not there. The emperor frowned. Messengers were despatched to summon him at once. They returned with a message from Birbal to say he was waiting for his meal of *khichchri* to be ready, and would join them shortly. An hour went by. The time for the durbar was drawing close and the emperor wanted Birbal to be present. More messengers were sent to call him. They returned with the same message. Birbal was waiting for his *khichchri* to be cooked. "*Khichchri* does not take so long!" the Emperor said angrily. He decided to go to Birbal's house himself to find out what the matter was. He found Birbal on the terrace of his house. In front of him was a pot, filled to the brim with water, rice and lentils. The pot was set in a wooden frame which was tilted so that the bottom of the pot faced the Emperor's palace.

"Birbal, have you gone completely mad?" Emperor Akbar roared as Birbal rose to greet him.

"Huzoor, if the poor stonemason was able to warm himself by the light of the lamps in the royal palace, then surely that same heat will cook my *khichchri*, especially since I am so much closer to the royal lamplight", Birbal said quietly.

In reply, the emperor put his arm around Birbal and asked the treasurer to hand him the bag of gold coins. "You shall have the honour of holding the award when I present it to the stonemason this evening", he said. Then, pulling off the rope of perfectly matched pearls which he wore around his neck, he slid it over

Birbal's head. "And now, shall we proceed to the durbar?" he said, leading the way down the stairs.

"Huzoor", Birbal murmured in gratitude as he followed his emperor down the stairs. Together they walked towards the Diwan-i-Am where the stonemason was waiting.

A Hairy Tale

It was a hot summer morning. Emperor Akbar had not slept very well the previous night. It was clear to everyone that the emperor was not in a very good mood. "I've asked the keeper of the royal forests to prepare for a tiger hunt", Raja Man Singh whispered to Birbal. "At such a time, what cheers the emperor most is to be out riding and camping in the forest away from the palace and the fort and the cares of government." Birbal nodded. But in the meanwhile he knew he had to keep the emperor in good humour. So, when Emperor Akbar asked abruptly, "Who can answer this? Why is it that no hair grows on the palms of my hand?" Birbal stepped forward at once. "Huzoor", he replied, "How can hair grow on the palms of your hand? It is just not possible, because your munificence, your generosity is so great that the constant flow of gold and gifts that slip from your hands into the hands of your worthless servant wears away any hair that might grow there."

Akbar nodded and even smiled, but he was still a little irritable. "Is that so?" he said. "In that case, how is it that no hair grows on the palms of *your* hands, Birbal?"

Birbal held out his hands to the emperor. "Jahan-panah, your generosity in filling these worthless hands with gold and gifts wears away every last hair that might grow there."

"And the others?" Emperor Akbar pointed to all the courtiers who stood around them, filling the hall. "What about them? Am I so generous to each and every person gathered here? I'd soon have an empty treasury if I were as generous as you say." Several of those standing nearby smiled at each other. Even Birbal, clever Birbal would find it difficult to answer that one, they thought, and waited expectantly to hear him admit that he was at a loss for words.

But Birbal smiled back at them and replied without a moment's hesitation, "Huzoor, when my fellow servants see the magnificence that your generosity bestows on my worthless being, they cannot stop wringing their hands in jealousy. In doing this, they have rubbed away every single of hair that might have grown on their palms!"

At this, even Emperor Akbar burst out laughing. Soon others joined in the laughter and a wave of merriment filled the hall. "Well done, Birbal Bhaiya!" Raja Man Singh whispered to him. "You've saved the day!"

The Reader of Minds

Some years after Birbal had come to the imperial court at Agra, Emperor Akbar had a magnificent new capital built at Fatehpur Sikri, about twenty kilometres outside the city. The emperor and his queens moved into exquisite stone palaces in the new capital and some of the more important courtiers were given houses close to the emperor's palace. Among them was Birbal. Many of the other courtiers had to build their own havelis below the hill on which Fatehpur Sikri was built. Some built their homes in the village of Sikri. They could not understand why Raja Birbal had been shown such special favour. It made them feel very envious indeed. They wished there was some way to make Birbal look foolish in front of the emperor. But Birbal was too clever for them. So they grumbled to each other and longed for the day that the emperor would ask him a question that he would be unable

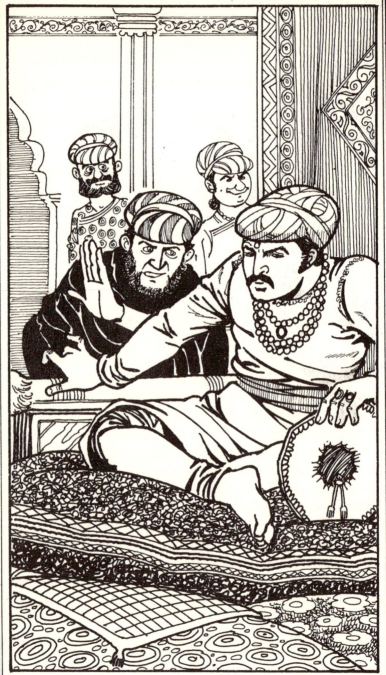

to answer.

One of these courtiers, a man called Yusuf Khan, went a step further. One day, when Birbal was away to a distant kingdom, on a special mission for the emperor, Yusuf Khan thought of a plan. That evening, at the durbar, he said to Emperor Akbar, "Jahanpanah, it is said that Raja Birbal now claims that he can even read the thoughts of others. Is he not extraordinarily clever?"

"Oh, he is a genius, of that there is no doubt", commented another jealous. courtier. "There is surely nothing that he does not know."

"Is he so clever?" the Emperor asked, reacting just as Yusuf Khan hoped he would. "We shall soon find out."

Some days later, when Raja Birbal returned from his mission, he attended the small private durbar in the emperor's palace. Yusuf Khan and his friends waited anxiously for the emperor to ask the fateful question. They were sure it would put Birbal in a spot. How would he answer? Would he protest and deny that he had ever said such a thing? Would he try to bluff his way out? Could he? Yusuf Khan was certain it was not possible to do so. He waited gleefully for the business part of the durbar to end. Birbal made his report on his successful mission to end the rebellion of a minor ruler and Emperor Akbar congratulated him warmly. Other reports were heard and decisions given to commanders of the army and to various officials. Then, when all the work was done, Emperor Akbar asked Birbal, "It is said, my friend, that you can even read minds now. Is this true?"

Raja Birbal glanced around the hall and saw the nasty smiles on the faces of Yusuf Khan and his group.

He turned back to the emperor and answered calmly, "Jahanpanah, I would not dare to presume enough to think that I could ever read the subtle mind of Your Highness. However, I can certainly tell you the thought that fills the minds of each and every other person present here this evening." He paused and smiled at Yusuf Khan. "Each of Jahanpanah's servants who are gathered here today has but one thought in his mind. They are thinking: May God bless our emperor in his mercy and wisdom and allow him good health so that he may rule over us for ever and ever!" Then, turning to Yusuf Khan, he asked, "Am I not right, my dear friend?"

Yusuf Khan met Birbal's bright eyes and knew that he was beaten. He didn't dare deny that he was thinking only of the emperor's welfare and nothing else. Forcing a smile upon his lips, he bowed and said, "Shahanshah, he is absolutely right!" A murmur of agreement rose from all who were gathered there. Not one dared to admit that he was thinking of anything else but the emperor.

Birbal turned to the emperor with a look of immense amusement on his face. He and the emperor both understood exactly what had happened. Emperor Akbar began to laugh. "Birbal, you are incomparable!" he cried, while Birbal's enemies fumed in helpless silence.

Greater Than Gods

Emperor Akbar enjoyed listening to stories and poems from distant lands, and travellers to Fatehpur Sikri were welcome and treated kindly. One day, two poets from a faraway kingdom arrived at the court. They delighted all who listened with songs and poems and the emperor, with his customary generosity, rewarded them well. The poets had seldom seen so much gold before. They had certainly never been given a whole bag of gold coins each in their entire lives. They were overwhelmed. And, when the emperor ordered the treasurer to give them a set of clothes each, one of the poets begged permission to offer a poem of thanks. Emperor Akbar nodded and the poet began his recitation. He spoke of the emperor's bravery and kindness. He praised the emperor's learning and wisdom and in the final verse, inspired beyond sensible limits, he ended by declaring that Emperor

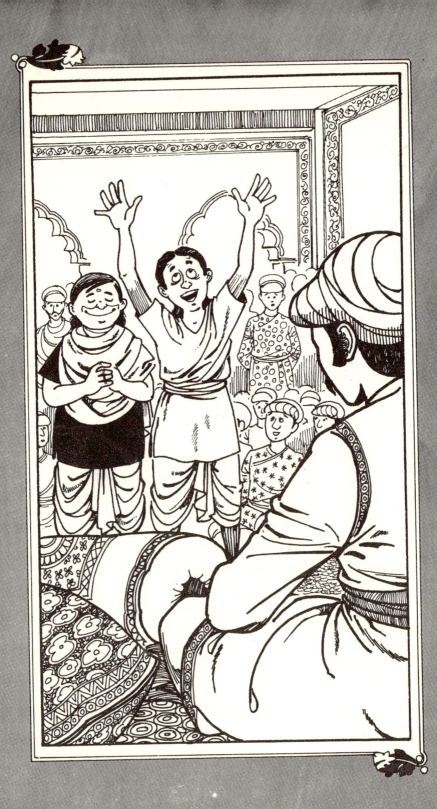

Akbar was the greatest king that had ever ruled "over this world or any other. He is greater than Lord Indra himself!" cried the poet as he bowed and left the hall.

There was a moment's silence. Many of those in the hall were absolutely shocked that the poet had compared a mortal to a god. Emperor Akbar looked around and his eyes began to twinkle mischievously. "So", he said, "it appears that I am now even greater than the God Indra!"

All the people in the hall looked at their emperor in horror. Had he really believed the poet's word? Surely not! And yet, they weren't entirely sure. Emperor Akbar looked back at his ministers and commanders, his nobles and his counsellors, wondering if any of them would have the courage to speak the truth. The ministers, commanders, nobles and counsellors looked back at him. Nobody stirred. "In that case", said the emperor, beginning to feel irritated, "You all agree, then. Your emperor is greater than the God Indra himself!"

Nobody dared to disagree. Slowly, one by one, the courtiers bowed to show that they agreed. A low, ashamed murmur of "Ji, Huzoor. It is so, Jahanpanah", filled the hall.

Emperor Akbar thought that the foolishness had gone far enough. He turned to Birbal with a frown. "And you, Birbal. Do you agree?" he asked.

"Oh yes", Birbal replied immediately. The emperor's frown grew. "Huzoor, you can do something even God cannot!" Birbal said. "If any of your subjects displeases you, Jahanpanah, you can send him on a pilgrimage, or banish him from your empire, never to return. But God cannot. For God rules over the entire earth and the sky and the heavens. There is no place in this world or any other that does not belong to God. So he cannot banish any one of his creatures!" Emperor Akbar's frown vanished. "Well said, Birbal", he cried delightedly. And, from every corner of the court, relieved courtiers began to smile weakly and then to laugh. Birbal had done it again!

Temper

In the village below Emperor Akbar's capital at Fatehpur Sikri, there lived a quick-tempered priest and his wife. The priest used to eat only one meal a day and his wife took a great deal of trouble to cook something delicious. Wonderful aromas would drift out of the kitchen, so when afternoon came and the priest sat down to eat, he would be very hungry indeed. One day, as he broke off a piece of freshly made *roti* and dipped in into the bowl of fragrant, steaming *dal,* the priest noticed a hair floating on the dal. He flung the food away in a rage, shouting to his wife. "This food is bad! It's been ruined! There's a hair in the *dal* and it's not fit to eat!"

The priest's wife came running when she heard her husband. She wept when she saw the *dal* and *rotis* scattered all over the courtyard. There was no time to make a fresh meal and the priest had to go without

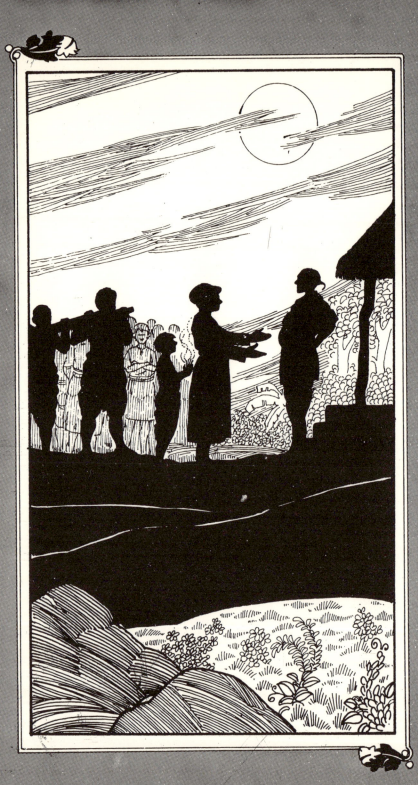

his food that day. He got angrier and angrier and when evening came, he said, "Beware, wife. If ever I find a hair in my food again, I will shave off every last hair on your head."

This frightened his wife and she became even more careful, pulling her hair back tightly and covering her head with her sari. A week went by. The priest ate his daily meal with all his usual enjoyment. And then, one day, as he was about to bite into a morsel of brinjal and *roti*, he saw another hair. It was embedded in the *roti*. The priest sprang to his feet with a terrible roar and rushed towards the kitchen, shouting, "Bring me a razor. Now I shall have to shave off your hair!" His wife gave a howl of terror and, before he could reach the kitchen, she sprang up and slammed the door shut.

"Open this door at once!" shouted the enraged priest.

"Oh, no, no, no, no!" wailed his wife. "Punish me, starve me, only promise you won't cut off my hair. Oh, forgive me, forgive me!"

The woman's heart-rending cries and the priest's bellowing voice could be heard all over the village. People came running to see what disaster had befallen them. When they understood what had happened, some began to laugh and others began to argue. A few tried to reason with the priest. He turned upon them with a snarl. The crowd grew bigger and bigger as more and more people arrived. And all the while, the priest's wife wailed and wept unceasingly from behind the locked kitchen door.

Finally, one very old woman murmured to her grandson. "Only Raja Birbal can solve this problem, *beta*. Run as quickly as you can and beg him to come to the rescue of this wretched woman. The boy nodded and ran up the hill to the double-storied red-stone house in which Birbal lived. Birbal listened to the tale and nodded. Then he gave the boy certain instructions. The boy smiled and hurried away to do as Birbal had asked.

Half an hour later, Birbal led a small procession towards the priest's house. It looked like a funeral procession. Two men carried a bamboo bier. It was empty, however. Another man carried some logs of wood. The boy carried some flowers and incense. They arrived at the priest's house and stopped beside the priest. He turned and asked angrily, "What's going on? Has somebody died? Why have you brought the bier here?"

"I heard that someone had died here", said Birbal. "Only widows shave their heads, don't they? I heard your wife was about to shave her head and so I thought you must have died. Are you about to die? We've made all the preparations for your funeral."

"He'll have to die first, won't he?" cried a cheeky little boy in the crowd.

"But then who'll shave his wife's head? He wants to do it himself!" cried another. People began to laugh. The priest hung his head in shame. He understood what Birbal was trying to show him. Slowly, he went towards the kitchen. "Come out, wife", he said quietly. "I will try never to be so foolish again." His wife unlatched the kitchen door and came to stand beside him. "And I'll be even more careful when I cook, from now on."

Smiling, Birbal and the village people went home in cheerful good humour.

The Sadhu

Akbar came to the throne when he was only thirteen years old. In the years that followed, he built one of the greatest empires of his time. He lived in unimaginable splendour. He was surrounded by courtiers who agreed with every word he said, who flattered him and treated him as if he were a god. Perhaps it was not surprising that Emperor Akbar was sometimes arrogant and behaved as if the whole world belonged to him. One day, Birbal decided to make the great emperor stop and think about life.

That evening as the emperor was going towards his palace, he noticed a sadhu lying in the centre of his garden. He could not believe his eyes. A strange sadhu, in ragged clothes, right in the middle of the palace garden? The guards would have to be punished for this, thought the emperor furiously as he walked over to the sadhu and prodded him with the tip of his

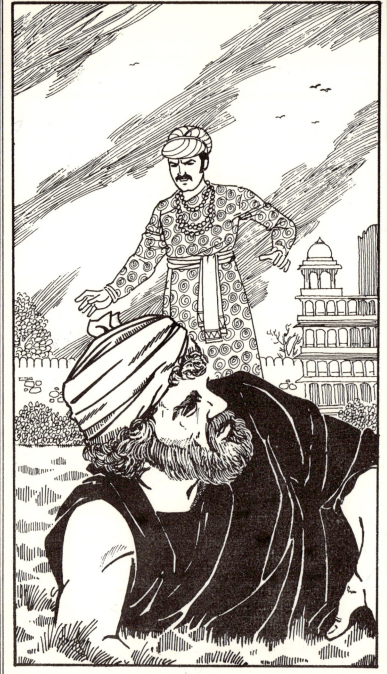

embroidered slipper. "Here, fellow!" he cried. "What are you doing here? Get up and go away at once!"

The sadhu opened his eyes. Then he sat up slowly. "Huzoor," he said in a sleepy voice. "Is this your garden, then?"

"Yes!" cried the Emperor. "This garden, those rose bushes, the fountain beyond that, the courtyard, the palace, this fort, this empire, it all belongs to me!"

Slowly the sadhu stood up. "And the river, Huzoor? And the city of Agra? And Hindustan?"

"Yes, yes, it's all mine", said the Emperor. "Now get out!"

"Ah", said the sadhu. "And before you, Huzoor. Who did this garden and fort and city belong to then?"

"My father, of course", said the emperor. In spite of his irritation, he was beginning to get interested in the sadhu's questions. He loved philosophical discussions and he could tell, from his manner of speaking, that the sadhu was a learned man.

"And who was here before him?" the sadhu asked quietly.

"His father, my father's father, as you know."

"Ah", said the sadhu. So this garden, those rose bushes, the palace and the fort — all this has only belonged to you for your lifetime. Before that they belonged to your father, am I right? And after your time they will belong to your son, and then to his son?

"Yes", said Emperor Akbar wonderingly.

"So each one stays here for a time and then goes on his way?"

"Yes."

"Like a *dharmashala*?" the sadhu asked. "No one owns a *dharmashala*. Or the shade of a tree on the side of a the road. We stop and rest for a while and then go on. And someone has always been there before us and someone will always come after we have gone. Is that not so?"

"It is", said Emperor Akbar quietly.

"So your garden, your palace, your fort, your empire . . . these are only places you will stay in for a time, for the span of your lifetime. When you die, they will no longer belong to you. You will go, leaving them in the possession of someone else, just as your father did and his father before him."

Emperor Akbar nodded. "The whole world is a *dharmashala*", he said slowly, thinking very hard. "In which we mortals rest awhile. That's what you are telling me, isn't it? Nothing on this earth can ever belong to a single person, because each person is only passing through the earth and must die one day?"

The sadhu nodded solemnly. Then, bowing to the ground, he removed his white beard and saffron turban and his voice changed. "Jahanpanah, forgive me!" he said, in his normal voice. "It was my way of asking you to think about . . ."

"Birbal, oh, Birbal!" the emperor exclaimed. "You are wiser than any philosopher. Come, come at once to the royal chamber and let us discuss this further. Even emperors are but wayfarers on the path of life, it is clear!"